Pathology of Emerging Infections 2

EDITED BY

Ann Marie Nelson
C. Robert Horsburgh, Jr.

ASM PRESS • WASHINGTON, D.C.

Copyright © 1998   American Society for Microbiology
                   1325 Massachusetts Ave., NW
                   Washington, DC 20005-4171

Pathology of emerging infections 2 / edited by Ann Marie Nelson and C.
    Robert Horsburgh, Jr.
          p.   cm.
      Includes index.
      Sequel to: Pathology of emerging infections. c1997.
      ISBN 1-55581-140-X
      1. Communicable diseases.   2. Communicable diseases-
    -Pathophysiology.   I. Nelson, Ann Marie.   II. Horsburgh, C. Robert.
      [DNLM: 1. Communicable Diseases—pathology.   2. Communicable
    Diseases—epidemiology.   3. Disease Outbreaks.   WC 100P296 1998]
    RC111.P393   1998
    616.9'047—dc21
    DNLM/DLC
    for Library of Congress   98-8770
                                                           CIP

Contents

Contributors

David G. Addiss
Division of Parasitic Diseases, National Center for Infectious Diseases, Centers for Disease Control and Prevention, Mailstop F-22, 4770 Buford Highway, Atlanta, Georgia 30341

Peter B. Bloland
Malaria Epidemiology Section, Division of Parasitic Diseases, National Center for Infectious Diseases, Centers for Disease Control and Prevention, Mailstop F-22, 1600 Clifton Road, Atlanta, Georgia 30333

Henry M. Blumberg
Division of Infectious Diseases, Department of Medicine, Emory University School of Medicine, 69 Butler Street, S.E., Atlanta, Georgia 30303

Corrie Brown
Department of Veterinary Pathology, College of Veterinary Medicine, The University of Georgia, D. W. Brooks Drive, Athens, Georgia 30602-7388

Donald S. Burke
Center for Immunization Research, School of Hygiene and Public Health, Johns Hopkins University, Hampton House, Room 241, 624 North Broadway, Baltimore, Maryland 21205

Francis W. Chandler
Department of Pathology - BF230, Medical College of Georgia, Augusta, Georgia 30912-3605

Carlos del Río
Division of Infectious Diseases, Department of Medicine, Emory University School of Medicine, 69 Butler Street, S.E., Atlanta, Georgia 30303

Gerusa Dreyer
Departamento de Parasitologia, Centro de Pesquisas Aggeu Magalhães-FIOCRUZ, Av. Moraes Rego S/N, Ciudade Unversitaria, Recife, PE, Brazil 52020-200

José Figueredo-Silva
Laboratorio de Immunopatologia Keiso Asami, Universidade Federal de Pernambuco, Recife, Brazil

Patricia Griffin
Foodborne and Diarrheal Diseases Branch, Division of Bacterial and Mycotic Diseases, National Center for Infectious Diseases, Centers for Disease Control and Prevention, Mailstop A-38, 1600 Clifton Road, N.E., Atlanta, Georgia 30333

Jeannette Guarner
Infectious Disease Pathology Activity, National Center for Infectious Diseases, Centers for Disease Control and Prevention, Mailstop D-17, 1600 Clifton Road, N.E., Atlanta, Georgia 30333

Duane J. Gubler
Division of Vector-Borne Infectious Diseases, Centers for Disease Control and Prevention, P.O. Box 2087 (Foothills Campus), Fort Collins, Colorado 80520

C. Robert Horsburgh, Jr.
Emory University School of Medicine, 69 Butler Street, S.E., Atlanta, Georgia 30303

Leo Kaufman
Division of Bacterial and Mycotic Diseases, Centers for Disease Control and Prevention, Mailstop G-11, 1600 Clifton Road, Atlanta, Georgia 30333

Mary Klassen
Department of Infectious and Parasitic Disease Pathology, Armed Forces Institute of Pathology, Washington, DC 20306-6000

James W. LeDuc
National Center for Infectious Diseases, Centers for Disease Control and Prevention, NCID/OD, Mailstop C-12, 1600 Clifton Road, N.E., Atlanta, Georgia 30333

Jeffrey Lennox
Department of Medicine, Emory University School of Medicine, Atlanta, Georgia 30303

William H. Lyerly, Jr.
United States Agency for International Development, 1300 Pennsylvania Avenue, N.W., RRB, Room 4.06-044, AFR/SD/HRD, Washington, D.C. 20523-3700

Jo Marie Lyons
Department of Anatomical Pathology, Emory University School of Medicine, Grady Memorial Hospital, Box 268, 80 Butler Street, S.E., Atlanta, Georgia 30335

Aileen M. Marty
Infectious Disease Pathology, Department of Infectious and Parasitic Disease Pathology, Armed Forces Institute of Pathology, Washington, DC 20406-6000

John E. McGowan, Jr.
Department of Epidemiology, Rollins School of Public Health, and Department of Pathology and Laboratory Medicine, Emory University, Atlanta, Georgia 30322

Tracey S. McNamara
Department of Pathology, Wildlife Conservation Society, 2300 Southern Boulevard, Bronx, New York 10460

Michael M. McNeil
Division of Bacterial and Mycotic Diseases, Centers for Disease Control and Prevention, Mailstop C-23, 1600 Clifton Road, Atlanta, Georgia 30333

Frederick A. Meier
Clinical and Anatomic Pathology, DuPont Hospital for Children, P.O. Box 269, 1600 Rockland Road, Wilmington, Delaware 19899-0269, and Jefferson Medical College, Philadelphia, Pennsylvania

Ronald C. Neafie
Parasitic Disease Pathology Branch, Geographic Pathology Division, Department of Infectious and Parasitic Disease Pathology, Armed Forces Institute of Pathology, Washington, DC 20306-6000

Ann Marie Nelson
Division of AIDS Pathology, Department of Infectious and Parasitic Disease Pathology, Armed Forces Institute of Pathology, Washington, DC 20306-6000

Kurt B. Nolte
Office of the Medical Investigator, University of New Mexico School of Medicine, 700 Camino de Salud, Albuquerque, New Mexico 87131-5091

R. Gibson Parrish
Division of Environmental Hazards and Health Effects, National Center for Environmental Health, Centers for Disease Control and Prevention, Mailstop F-35, 4770 Buford Highway, N.E., Atlanta, Georgia 30341-3714

Robert W. Pinner
National Center for Infectious Diseases, Centers for Disease Control and Prevention, Building 1, Room 6029, Mailstop C-12, 1600 Clifton Road, N.E., Atlanta, Georgia 30333

George P. Schmid
Division of STD Prevention, National Center for HIV, STD, and TB Prevention, Centers for Disease Control and Prevention, Mailstop E-27, 1600 Clifton Road, N.E., Atlanta, Georgia 30333

David A. Schwartz
Departments of Pathology and Medicine (Infectious Diseases), Emory University School of Medicine, 69 Butler Street, S.E., Atlanta, Georgia 30303

Gary L. Simpson
Public Health Division, New Mexico Department of Health, 1190 St. Francis Drive, Santa Fe, New Mexico 87502

Lawrence Slutsker
Foodborne and Diarrheal Diseases Branch, Division of Bacterial and Mycotic Diseases, National Center for Infectious Diseases, Centers for Disease Control and Prevention, Mailstop A-38, 1600 Clifton Road, N.E., Atlanta, Georgia 30333

Richard A. Spiegel
Division of Bacterial and Mycotic Diseases, National Center for Infectious Diseases, Centers for Disease Control and Prevention, Mailstop C-23, 1600 Clifton Road, Atlanta, Georgia 30333

Fred C. Tenover
Nosocomial Pathogens Laboratory Branch, Hospital Infections Program, Centers for Disease Control and Prevention, Mailstop G-08, 1600 Clifton Road, Atlanta, Georgia 30333

Melinda Wharton
National Immunization Program, Centers for Disease Control and Prevention, Mailstop E-61, 1600 Clifton Road, N.E., Atlanta, Georgia 30333

Sherif R. Zaki
Infectious Disease Pathology Activity, Division of Viral and Rickettsial Diseases, National Center for Infectious Diseases, Centers for Disease Control and Prevention, Mailstop G-32, 1600 Clifton Road, Atlanta, Georgia 30333

Acknowledgments

The editors are grateful for the encouragement and support of Florabel G. Mullick, Director, Center for Advanced Pathology, Armed Forces Institute of Pathology (AFIP), and James M. Hughes, Director, National Center for Infectious Diseases, Centers for Disease Control and Prevention. We also thank Sunny Walton for her secretarial assistance, excellent organizational skills, and dedication.

Emerging Infectious Diseases: An Introduction

William H. Lyerly, Jr., and James W. LeDuc

In many countries, escalating post-Cold War civil strife and failing economies have significantly increased the number of humanitarian and transitional crises. Emerging diseases and deplorable health situations are exacerbated by migration, displaced populations, internal conflict, and collapsing civil infrastructures. As a consequence, rapid international responses are needed to mitigate human suffering and restore regional stability. Resolution of the social and economic conditions arising from these complex humanitarian emergencies will require coordinated multidisciplinary and interagency approaches that span the relief-to-development continuum (i.e., disaster relief, transition, and follow-on nation building). As a case in point, it is estimated that during the nearly two decades of civil war in Mozambique, more deaths resulted from the collapsed health infrastructure than from the actual fighting.

Infectious diseases are the most common cause of death during these complex humanitarian emergencies, and numerous geopolitical considerations affect, or are affected by, emerging infectious diseases. Wars in numerous countries have been bilaterally interrupted to allow for polio

William H. Lyerly, Jr., United States Agency for International Development, 1300 Pennsylvania Avenue, N.W., RRB, Room 4.06-044, AFR/SD/HRD, Washington, DC 20523-3700. **James W. LeDuc,** National Center for Infectious Diseases, Centers for Disease Control and Prevention, NCID/OD, Mailstop C-12, 1600 Clifton Road, N.E., Atlanta, GA 30333.

Pathology of Emerging Infections 2
Edited by Ann Marie Nelson and C. Robert Horsburgh, Jr.

immunization of children during "Days of Tranquility," and military forces helped to implement civilian immunization campaigns during the Angolan civil war. In contrast, the high rates of HIV infection and AIDS among military and security forces (e.g., sub-Saharan Africa) threaten internal security and regional stability. Increases in HIV transmission occur during periods of social disruption and in post-conflict settings. The AIDS epidemic saps the economic strength of affected countries. The international political goal of smaller, more economical defense structures requires the demobilization of military and security forces in many developing countries. This demobilization may augment the spread of HIV as infected soldiers return to civilian life.

Infectious diseases and other environmental issues influence the balance of the global economy, the stability of the international political situation, and the future health of the world environment. Communicable disease epidemics and pandemics have threatened human health and productivity throughout history. Compared to other regions of the world, an extremely high prevalence of infectious and parasitic diseases exists in Africa, where tropical and infectious diseases are the most important causes of morbidity and mortality. Although the most serious impact is on young children, death rates in adolescents and adults are also higher in sub-Saharan Africa than in other regions of the world. In recent years, the human population has experienced rapid growth and increased mobility, resulting in intrusion into new ecological settings. This increased interaction between infectious agents and human populations favors exposure to new pathogens as well as more efficient transmission of recognized ones.

Many studies predict that, despite health advances, infectious disease threats will continue and even intensify in coming years. Recent reports by the World Health Organization (WHO) (9), the Institute of Medicine (IOM) of the National Academy of Sciences (6), the National Institutes of Health (NIH) (7), and the Centers for Disease Control and Prevention (CDC) (2) warn of the increased global threat of "new" diseases such as HIV/AIDS which are emerging, and "old" diseases such as tuberculosis which are newly advancing or reemerging. The IOM defines emerging infectious diseases as "new, resurgent, or drug resistant infections of which the incidence in humans has increased within the past two decades or threatens to increase in the near future" and lists the following as determinants or risk factors for the emergence of these new threats: increasing population density/urbanization, immunosuppression (due to aging, pregnancy, malnutrition, or HIV and other infections), changes in agricultural conditions and practices, economic development and land use (e.g., reforestation), global warming, international travel and commerce, microbial/vector adaptation and change (e.g., development of microbial drug resistance and vector resistance to pesticides), and the breakdown of public health measures due to complacency or war (6).

The international community faces the challenge of effectively responding to epidemic outbreaks while concurrently addressing the underlying conditions that contribute to the emergence and reemergence of infectious

Compared to other regions of the world, an extremely high prevalence of infectious and parasitic diseases exists in Africa

diseases. Factors, both old and new, affecting global public health today include population pressures, haphazard human settlement patterns, irrational land and water management, and socioeconomic conditions that exacerbate risk of infection. Development programs must invest in strengthening national health systems so that they can function at the front line in monitoring and reacting to disease threats.

A close relationship exists between disease and development (5); prevalent diseases can stimulate development activities as well as inhibit economic development. Many development programs have both intended and unintended outcomes, with disease an important unintended consequence of development interventions. Because of these complex sociocultural interactions between disease and economic development, control strategies for the developing world should be based on sound interdisciplinary analyses and must be cross-sectorial in implementation.

Political instability, conflict, and inadequate health resources contribute to the breakdown of public health delivery systems and the resulting resurgence in previously "controlled" diseases (e.g., measles, diphtheria, tuberculosis, malaria, and dengue). These factors account for a large proportion of the reemerging disease burden in many developing and transitional countries. Increased rates of urbanization with higher population densities and shared resources (e.g., water) enhance transmission of communicable diseases. Further, migration can either bring infections to an immunologically naive population or impose endemic infections on the migrating population. This is particularly true of refugees in overcrowded camps with poor infrastructure, exemplified by the cholera outbreaks in the Rwandan refugee camps in Tanzania.

Economic development and rapid population growth lead to dramatic increases in rates of urbanization, population density, and exploitation of undisturbed land. This may bring people into closer physical contact with previously isolated vectors. As countries develop economically, intensive utilization of land and the need for additional land increase dramatically, leading to exploration and development of areas that had been relatively untouched. This increases exposure of populations to new agents or to those that had been previously contained (e.g., Lyme disease due to greater exposure to ticks). Widespread use and misuse of antibiotics in humans and in the agricultural sector contribute to the development of resistant strains of microorganisms, making common, previously treatable infections more difficult to control. Population movement by way of urbanization (i.e., economic development), displacement of populations (e.g., refugees from regions of conflict), circular migration, or international travel and commerce increases the likelihood of spreading resistant strains (3).

The world community has been made acutely aware of the risks and consequences of infectious diseases by such recent outbreaks as Ebola hemorrhagic fever in the former Zaire, hantavirus pulmonary syndrome in the southwestern United States, and epidemic plague in India. Previously unknown or obscure infectious diseases are emerging, and ones thought to be under control are reemerging or becoming resistant to

A close relationship exists between disease and development

therapy. Public health officials have been monitoring these situations over several decades, but only recently have the media given extensive coverage to acute outbreaks. Thus increasing attention has been focused on the broader issues of emerging and reemerging infections.

In response to growing concerns about emerging and reemerging diseases, the United States Congress has stated that federal agencies should do more to address infectious disease issues, both domestically and internationally. Considerable interest in the international dimension stems from the visibility of "high-profile" outbreaks and the recognition that disease transmission anywhere is a direct threat to the United States population, both at home and abroad. The White House responded with the creation of an interagency Working Group on Emerging and Re-emerging Infectious Diseases under the auspices of the National Science and Technology Council Committee on International Science, Engineering, and Technology (CISET). The 1995 publication of the CISET Working Group's recommendations for future action resulted in a June 1996 Presidential Decision Directive on "U.S. Policy on Emerging Infectious Diseases" (8). The directive declared that "emerging infectious diseases present one of the most significant health and security challenges facing the global community." This expanded focus on emerging diseases has resulted in an increase in domestic and international programs in such organizations as the United States Agency for International Development, CDC, NIH, Food and Drug Administration, Department of Defense, National Oceanic and Atmospheric Administration, and NASA. The emerging disease issue has also been incorporated into the U.S.-Japan "Common Agenda" and the U.S.-European Union "Trans-Atlantic Agenda" agreements and other diplomatic activities of the Department of State.

Bioterrorism is another emerging concern related to infectious diseases. Another Presidential Decision Directive (PDD-39) discusses "Consequence Management," or the measures needed to anticipate, prevent, and resolve a threat or act of terrorism involving "weapons of mass destruction." A prestigious foreign affairs journal argued in a cover story that the potential use of infectious agents as such weapons is of greatest concern (1). Biological warfare has been referred to for many years as "the poor man's atomic bomb." With the current ease of air travel and ability to transport exotic pathogens (or people infected with them) intercontinentally, it may become difficult to differentiate a natural from an artificial outbreak of a pathogenic microorganism. The 1995 Tokyo subway attack with sarin nerve gas has revealed our vulnerability to bioterrorist threats and the need for the international infectious disease community to prepare for such a contingency.

Major issues related to monitoring disease patterns and the progression of emerging infectious diseases include the paucity of effective national and inter-regional infectious disease surveillance systems, rapid response methods, and trained laboratory scientists and epidemiologists. Additional challenges include inadequate field laboratory facilities to detect and rapidly identify pathogens and the need for consistent research efforts in disease transmission prevention, antimicrobial resistance, and vaccine technology.

The United States Congress has stated that federal agencies should do more to address infectious disease issues, both domestically and internationally

The development of an adequate global epidemic preparedness and response capability is a significant challenge that will require effective partnerships from all corners of the health sector. This should include an active, ongoing interchange of information and ideas among clinicians, epidemiologists, pathologists, veterinarians, and development agencies.

The symposium on Emerging Infections: Clinical and Pathologic Update II and this book, an outgrowth of the presentations made during that meeting, illustrate the key contributions made by the pathology community in addressing the challenges of new, emerging, and reemerging infectious diseases. Important and informative updates are presented that highlight the threat of classic infectious diseases now threatening resurgence: yellow fever, dengue, leptospirosis, diphtheria, lymphatic filariasis, meningitis, tuberculosis, chancroid, and malaria. Complementing these are summaries of newly recognized challenges such as human immunodeficiency virus, *Mycobacterium avium*, emerging fungal diseases, *Escherichia coli* O157, bovine spongiform encephalopathy, and the growing problem of antibiotic resistance among bacterial infections. In addition, discussions of the evolvability of emerging viruses, infections among captive wildlife, and the role of the forensic pathologist in emerging infectious diseases illustrate the breadth of those challenges. An insightful collection of relevant and practical papers emerges which offers the reader a glimpse of the diversity of pathogens of importance and the complexity of the challenges to be faced. This volume and its companion, *Pathology of Emerging Infections* (4), together provide a comprehensive overview of the spectrum of emerging infections today. While the enormity of the challenges ahead is apparent, it is clear from these contributions that significant progress is being made.

The development of an adequate global epidemic preparedness and response capability is a significant challenge

References

1. **Betts, R. K.** 1998. The new threat of mass destruction. *Foreign Affairs* **Jan./Feb:**26–41.

2. **Centers for Disease Control and Prevention.** 1994. *Addressing Emerging Infectious Disease Threats: a Prevention Strategy for the United States.* U.S. Department of Health and Human Services, Public Health Service, Atlanta, Ga.

3. **Garrett, L.** 1996. The return of infectious disease. *Foreign Affairs* **Jan./Feb.:**66–79.

4. **Horsburgh, C. R., Jr., and A. M. Nelson (ed.).** 1997. *Pathology of Emerging Infections.* ASM Press, Washington, D.C.

5. **Hughes, C. C., and J. M. Hunter.** 1970. Disease and "development" in Africa. *Soc. Sci. Med.* **1970(3):**443–493.

6. **Institute of Medicine.** 1992. *Emerging Infections: Microbial Threats to Health in the United States.* National Academy of Sciences, Washington, D.C.

7. **National Institutes of Health.** 1996. *The NIAID Research Agenda for Emerging Infectious Diseases.* U.S. Department of Health and Human Services, Public Health Service, Bethesda, Md.

8. **National Science and Technology Council Committee on International Science and Technology.** 1995. *Infectious Diseases—a Global Health Threat.* Report of the Working Group on Emerging and Reemerging Infectious Diseases. Publication no. 400–451/40284. U.S. Government Printing Office, Washington, D.C.

9. **World Health Organization.** 1994. Emerging infectious diseases. *Weekly Epidemiol. Rec.* **31:**234–236.

chapter 1

Evolvability of Emerging Viruses

Donald S. Burke

RNA viruses are, by several orders of magnitude, the most genetically labile "life forms" (15, 23). Mutation rates for RNA viruses are typically on the order of one error per 10,000 nucleotides replicated, compared to one per 10 million nucleotides for larger DNA-based life forms like vertebrates (8) (Table 1.1). Since the average genome length of RNA viruses is only 10,000 nucleotides, and all are shorter than 40,000 nucleotides, almost all new viral RNA strands differ from their parent strand by one or more nucleotides. Indeed, the error rate of one mutation per progeny genome poises RNA viruses at the edge of "error catastrophe," error rates so fast that genetic information degenerates into replication incompetence. Viruses can also recombine with other related viruses to effectively "shuffle" newly evolved genes. Recombination serves both to hybridize highly fit variants and to replace defective and incompetent genes. This general strategy of repeated iterations of random variation, selection, and recombination between the best solutions ("most fit progeny") has been found to have widespread applications in problem solving,

Donald S. Burke, Center for Immunization Research, School of Hygiene and Public Health, Johns Hopkins University, Hampton House, Room 241, 624 North Broadway, Baltimore, MD 21205.

Pathology of Emerging Infections 2
Edited by Ann Marie Nelson and C. Robert Horsburgh, Jr.

Table 1.1 Error rates and genome sizes of RNA viruses as compared to autonomous organisms

Virus	Genome size: ν (number of nt or bp)	Error rate: $(1 - q)$ (per replication round and per nt)	Error rate: $\nu (1 - q)$ (per replication round and per genome)
RNA			
Bacteriophage Q_β	4,200	3×10^{-4}	1.3
Poliovirus type 1	7,400	3×10^{-4}	0.2
Vesicular stomatitis virus	11,000	1×10^{-4}	1.1
Foot and mouth disease virus	8,400	1×10^{-4}	0.8
Influenza A virus	14,000	6×10^{-5}	0.8
Sendai virus	15,000	3×10^{-5}	0.5
HIV-1 (AIDS virus)	10,000	1×10^{-4}	1.0
Avian myeloblastosis virus	7,000	5×10^{-5}	0.4
DNA			
Bacteriophage M13	6,400	7×10^{-7}	4.6×10^{-3}
Bacteriophage γ	48,500	8×10^{-8}	3.8×10^{-3}
Bacteriophage T4	166,000	2×10^{-8}	3.3×10^{-3}
Escherichia coli	4.7×10^{6}	7×10^{-10}	3.3×10^{-3}
Yeast (*Saccharomyces cerevisiae*)	13.8×10^{6}	3×10^{-10}	3.8×10^{-3}
Neurospora crassa	41.9×10^{6}	1×10^{-10}	4.2×10^{-3}
Human	3×10^{6}	$\sim10^{-12}$	$\sim3 \times 10^{-3}$

[a]Reprinted from reference 8 with permission from Elsevier Science.

> *"Genetic algorithm" strategies are widely used to rapidly calculate solutions to complex problems*

even in fields far removed from biology. Such strategies are now central to many artificial intelligence systems, from database searching to machine learning. "Genetic algorithm" strategies are widely used to rapidly calculate solutions to complex problems (5, 12, 14).

This chapter will (i) review basic evolutionary theory, particularly as it relates to viruses; (ii) summarize recent viral epidemics of global significance; (iii) present a computational model of viral evolution; and (iv) offer some thoughts about how future epidemics of emerging viruses might be predicted and prevented.

Evolutionary Theory

The nucleotide sequence of a viral genome can be thought of as an information string of 10,000 bits with four alternative states (A, C, G, and U or T) per bit. The total evolutionary potential for such a system is the universe of all possible 10,000-bit strings. These can be hypothetically arranged in a "sequence space" so that each string is adjacent to its 30,000 one-step-nearest neighbors. The total dimension of this space is 4 to the 10,000th power, a number that is greater than all atoms in the universe. Obviously, many regions in this hypothetical RNA sequence space [for example, the fringe region around a pure 10,000-poly(C) sequence] are out of bounds for replication. However, many regions of RNA sequence space do permit replication, and within these there are local optima. These optima can be conceptualized as peaks on a fitness landscape in nucleotide sequence space (25, 34).

Similarly, *evolution* can be thought of as the process whereby sequence space is explored, with successful variants colonizing the fitness peaks. Because the mutation rate of RNA replication is so high, evolutionary time for exploration of sequence space for RNA-based life can be measured in weeks and years, compared to the millennia required for DNA-based life. Rephrased, evolution of RNA life occurs on a scale that can be comprehended and studied within human dimensions. The disparity between rates of RNA and DNA evolution, the difference in RNA and DNA "evolvability," probably accounts for the fact that most of the new emerging diseases are caused by RNA viruses; RNA-based genomes have sufficient plasticity to permit rapid host switching.

This high evolvability of RNA may also account for the fact that almost all known arthropod-borne viruses (viruses that alternately replicate within vertebrate and arthropod cells) have RNA genomes. Although there are numerous DNA viruses of vertebrates and numerous DNA viruses of arthropods, remarkably there is only a single known DNA arbovirus (African swine fever virus) (24). It is likely that for most arthropod-borne viruses the sequence space fitness peak for growth in arthropod cells is close to, but not perfectly congruent with, that for growth in vertebrate cells, and mutation is required to trampoline back and forth through sequence space between the two host-specific optima.

Mutation alone may be insufficient to permit movement through some regions of sequence space (9, 10, 19). By definition, even single-step mutations from a local fitness optimum are less fit than their parents. Particularly in rugged fitness landscapes, genomes only slightly removed from the local optimum may be totally unfit, so that exploration of the surrounding space becomes impossible. Recombination between genomes on separated fitness optima permits such an "evolutionary broad-jumping" type of sequence space exploration; recombinant progeny may fall on previously totally unexplored fitness peaks (18). Naturally occurring recombination (or reassortment) has been closely studied in RNA viruses with segmented genomes such as influenza virus. Recombination has also recently been shown to occur commonly among HIV strains (2, 3). The role of recombination in nature is less well studied for other RNA viruses, but convincing examples have been found wherever they have been sought (1, 4).

The biological consequences of such recombination, whether by reassortment of segmented genomes or by true recombination through crossing over, may be the generation of novel variants with new epidemiological properties. For influenza, change by mutation, widely known as "drift," is of minor epidemiological significance, while change by recombination often results in a "shift" with an epidemiological impact felt on a global scale (20). It is now clear that "shifts" in influenza come about through recombination (reassortment) of RNA sequences from bird and pig influenza viruses with sequences from human viruses. Bird (and pig) influenza RNA explores certain regions of fitness space far from that occupied by human influenza RNA (21). Coinfection of a single host (the pig usually serves as the "mixing vessel" for avian and human influenza viruses) allows widely divergent sequences to coinfect the same cell and recombine (30). Many such progeny

Evolution of RNA life occurs on a scale that can be comprehended and studied within human dimensions

are nonviable and never reproduce, but occasionally a new variant emerges (11, 31). The same model may be applicable to many other RNA viruses. All RNA viruses apparently can and do recombine, but the epidemiological significance of recombination is less clear. Recent studies of the nucleotide sequences of HIV strains from around the world have shown that recombination may be just as dominant an evolutionary force for this virus as it is for influenza (27, 28). Non-human primate lentiviruses may contribute to the human HIV gene pool (17).

> *Recombination may be just as dominant an evolutionary force for HIV as it is for influenza*

Existing RNA viruses occupy only a tiny fraction of the available RNA sequence space. Clearly a dominant constraint is the ability of the proteins encoded by the viral RNA to functionally interact with host cell constituents. However, there are probably several other structural (protein/protein, protein/RNA, etc) constraints on sequence space exploration.

In addition, models from the new scientific field of "complexity" suggest that genomes in whole galaxies of sequence space may be inherently unfit not because of protein structural constraints but because of deeper constraints on the evolvability of their informational content (18). Some sequence sets may fail to evolve and remain frozen in sequence space (analogous to a solid). Others may expand through sequence space too rapidly and degenerate to chaos (analogous to a gas). If the concept of "life at the edge of chaos" has merit, perhaps only certain regions of sequence space encode the "liquid" information evolvability necessary to explore and then stably colonize new fitness peaks.

Real Viruses, Real Pandemics

In the past 30 years there have been at least seven "new" viruses that have caused global epidemics involving millions of humans (Table 1.2). All of the recent global pandemics have been of RNA viruses with an ability to recombine or reassort genetic material between viruses. For the influenza A viruses (H3N2 and H1N1) there is solid evidence that the new epidemic strains arise through mixing of genes from animal influenza viruses with genes from preexisting human influenza virus. For the retroviruses (HIV and HTLV) there is suggestive evidence that these viruses crossed the species barrier from non-human primates into humans. The recent pan-

Table 1.2   Recent viral pandemics (Ro >> 1) in human populations

Disease	Year	Location	Family	Virus
Influenza	1968	Hong Kong	*Orthomyxoviridae*	Influenza A (H3N2)
Hemorrhagic conjunctivitis	1969	Ghana	*Picornaviridae*	Enterovirus 70
Meningitis	1969	United States	*Picornaviridae*	Enterovirus 71
Hemorrhagic conjunctivitis	1970	Singapore	*Picornaviridae*	Coxsackievirus A24/variant
Influenza	1977	Russia	*Orthomyxoviridae*	Influenza A (H1N1)
AIDS	1981	United States, Zaire	*Retroviridae*	HIV-1
Leukemia, lymphoma	1982	Japan	*Retroviridae*	Human T-cell lymphotropic virus

Table 1.3 Recent localized (Ro < 1) new viral epidemics in human populations

Disease	Year	Location	Family	Virus
Neuropsychosis	1985	Germany	*Paramyxoviridae*	Borna disease virus
AIDS-like	1986	West Africa	*Retroviridae*	HIV-2
Hemorrhagic fever	1989	Venezuela	*Arenaviridae*	Guanarito virus
Influenza	1993	Netherlands	*Orthomyxoviridae*	Influenza A virus (H3N2, avian)
Pulmonary syndrome	1993	Western United States	*Bunyaviridae*	Sin Nombre virus
Hemorrhagic fever	1995	Zaire	*Filoviridae*	Ebola virus

demic picornaviridae (enterovirus 70, enterovirus 71, and coxsackievirus A24/variant) probably derived directly from preexisting human viruses, but a genetic contribution from an animal picornavirus gene pool cannot be ruled out.

Outbreaks and epidemics of new viruses in humans are continually being observed around the world. Some very recent examples are shown in Table 1.3; all are RNA viruses. As compared to the viruses causing global pandemics (above and Table 1.2), these viruses show no or only a limited capacity for human-to-human transmission. For four of the six viruses shown in Table 1.3, humans are known to become infected directly with a virus that is native to animals. In one case (Borna) an animal reservoir is suspected, and in one (Ebola) the reservoir is unknown.

New viral epidemics are also continually being observed around the world in animal populations. Table 1.4 shows some very recent examples. All but one of these recent epidemic viruses are RNA viruses; the canine parvovirus is the only example of a new epidemic animal DNA virus. Four of these viruses are thought to have arisen through interspecies transfer (canine parvovirus, lion paramyxovirus, dolphin paramyxovirus, equine paramyxovirus), while the other two are thought to have arisen through mutation of a virus already endemic in the species (pig coronavirus, chicken influenza virus).

Collectively, these new epidemics demonstrate the ability of viruses in many RNA virus families to cross species barriers where they can cause disease and become serially transmitted within the new host species.

These new epidemics demonstrate the ability of viruses in many RNA virus families to cross species barriers

Table 1.4 Some important recent viral epidemics in animal populations

Host	Disease	Year	Location	Family	Virus
Zoo	Pox/pulmonary	1973	Russia	*Poxviridae*	Cowpox (rodent) virus
Chicken	Influenza	1983	United States	*Orthomyxoviridae*	Influenza A virus (H5N2)
Pig	Respiratory	1984	Europe	*Coronaviridae*	Porcine respiratory coronavirus
Dog	Enteritis	1987	Worldwide	*Parvoviridae*	Canine parvovirus
Dolphin	Respiratory	1988	United States	*Paramyxoviridae*	Dolphin and porpoise morbillivirus
Lion	Encephalitis	1994	Tanzania	*Paramyxoviridae*	Canine distemper virus
Horse	Respiratory	1994	Australia	*Paramyxoviridae*	Equine morbillivirus
Rabbit	Hemorrhagic	1995	Australia	*Caliciviridae*	Rabbit hemorrhagic disease virus

Virtual Viruses

My colleagues at the Navy Center for Applied Research in Artificial Intelligence and I have recently been working on a computational model of viral evolution, a "virtual virus" that we call "VIV." The effort to construct a computer simulation of virus evolution was inspired by the observation that the evolutionary strategy of HIV, a diploid virus with a high mutation rate and a high recombination rate, was remarkably similar to the evolutionary computation strategies known as "genetic algorithms" used for machine learning and robotics.

Genetic algorithms (GAs) are heuristic learning (problem-solving) models based on principles drawn from natural evolution and selective breeding (5, 12). In a typical GA a *population of structures* (a population of bit strings or programs) is established that can be interpreted as a pool of candidate solutions to the given problem. *Competitive selection* is employed to allow these structures to reproduce, based on each structure's fitness as a solution to the given problem. Idealized *genetic operators*, such as mutation or recombination, are applied to the selected structures in order to create a new generation of structures. In many applications in optimization and search, these features enable the genetic algorithm to rapidly improve the average fitness of the population and to quickly identify the high-performance regions of very complex search spaces (6, 13, 29).

For the VIV computational model we constructed an artificial genetic system (33). In this system arbitrary "nucleotide" triplets encode English letters rather than amino acids, and sequences are translated into words or groups of words rather than into polypeptides or proteins. The standard target phenotype in VIV is the words "COREPROTEIN," "POLYMERASE," and "ENVELOPE," which can be present in any order along the string. Run-on and overlapping reading frames are permitted. Fitness is assigned to each string according to the encoded spelling score. Perfect spelling of all three words is assigned a fitness of 1.0, while random gibberish is assigned a fitness score of 0.0. Although redundancies and noncoding regions are not directly scored, string brevity is rewarded with higher fitness. In a typical VIV simulation experiment, a single population of 500 random strings of lengths distributed between 100 and 500 nucleotides is permitted to evolve for 2,000 generations. Evolutionary operators such as the frequency of mutation or recombination are then systematically varied, and "adaptation curves" (plots of population fitness per generation) are analyzed.

We have drawn several conclusions from our preliminary VIV simulations, as follows: (i) the optimal point mutation rate is close to one mutation per genome per replication cycle; (ii) when added to mutation, recombination in any form speeds adaptation; (iii) homologous recombination is superior to random crossover recombination; and (iv) adaptation speed increases with homologous recombination rates up to 0.4 recombination events per replication cycle, but little more at higher recombination rates. These results suggest that HIV, a real "diploid" virus with a measured mutation rate of about one mutation per genome per replication cycle and a measured high recombination rate, may search sequence space with near-optimal efficiency (16, 26, 32, 35).

For the VIV computational model we constructed an artificial genetic system

The basic VIV model can be modified to incorporate a variety of evolutionary operators, such as genome segmentation, genomic secondary structures, insertions and deletions, and feedback loops and hypercycles. Such studies are in progress.

Predicting and Preventing Viral Pandemics

Given the considerable attention focused on emerging diseases, it is striking how little discussion there has been on how we, the human species, might predict and prevent, rather than simply detect and react to, future pandemics. To do so requires a rational approach to risk assessment. I propose three criteria to identify the set of virus families that pose the greatest risk for a new global pandemic.

It is striking how little discussion there has been on how we, the human species, might predict and prevent future pandemics

The first criterion is the most obvious: recent pandemics in human history. Those viruses already proven to cause human pandemics are clearly able to do so again. These would include the *Orthomyxoviridae* (influenza), the *Lentiviridae* (HIV-1), and the *Picornaviridae* (enterovirus 70).

The second criterion is proven ability to cause major epidemics in non-human animal populations. Here a different but overlapping set of virus families is identified, including the *Orthomyxoviridae*, the *Paramyxoviridae*, and the *Coronaviridae*.

The third criterion (which may be less obvious) reflects the thesis that I have tried to build in this chapter, that intrinsic evolvability confers on a virus the potential to emerge into and to cause pandemics in human populations. Virus families with proven high mutation rates and which have genomic organizational features that foster recombination meet this criterion. These include the *Orthomyxoviridae*, *Retroviridae*, *Coronaviridae*, and *Reoviridae*.

Some of these viruses, particularly those like the *Coronaviridae* and the related *Arteriviridae*, should be considered as serious threats to human health. These are viruses with high evolvability and proven ability to cause epidemics in animal populations.

Whence and when will new viruses emerge? Of the 68 virus genera that are known to infect vertebrates, 47 are already known to infect humans. The remaining 21 virus genera are thought to infect only non-human vertebrates. Of these, 10 are large DNA viruses not likely to successfully cross species into humans; 2 are small DNA viruses; and 3 are RNA viruses known to infect only fish and fowl. This leaves six genera of RNA viruses that routinely infect other mammals but are not known to infect humans. Among these, the *Arteriviridae* (particularly simian hemorrhagic fever virus) are particularly worrisome.

Serious consideration must also be given to the geographic location of research laboratories for the study of emerging viruses (22). Two observations should guide the placement of study sites. First, viruses easily cross species boundaries between closely related host species but are less able to do so between more distantly related hosts: humans are more susceptible to viruses of monkeys than to viruses of fish. Second, for any given viral taxon the pool of viral variation is greatest in those geographic regions where host variation is greatest. For these reasons, any effective global program to predict and prevent emerging viral pandemics should systematically study viruses in those parts of the world where the number and diversity of mammalian species, and in particular the diversity of primate species, is the greatest, such as the tropical rain forests of Africa and South America. The current complete lack of sustained United States-supported research efforts in these important regions should be corrected.

A Closing Thought

This chapter has presented a fairly abstract, conceptual approach to viral evolution and emergence. Indeed, the skeptical reader might liken it to William James's view, offered over a century ago (7):

Evolution is a change . . .

Evolution is a change
from a nohowish, untalkaboutable,
all-alikeness,
to a somehowish and in-general-talkaboutable,
not-all-alikeness,
by continuous
somethingelsifications and sticktogetherations.

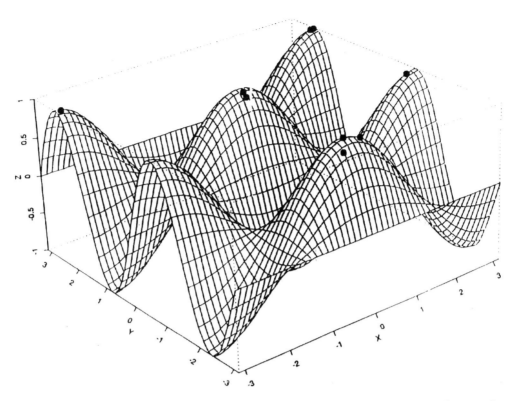

Figure 1.1 Representation of evolving bit strings in sequence space. Here the sequence space is shown only in two dimensions, the *x* and *y* axes. For a string of length *L*, the strings would evolve through an *L*-dimensional sequence space, but this is impossible to draw on a two-dimensional paper surface. Fitness is represented as the height on the *z* axis. In this example populations of strings are colonizing several local fitness optima.

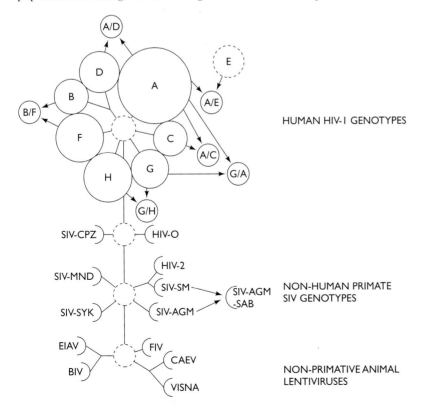

Figure 1.2 Cartoon of the lentivirus phylogenetic tree, showing the relationship between major virus groups. The dotted circles at nodes represent branch points for which relationships are not entirely certain. Viruses branching from the bottom node are the lentiviruses of horses, equine infectious anemia virus (EIAV); of cows, bovine immunodeficiency viruses (BIV); of cats, feline immunodeficiency virus (FIV); and of goats and sheep, caprine arthritis encephalitis virus (CAEV) and visna virus. Viruses from the second node are the simian immunodeficiency viruses (SIVs) of African green monkeys (AGM), mandrills (MND), Syke's monkeys (SYK), sooty mangabeys (SM), and sabeus monkeys (SB). The SIV of chimpanzees branches from the next node along with the HIV-1 outlier strains (HIV-O) and the standard genotypic variants of HIV-1, shown as letters A through H. Diameter size for each variant is roughly proportional to the genetic variation within that genotype. HIV-2 is genetically very similar to SIV-SM. Known recombinant lentiviruses are shown as the juncture of two arrows from their parent genotypes.

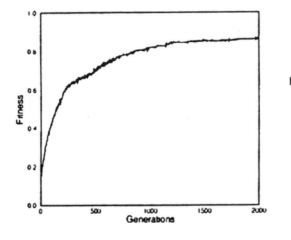

Experimental parameters:
- Population size: 500
- Initial length: 512
- Length of Run: 2000 generations
- 1-point homologous crossover
- Best of generation, avg over 10 runs

```
Generation 0:   Fitness: 0.118
        -----------_CFGOMFLSAR.-----------------------------------------
        -------_POLFHCTWNMEPQ.----------------------------------------
        ------:-------------------------------------------_EIEPJUHME.---

Generation 500:   Fitness: 0.856
        -------------------------------------_COREPROF_LTKREIN.-------
        ----------------------
        -------_POLYMERASE.-------------------------------------------
        ----------------------
        ----------------------_ENVEBQNLOPE.--------------------------
        ----------------------

Generation 2000:   Fitness: 0.930
        -----------------------------------_COREPROVEJTEIN.-
        ---_POLYMERASE.-----------------------------------------
        --------------------_ENVEWLOPE.-----------------------
```

Figure 1.3   "Learning curves" for evolving populations of strings in the virtual virus (VIV) model. Generations (replication cycles) are shown on the *x* axis, and fitness (a value based on the spelling score and adjusted for string length; see text) is shown on the *y* axis. In this experiment the population sizes = 500; generations = 2,000; initial genome lengths = 100 to 500; and mutation rate = 0.003 per site per replication. Curve shows a population replicating with homologous recombination at every replication.

References

1. **Ahmen, R., C. S. Hahn, T. Somasundaram, L. Villarete, M. Matloubian, and J. H. Strauss.** 1991. Molecular basis of organ-specific selection of viral variants using chronic infection. *J. Virol.* **65:**4242–4247.

2. **Burke, D. S.** 1997. Recombination in HIV: an important viral evolutionary strategy. *Emerg. Infect. Dis.* **3:**253–259.

3. **Burke, D. S., and F. E. McCutchan.** 1996. Global distribution of human immunodeficiency virus-1 clades, p. 119–126. *In* V. T. Devita, Jr., S. Hellman, and S. A. Rosenberg (ed.), *AIDS: Biology, Diagnosis, Treatment and Prevention,* 4th ed. Lippincott-Raven Publishers, Philadelphia.

4. **Clarke, D. K., E. A. Duarte, A. Moya, S. F. Elena, E. Domingo, and J. Holland.** 1993. Bottlenecks and population passages cause profound fitness differences in RNA viruses. *J. Virol.* **67:**222–228.

5. **DeJong, K. A.** 1990. Genetic-algorithm-based learning. *In* Y. Kodratoff and R. Michalski (ed.), *Machine Learning: an Artificial Intelligence Approach,* vol. 3. Morgan Kaufmann, San Francisco.

6. **DeJong, K. A., and W. M. Spears.** 1992. A formal analysis of the role of multipoint crossover in genetic algorithms. *Ann. Math. Artificial Intelligence* **5:**1–26.

7. **Dennett, D. C.** 1995. *Darwin's Dangerous Idea: Evolution and the Meanings of Life,* p. 393. Simon & Schuster, New York.

8. **Eigen, M.** 1993. The origin of genetic information: viruses as models. *Gene* **135:**37–47.

9. **Felsenstein, J.** 1974. The evolutionary advantage of recombination. *Genetics* **78:**737–756.

10. **Felsenstein, J., and S. Yokoyama.** 1976. The evolutionary advantage of recombination. II. Individual selection for recombination. *Genetics* **83:**845–859.

11. **Gammelin, M., A. Altmuller, U. Reinhardt, and J. Mandler.** 1990. Phylogenetic analysis of nucleoproteins suggests that human influenza A viruses emerged from a 19th-century avian ancestor. *Mol. Biol. Evol.* **7:**194–200.

12. **Goldberg, D. E.** 1989. *Genetic Algorithms in Search, Optimization, and Machine Learning.* Addison-Wesley Publishing Co., Reading, Mass.

13. **Grefenstette, J. J.** 1988. Credit assignment in rule discovery systems based on genetic algorithms. *Mach. Learning* **3**(2/3)**:**225–245.

14. **Holland, J. H.** 1975. *Adaptation in Natural and Artificial Systems.* University of Michigan Press, Ann Arbor, Mich.

15. **Holland, J., K. Spindler, F. Horodyski, E. Grabau, S. Nichol, and S. VandePol.** 1982. Rapid evolution of RNA genomes. *Science* **215:**1577–1585.

16. **Hu, W.-S., and H. M. Temin.** 1990. Genetic consequences of packaging two RNA genomes in one retroviral particle: pseudodiploidy and high rate of genetic recombination. *Proc. Natl. Acad. Sci. USA* **87:**1556–1560.

17. **Jin, M. J., H. Hui, and D. L. Robertson.** 1994. Mosaic genome structure of simian immunodeficiency virus from West African green monkeys. *EMBO J.* **13:**2935–2947.

18. **Kauffman, S. A.** 1993. *The Origins of Order,* p. 114–117. Oxford University Press, New York.

19. **Kondrashov, A. S.** 1984. Deleterious mutations as an evolutionary factor. I. The advantage of recombination. *Genet. Res.* **44:**199–217.

20. **LaForce, F. M., K. L. Nichol, and N. J. Cox.** 1994. Influenza: virology, epidemiology, disease, and prevention. *Am. J. Prev. Med.* **10**(Suppl.):31–44.

21. **Ludwig, S., U. Schultz, J. Mandler, W. M. Fitch, and C. Scholtissek.** 1991. Phylogenetic relationship of the nonstructural (NS) genes of influenza A viruses. *Virology* **183**:566–577.

22. **Morse, S.** 1991. Emerging viruses: defining the rules for viral traffic. *Perspect. Biol. Med.* **34**:387–409.

23. **Morse, S., and A. Schluederberg.** 1990. Emerging viruses: the evolution of viruses and viral diseases. *J. Infect. Dis.* **162**:1–7.

24. **Murphy, F. A., C. M. Fauquet, D. H. L. Bishop, S. A. Ghabrial, A. W. Jarvis, G. P. Martelli, M. A. Mayo, and M. D. Summers (ed.).** 1995. *Virus Taxonomy: Classification and Nomenclature of Viruses: Sixth Report of the International Committee on Taxonomy of Viruses*, p. 586. Springer-Verlag, New York.

25. **Provine, W. B.** 1986. *Sewall Wright and Evolutionary Biology*, p. 307–317. University of Chicago Press, Chicago.

26. **Roberts, J. D., K. Bebenek, and T. A. Kunkel.** 1988. The accuracy of reverse transcriptase from HIV-1. *Science* **242**:1171–1173.

27. **Robertson, D. L., B. H. Hahn, and P. M. Sharp.** 1995. Recombination in AIDS viruses. *J. Mol. Evol.* **40**:249–259.

28. **Robertson, D. L., P. M. Sharp, F. E. McCutchan, and B. H. Hahn.** 1995. Recombination in HIV-1. *Nature* **374**:124–126. (Letter.)

29. **Ross, J.** 1993. Learning Boolean function with genetic algorithms: a PAC analysis. *In* D. Whitley (ed.), *Foundations of Genetic Algorithms-2*. Morgan Kaufmann, San Francisco.

30. **Schultz, U., W. M. Fitch, S. Ludwig, J. Mandler, and C. Scholtissek.** 1991. Evolution of pig influenza viruses. *Virology* **183**:61–73.

31. **Shu, L. L., W. J. Bean, and R. G. Webster.** 1993. Analysis of the evolution and variation of the human influenza A virus nucleoprotein gene from 1933 to 1990. *J. Virol.* **67**:2723–2729.

32. **Temin, H. M.** 1991. Sex and recombination in retroviruses. *Trends Genet.* **7**:71–74.

33. **Woese, C.** 1969. Models for the evolution of codon assignments. *J. Mol. Biol.* **43**:235–240.

34. **Wright, S.** 1932. The roles of mutation, inbreeding, crossbreeding, and selection in evolution, p. 356. *In Proceedings of the Sixth International Congress of Genetics*.

35. **Zhang, J., and H. M. Temin.** 1994. Retrovirus recombination depends on the length of sequence identity and is not error prone. *J. Virol.* **68**:2409–2414.

chapter 2

Yellow Fever

Carlos del Río and Frederick A. Meier

In the past decade there has been a reemergence of yellow fever (68), a disease which appeared well controlled and for which an effective vaccine has been available for over 50 years (2). The disease occurs only in Central America, the northern half of South America, and Central Africa (52, 54). Yellow fever is a viral disease transmitted by a mosquito and is one of the "viral hemorrhagic fevers." In its most severe form the disease is characterized by fever, jaundice, and hemorrhagic manifestations, with a case-fatality rate for adults who are not immune of over 50% (52).

The yellow fever virus is a group B arbovirus and the prototype of the Flavivirus genus of the family *Flaviviridae*, which includes 29 other viruses that cause human disease including other hemorrhagic fevers like dengue, Kyasanur Forest disease, and Omsk hemorrhagic fever (54). The yellow fever virus is a spherical, enveloped, single-stranded RNA particle approximately 38

Carlos del Río, Division of Infectious Diseases, Department of Medicine, Emory University School of Medicine, 69 Butler Street, S.E., Atlanta, GA 30303. **Frederick A. Meier,** Clinical and Anatomic Pathology, DuPont Hospital for Children, P.O. Box 269, 1600 Rockland Road, Wilmington, DE 19899-0269, and Jefferson Medical College, Philadelphia, PA.

Pathology of Emerging Infections 2
Edited by Ann Marie Nelson and C. Robert Horsburgh, Jr.
© 1998 American Society for Microbiology, Washington, D.C.

nm in diameter. The viral genome is 11,000 nucleotides in length and encodes 10 gene products. The nucleotide sequence of the 17D vaccine strain was described in 1985 (66), and 2 years later the entire sequence of the parental virulent Asibi strain was described (53). The virulent strain differs from strain 17D by 32 amino acids, primarily in the E glycoprotein gene. The flaviviruses share many antigenic determinants, and frequent cross-reactions make the serologic diagnosis difficult.

Yellow fever has two types of transmission cycles, determined on the basis of different mosquito vectors and hosts involved. However, the disease is clinically and pathologically the same (52). "Jungle yellow fever" is a zoonotic infection in which the virus is transmitted among non-human primates by wild (usually tree-hole-breeding) mosquitoes, and humans become infected incidentally; in "urban yellow fever" the virus is transmitted from infected to susceptible humans by *Aedes aegypti* mosquitoes which breed in household containers and refuse (51, 52, 54).

> *Yellow fever has two types of transmission cycles, determined on the basis of different mosquito vectors and hosts involved*

History

Yellow fever was first described in 1684 and caused significant economic and human losses for many years. Dr. Carlos Finlay in Cuba proposed in 1881 that yellow fever was transmitted by mosquitoes, a theory proven to be correct in 1900 by Major Walter Reed and colleagues, who demonstrated transmission by *Aedes aegypti* and also suggested a viral etiology for the disease. The virus was not isolated until 1927, when blood from a Ghanaian man was inoculated into rhesus monkeys (21, 53). Within the next few years a vaccine was developed, and wide-scale use of the vaccine and efforts to eradicate the vector brought yellow fever under control. Indeed, by 1951 a book on yellow fever by George Strode described the remarkable achievements of the past and optimistically considered the "conquest of yellow fever" (the title of the book's first chapter) a reality (77).

Epidemiology

Yellow fever is endemic exclusively in equatorial Africa and South America. For reasons that are unclear, the disease does not occur in Asia. Between 1987 and 1991 a total of 18,735 cases and 4,522 deaths were reported worldwide. In 1994, 1,439 cases were reported to the World Health Organization (WHO) (94% in Africa), with 491 deaths. In contrast, in 1995, 974 (47% in Africa) cases and 247 deaths were reported to WHO (92); however, these numbers do not accurately reflect the true incidence of yellow fever because only a small fraction of cases are recognized or reported. Some estimates suggest that over 200,000 cases of yellow fever now occur yearly in the 33 endemic African countries alone (93). Rural populations are at greatest risk, with most adult cases occurring among young men who enter forests as part of their work. Male cases normally outnumber female by a ratio of about 2:1

(93). Outbreaks of yellow fever were reported in 1994 in Cameroon, Gabon, Ghana, and Nigeria. Nigeria reported 91% of all cases from Africa and 85% of cases in the world for that year. Some countries, like Liberia and Kenya, which had not reported yellow fever since 1950 have experienced recent outbreaks which suggest that yellow fever not only is prevalent in equatorial Africa but may be expanding its range to previously unaffected areas (Table 2.1).

In South America less than 200 cases per year were reported from 1990 to 1994. The number of cases increased dramatically in 1995 to 515 with 213 deaths. Of all countries in South America which reported yellow fever, Peru has experienced the largest increase in the number of cases, from less than 100 each year from 1991 through 1994 to 492 cases and 192 deaths in 1995 (92). In fact, in 1995 Peru reported 96% of yellow fever cases in South America and 51% of world cases (Table 2.2).

Since yellow fever usually occurs in remote areas with few medical services, recognition of cases is frequently delayed, which delays the initiation of control measures. In Africa, delays of 2 months or more are not uncommon between the onset of epidemics and their recognition (93). For this reason a system for surveillance of hemorrhagic fevers has been suggested for countries at risk for yellow fever outbreaks. Such a system, if implemented, could potentially improve case recognition as well as the implementation of public health interventions to control outbreaks (71).

Imported yellow fever was not reported in the United States from 1924 until 1996, when an American tourist returning from Brazil died of yellow fever (49). *Aedes aegypti* is well established in the southern United States, from Texas to South Carolina, and recently this mosquito has also been found as far north as Maryland and New Jersey and as far west as Arizona; thus, the potential exists for transmission in the United States (29).

Imported yellow fever was not reported in the United States from 1924 until 1996

Table 2.1 Yellow fever cases notified from Africa to WHO, 1991–1996[a]

Country	No. of cases per year:					
	1991	1992	1993	1994	1995	1996
Burkina Faso	0	0	0	0	0	114
Cameroon	0	0	0	10	0	0
Gabon	0	0	0	28	16	0
Ghana	0	0	39	79	0	27
Kenya	0	27	27	7	3	0
Liberia	0	0	0	0	360	0
Nigeria	2,561	149	152	1,227	0	0
Senegal	0	0	0	0	79	0
Sierra Leone	0	0	0	0	1	0
Total	2,561	176	218	1,351	459	141
Deaths	661	21	38	452	34	N.A.

[a]Last update, May 16, 1997. N. A., not available.

Table 2.2 Yellow fever cases notified from South America to WHO, 1991–1996[a]

Country	No. of cases per year:					
	1991	1992	1993	1994	1995	1996[b]
Bolivia	91	22	18	7	15	30
Brazil	15	12	66	18	4	0
Colombia	4	2	1	2	3	0
Ecuador	14	16	1	0	1	0
Peru	27	67	89	61	492	0
Total	151	119	175	88	515	30
Deaths	90	81	79	39	213	N.A.

[a]Last update, May 16, 1997.

[b]United States and Switzerland: one imported and one fatal case each.

Clinical Features

Yellow fever is an acute disease characterized by sudden onset of fever, chills, head, back, and muscle pain, nausea, and vomiting. These symptoms may progress to the icteric phase, which involves jaundice with hemorrhagic signs, but the spectrum ranges from mild, nonspecific febrile illness to fulminating disease (51). The incubation period is usually 3 to 6 days but occasionally may be longer.

Most infected persons (80 to 90%) have a mild, nonspecific febrile illness, but 10 to 20% develop classic yellow fever. The early phase ("period of infection") is characterized by fever, chills, headache, generalized malaise, and myalgias. On physical examination, fever with relative bradycardia (Faget's sign) and conjunctival injection are the most common findings. Over the next few days the patient appears to recover ("period of remission") only to have the fever recur ("period of intoxication") associated with jaundice, oliguria, and hemorrhagic manifestations, including hematemesis ("black vomit") and diffuse oozing from mucous membranes. Delirium, stupor, acidosis, and shock then follow, with up to 50% of patients dying between days 7 and 10 after the onset of illness. On laboratory examination, yellow fever is characterized by leukopenia, thrombocytopenia, and albuminuria as well as elevated transaminases, bilirubin, blood urea nitrogen, and creatinine (51, 52, 54). Data regarding the coagulopathy observed in patients with severe yellow fever are conflicting, but in some cases it appears that it may be secondary to disseminated intravascular coagulation (23, 51, 55).

The differential diagnosis of severe yellow fever includes dengue and other flavivirus hemorrhagic fevers, Ebola and other non-flavivirus hemorrhagic fevers, acute viral hepatitis, leptospirosis and other hepatotropic bacterial infections, and malaria. The isolation of the yellow fever virus from blood or tissue specimens, the detection of viral antigen in serum by enzyme-linked immunosorbent assay (ELISA), or detection of viral RNA by PCR will provide a definite diagnosis (57, 59). The virus is most readily isolated from blood during the first 3 or 4 days of illness (period of infection), and proper handling of the specimens to preserve the virus is essential. Thus, attempts to isolate the virus during suspected outbreaks are frequently unsuccessful (71).

Serologic methods useful in the diagnosis of yellow fever include hemagglutination inhibition, complement fixation, neutralization, indirect immunofluorescence, and ELISA. The detection of immunoglobulin M (IgM) antibodies by ELISA is especially useful and appears to be more sensitive and specific than hemagglutination inhibition or complement fixation; these antibodies do not appear until 1 week after infection (25). When acute- and convalescent-phase sera are available, a rising antibody titer also provides a confirmatory diagnosis. Molecular techniques could certainly be developed for the diagnosis of yellow fever, but advances have been slow, reflecting the fact that yellow fever is a neglected disease. As described in detail below, histologic diagnosis from autopsy material still remains a useful approach to the detection of yellow fever.

Attempts to isolate the virus during suspected outbreaks are frequently unsuccessful

Diagnosis

The components of an integrated diagnostic approach to yellow fever can include (i) viral culture (either in tissue monolayers or, more frequently in the past, in rodent meningocephalitis models) (17, 48); (ii) serologic or nucleic acid amplification diagnosis (using, in the past, the then available methods of hemagglutination, complement fixation, and infection neutralization and now an IgM-ELISA and RNA amplification) (80); and (iii) histopathologic diagnosis. In clinical circumstances, however, culture diagnosis depends on the patient being viremic at the time that the sample is collected for inoculation into the tissue culture or animal model. As previously mentioned, in yellow fever viremia usually clears by day 4 of infection (40). This viremic period comprises the earlier, less specific, of the two clinical stages of this disease (55). In this initial stage, the signs and symptoms of yellow fever are essentially indistinguishable from those of dengue, also caused by a flavivirus spread by *Aedes aegypti* and other species of mosquitoes. In general, the signs and symptoms of the initial phase are also indistinguishable from those of other endemic fevers, including malaria, that are widely prevalent in areas where yellow fever may (re)appear (20). Because of this nonspecificity of clinical presentation, the window of opportunity to collect a blood sample appropriate for culture is frequently missed (20, 30).

In the past the serologic techniques available have been relatively nonspecific. Inapparent previous infection, waning vaccine-induced immunity, and cross-reactions due to other flaviviruses contribute to the nonspecificity of serodiagnosis. Yellow fever may reappear in populations where subclinical yellow fever infection is present and where incompletely successful yellow fever vaccination efforts have been attempted. In the same areas, not only dengue but also other endemic, typically simian, arthropod-borne flaviviruses, the latter usually nonpathogenic to humans, are often part of the ecosystem and produce antibodies that cross-react in yellow fever sero-

Characteristic histopathologic changes appear at a time that is "just right"

diagnostic tests. Unless the yellow fever IgM-ELISA is available, serodiagnosis of yellow fever requires the comparison of acute- and convalescent-phase antibody titers, the latter titers coming from blood samples collected weeks after the usual period of acute illness. This, at the very least, requires that the patient survive and be available for blood collection weeks after the clinical episode of disease.

In contrast to "too-early" culture diagnosis and frequently "too-late" serological diagnosis, characteristic histopathologic changes appear at a time that is "just right," between day 3 and day 7 of infection. This time span usually corresponds to the height of the clinical syndrome and the greatest incidence of mortality. By then, in the second clinical phase of the illness, coagulopathic hemorrhage, especially of the upper gastrointestinal tract, has produced the characteristic "black bile." At about the same point in the time course, liver failure has produced the characteristic, surprisingly mild jaundice that separates "yellow" from the rest of the "hemorrhagic" fevers. Acute renal failure is often a third, and the most ominous, component of this second clinical phase. In this phase of highest mortality, diagnostic material becomes immediately available postmortem (from patients among whom the development of convalescent immunity is definitely precluded). So, in this epidemiological and clinical setting, a series of features focus attention on histopathology: frequent unavailability of culture, problems with the specificity and availability of serology, and a temporal connection between relatively specific clinical findings, which raise the diagnostic question of yellow fever, and the highly specific histopathologic appearances that confirm that diagnosis.

On a practical level, histopathology can be of central importance because the technical capacity to produce interpretable histologic sections and the professional ability to recognize the characteristic histologic appearances of yellow fever in those sections may be more "exportable" than the techniques and expertise of tissue culture, both directly, for virological diagnosis, and indirectly, for the production of antigen for serologic diagnosis. The expense of animal and tissue culture models may preclude their use in many circumstances. In this context, during the middle third of this century, the relative ease and effectiveness of histopathologic diagnosis led, in some jurisdictions, to surveillance by necropsy of all persons dying of febrile illness in endemic areas, a tactic that regularly brought to light clinically unsuspected infections (76). Epidemiologically, these discoveries contributed sentinel cases that signaled where the wandering epizootic had ventured into a human population. Clinically, the results of these autopsies heightened practitioners' awareness of the nonspecificity, in the majority of patients, of yellow fever's clinical presentation: the biphasic pattern of sudden onset of fever and prostration, followed by liver (and kidney) failure with disproportionately mild to moderate jaundice as mentioned above. Most often malaria, but also other hemorrhagic fevers, viral hepatitides, typhoid fever, and the variety of other toxic and toxic-like (or "nutritional") conditions, the illnesses which make up the differential diagnosis of yellow fever, could also be diagnosed by necropsy techniques.

The impact of newer serodiagnostic and molecular diagnostic modalities on the timely, practical diagnosis of yellow fever remains unclear, partly because of the geographic mismatch between the technical ability to evaluate the newer modalities and the current distribution of yellow fever infection. As it stands, Strano's claim, advanced in the early 1970s, that "histopathology remains the most generally available way to diagnose yellow fever expeditiously," is still highly defensible (76).

The anatomic pathology of yellow fever on which this approach is based is made up of four components: gross pathology, histopathology of experimental simian infections, diagnostic histopathology of human infections, and the differential diagnosis of that histopathology (76).

Gross Pathology

The gross morbid anatomy of yellow fever seen at postmortem examination is shared with infections caused by other flaviviruses (9, 15, 28). In contrast to the generic gross findings, the microscopic characteristics in experimental infections of monkeys not only are specific to yellow fever (43), but also correlate with sequential stages of the infection (4). The experimental findings have, in turn, validated the consistent histopathologic presentation of human yellow fever (5, 51). In the usual clinical and epidemiological setting, the consistent, characteristic hepatic histopathology of yellow fever has proven useful in differentiating yellow fever from other similar but distinct entities (30, 76).

The gross morbid anatomy of yellow fever is shared with infections caused by other flaviviruses

Extrahepatic

Extrahepatic autopsy findings in yellow fever are nonspecific (1) but helpful with differential diagnosis (76). Despite the illness's name, jaundice of skin and sclera tends to be only moderate. Epithelial evidence of a hemorrhagic diathesis tends to be more prominent: oozing of blood from minute erosions in oral, gastric, proximal duodenal, and urinary bladder epithelia (39). This phenomenon in the stomach, worked upon by gastric acid, produces the "black vomit" stressed in historical descriptions of the disease (53). In the central nervous system the pattern of coagulopathic hemorrhage is typically petechial and localized in the meninges, mammillary bodies, and periventricular gray matter (76). These features demonstrated in patients dying from yellow fever—mild to moderate jaundice, epithelial oozing, and parenchymal petechial hemorrhage—are the gross appearances in most fatal flavivirus hemorrhagic fevers. For this reason, their appearance in combination should be regarded as raising this generic possibility rather than specifically implicating the yellow fever virus.

Some other findings in the gross examination of nonhepatic viscera are also potentially significant. An enlarged, greasy heart, especially if it correlates with clinical bradycardia, with or without hypotension, raises the question of a myocardiopathy as part of the presentation. Similarly, enlarged, congested, heavy kidneys, with or without yellow streaks in the medullary rays (especially if these findings correlate with clinical proteinuria and oliguria), increase the likelihood that acute tubular necrosis will be demonstrable microscopically (1, 76).

The gross appearance of the liver at autopsy is surprisingly subtle and nonspecific in yellow fever patients

Hepatic

Given the relative specificity of the microscopic hepatic findings, described below, the gross appearance of the liver at autopsy is surprisingly subtle and nonspecific in yellow fever patients (11). The size and weight of the liver tend to be within physiologic reference ranges. If the liver does not fall within reference measures, then it tends to be slightly enlarged, rather than shrunken (76). This usual gross appearance of the liver in yellow fever contrasts strikingly with the shrunken, underweight livers characteristically seen in fulminant viral hepatitis, e.g., due to acute hepatitis A, E, or B, this last especially with hepatitis D coinfection.

The color of the liver is variable, accentuated by red hues (taken to suggest congestion) and yellow tints (suggesting cholestasis); however, the hepatic parenchyma is very seldom strikingly bile stained (76). This absence of striking hepatic bile staining accords with the equally characteristic mild peripheral jaundice. The red and yellow areas sometimes swirl together in a "boxwood" or "chamois," mottled or marbled pattern across hepatic lobules. This swirl pattern at least hints at the striking zonality of involvement seen microscopically.

The consistency of the liver parenchyma upon gross cross-sectioning is characteristically bulging around retracted portal triads and depressed venous tracks (76). Although blood may exude from the liver's cut surface, parenchymal hemorrhages are not usually demonstrable grossly. The absence of parenchymal hemorrhages can be a useful negative finding in sorting through the differential diagnosis in a patient dying after a short clinical course characterized by acute liver failure. Finally, the texture of the cut surface tends to be greasy; this finding points toward another important histologic feature of yellow fever, the acute fatty metamorphosis of hepatocytes, which can be seen microscopically (76).

In summary, the significant gross autopsy findings in yellow fever patients are:

(i) the generic appearances of fatal hemorrhagic fever, i.e., (surprisingly) mild to moderate jaundice; oozing hemorrhage from epithelial surfaces, particularly of the (upper) gastrointestinal tract; and petechial hemorrhage in the parenchyma of organs, particularly of the central nervous system

(ii) the occasional appearance of enlarged and flabby nonhepatic viscera, e.g., the heart, suggesting the potential for a myocardiopathy, and the kidneys, raising the possibility of acute tubular necrosis

(iii) surprisingly subtle but diagnostically helpful hepatic changes, e.g., (a) the presence of a red-yellow mottling or marbling of the bulging, hepatic parenchyma, suggesting a zonality of disease; (b) the greasy texture of the parenchyma, suggesting acute fatty change; and (c) the significant absence of general parenchymal collapse. (d) Also strikingly absent are bile staining and areas of parenchymal hemorrhage. These latter negative findings argue against the "acute yellow atrophy" of fulminant viral hepatitis on the one hand (75) and against the toxic and vascular causes of acute liver failure, which produce parenchymal hemorrhage, on the other (38).

Experimental Pathology
of Simian Yellow Fever (4, 5, 47, 51, 76)

The availability and pertinence of yellow fever infection in non-human primate species have established the sequence of hepatic histopathologic changes in yellow fever and related that sequence to the presence and absence of demonstrable virus. The typical 6-day sequence divides itself, roughly, into an initial 24-h "eclipse" period, in which no histologic changes can be demonstrated, followed by two 48-h segments of "prehepatocytic" and "hepatocytic" localization of virus, followed by a final 24-h period of striking hepatocellular necrosis, due to subsequent hepatocytopathic effect. Only in this last phase do the characteristic histopathologic features of human yellow fever infection present themselves.

During the initial eclipse, no anatomic changes are observed; however, virus is demonstrable by immunofluorescence or immunoperoxidase techniques, not only in the liver, but also in blood vessels, bone marrow, spleen, lymph nodes, kidney, and brain in a viremic pattern. During the next, prehepatocytic phase, infection localizes to the liver, where the immunofluorescent or immunoperoxidase-positive viral particles are focused in the Kupffer cells (sinusoidal histiocytes or fixed macrophages). These professional phagocytes show the initial significant anatomic change of intracytoplasmic eosinophilic degeneration.

In the subsequent hepatocytic phase of infection, the Kupffer cells become necrotic, producing characteristic sinusoidal eosinophilic bodies. As the designation of the phase indicates, the hepatocytes themselves demonstrate a series of changes: depletion of intracytoplasmic glycogen; the appearance of transient cytoplasmic basophilia, associated with disappearance of the Golgi apparatus; and cytoplasmic vacuolization, associated with balloon degeneration of mitochondria. The nuclei of the affected hepatocytes further show nucleolar enlargement and margination of chromatin granules. These latter changes are followed by the appearance of intranuclear protein-containing structures, which demonstrate positive immunofluorescence for viral proteins.

In experimental infection, the next dramatically hepatocytopathic phase of liver infection occurs in susceptible monkeys, but not in resistant animals. Vesiculation of the endoplasmic reticulum is associated with the appearance of a characteristic parenchymal anatomic change, i.e., intracytoplasmic eosinophilic degeneration. Eosinophilic degeneration appears initially within the affected cells; after the cells break up, the contracted fragments of cytoplasm become extracellular. These extracellular fragments are the characteristic Councilman bodies. At the same time, mitochondria disappear as cytoplasmic packets of viral genome become demonstrable. Only in susceptible monkeys do mitochondria degenerate, packets of viral genome appear, and hepatocytes die; in resistant monkeys, at this juncture, mitochondria proliferate, only a few viral genomes are detected, and hepatocellular necrosis is limited. Among susceptible animals, in cells where necrosis does not immediately occur, the pivotal mitochondrial degeneration is associated with a second characteristic parenchymal anatomic change, cytoplasmic microvesicular fatty metamorphosis of hepatocytes.

In experimental infection, the next dramatically hepatocytopathic phase of liver infection occurs in susceptible monkeys, but not in resistant animals

Frequently in simian infection, but relatively rarely in its human counterpart, amphophilic condensations appear concurrently in the nuclei of the dying cells, from which nuclear chromatin has disappeared. These intranuclear Torres bodies, like the more frequent intracytoplasmic Councilman bodies introduced above, are not viral inclusions; they are, rather, products of viral cytopathic effect. Indeed, as this hepatocytopathic phase of the illness continues, intact viral particles become difficult to demonstrate in hepatocytes.

A third characteristic parenchymal anatomic change in this phase is seen in both simian and human infections: the coalescence of foci of hepatocellular necrosis into a midzonal (or zone 2)—that is, not periportal (zone 1) and not pericentral vein (zone 3)—hepatocellular necrosis. Despite the sometimes striking extent of this midzonal necrosis, experimental simian infections replicate three secondary, but useful, negative findings that help differentiate yellow fever infection from other infections producing rapid hepatocellular necrosis: the absence of reticulin collapse, the relative paucity of the inflammatory response (which, in the experimental infection, limits itself to a rare polymorphonuclear leukocyte [PMN] appearing in the hepatic sinusoids), and the absence of hepatic parenchymal hemorrhage.

Studies in the experimental pathology of yellow fever validate three major positive histologic findings of human yellow fever as characteristic of the disease

In summary, the main clinical utility of studies in the experimental pathology of yellow fever is to validate three major positive histologic findings of human yellow fever as characteristic of the disease: (i) eosinophilic degeneration/Councilman body formation, (ii) microvesicular fatty metamorphosis of hepatocytes, and (iii) a midzonal distribution of hepatocellular necrosis. These studies also validate three helpful negative findings not present in yellow fever: (i) reticulin collapse, (ii) an inflammatory infiltrate whose intensity is commensurate to the degree of hepatocellular necrosis, and (iii) hepatic parenchymal hemorrhage. Such findings would be characteristic of other viral infections or toxic or toxic-like conditions causing acute hepatocellular necrosis that are part of yellow fever's differential diagnosis:

Besides justifying the positive and negative criteria for histopathologic diagnosis, studies in experimental pathology also generate a pathogenic hypothesis, as follows. (i) Susceptible monkeys (and humans, it is argued) are unable to adapt to (or suppress) viral co-option of the host cell protein synthetic machinery. (ii) This inability leads to failure of the hepatocyte's energy supply system, indicated by glycogen depletion, mitochondrial degeneration, and fatty change. (iii) This combination of defects, probably along some metabolic gradient, concentrates hepatocellular necrosis in the middle zone of the hepatic lobule.

The experimental pathology studies also established two other findings of interest for the understanding of pathogenesis. First, the initial viral load (density of the viremia) is a major determinant of the extent of the subsequent histopathologic effects. This variability may, together with the effects of cross-immunity, account for the striking range of mortality rates attributed to yellow fever in different epidemiological settings. Second, spontaneous clearance of infection, without disease, is associated with up-regulation of the respiratory metabolic activity of hepatocytes, which is further associated with increased numbers of mitochondria. These responses appear in association with the reduction of viral replication.

Diagnostic Pathology of Human Yellow Fever (11, 28, 30, 43, 60, 76)

The characteristic histologic features of yellow fever present themselves, as mentioned above, between days 3 and 7 of infection. Histologic findings are scant before 72 h, and they become less specific in patients who succumb after more than a week's illness, when the central finding of midzonal necrosis, in particular, becomes obscured. Among those patients whose death is delayed, an inflammatory response, secondary to the more long-term hepatocellular necrosis itself, may also obscure one of the pertinent negative characteristics of yellow fever, i.e., the disproportionately little inflammation given the degree of necrosis.

The histopathologic diagnosis of yellow fever does not rest on individual pathognomonic features; it is, rather, based on a characteristic diagnostic pattern that fits together the three major, positive findings with three secondary but pertinent absences (Table 2.3). The positive findings, correlated with clinical presentation and viral culture results and validated by the controlled studies of simian infection as just described, are (i) eosinophilic (=acidophilic) degeneration, (ii) midzonal necrosis, and (iii) microsteatotic fatty change. The negative findings, similarly correlated and validated, are: (i) absence of reticulin framework collapse, (ii) paucity of inflammatory response, and (iii) absence of parenchymal hemorrhage. We next consider each component of this pattern individually.

The histopathologic diagnosis of yellow fever is based on a characteristic diagnostic pattern

Eosinophilic Degeneration

Eosinophilic degeneration (acidophilic degeneration) eventually forms Councilman (or "Councilman-like") bodies (86). The eosinophilic coagula are initially intracytoplasmic (intracellular) condensations of altered cytoplasm correlating, at a level of fine structure, with injury to the endoplasmic reticulin. As a parent cell becomes necrotic, the coagulum of condensed cytoplasm detaches itself from the wall of a sinusoid (in the case of a Kupffer cell), or detaches itself from the hepatocytic plate (in the case of a hepatocyte), sometimes carrying along a nuclear remnant. In the sinusoid, the Councilman body formed in this way either lies free or is phagocytosed by a (or another) Kupffer cell. The eosinophilic coagulum is round to oval, pink, and vacuolated, and varies greatly in density. In the sinusoids, Councilman bodies are associated with, at most, a scant polymorphonuclear inflammatory cell infiltrate.

Table 2.3 Characteristic histologic features of yellow fever

Positive	Negative
Eosinophilic degeneration	Absence of reticulin collapse
Midzonal hepatocellular necrosis	Paucity of inflammatory infiltrate
Microsteatotic fatty change	Absence of parenchymal hemorrhage

The Councilman body is not a viral inclusion; it is a consequence of cell injury

As mentioned above, the Councilman body is not a viral inclusion; it is a consequence of cell injury. It is also not pathognomonic of yellow fever virus, despite being highly characteristic of it. Eosinophilic inclusions, are, in fact, seen in most other flavivirus infections (44) including dengue and other causes of hemorrhagic fevers (38), vector-borne encephalitides (50), and hepatitis C (46). (Whether they can be associated with the putative hepatitis G flavivirus and its congeners, or with the non-flaviviruses that cause hepatitis A or hepatitis B ± D, is less certain.) Identical structures also appear in non-flavivirus hemorrhagic fevers (63, 88), as well as herpesvirus hepatitides, especially those due to Epstein-Barr virus (EBV) (41). Identical coagula can also be seen in some situations of apparently toxic injury, for example, in heat stroke patients (10).

Councilman bodies, however, can be clearly distinguished from a different eosinophilic structure, the Mallory body (31), seen in the most common form of acute hepatotoxic injury, alcoholic hepatitis (32). The Mallory body is intracytoplasmic in swollen hepatocytes. It is ameboid-angulated in shape, with dendritic edges, red-purple in color with a smooth hyaline consistency, and is associated histologically with intense, focal PMN infiltrates. By way of contrast, the yellow fever-associated Councilman body (76) is extracellular and arises from necrotic hepatocytes; it is round to oval in shape, with sharp edges, and pink in color, with an uneven, vacuolated consistency. It is not associated with an intense inflammatory infiltrate, attracting, at most, a rare sinusoidal PMN. Making this contrast, in fact, is a good exercise in defining the distinctive qualities of eosinophilic degeneration in yellow fever.

Midzonal Necrosis

Midzonal necrosis is the most variable of the three major pathologic features of yellow fever in the liver (30). It can range from (i) necrotic single cells, to (ii) occasional foci of necrotic cells, separated by expanses of physiologic-appearing hepatocytes, to (iii) a "salt-and-pepper" pattern of numerous foci of necrosis, to (iv) confluent sheets of necrotic cells (76). In the middle segment of this spectrum, numerous foci of necrosis disorganize the middle third of the hepatic parenchymal plates without stromal collapse and without distortion of the overall lobular architecture (that is, without distorting the arrangement of portal, midlobular, and central zones); this pattern constitutes the "classic" or typical hepatocellular necrosis of yellow fever. The less-involved segments of the spectrum, of single to multiple necrotic cells or islets to plaques of necrosis, however, also carry diagnostic weight, if they are most evident in the midzone of the lobule. Findings in this less-intense segment of the spectrum can be deceivingly subtle. In contrast, hepatocellular necrosis at the confluent end of the spectrum can become deceivingly florid and nonspecific by obscuring the pivotal, midzonal localization. In severely involved livers, however, although the necrosis spreads into portal (zone 1) and central (zone 3) areas, the other key findings of intact stroma and fatty change remain, as well as, often and interestingly, a preserved single row of cells around the central vein and another single row around the portal tract. These preserved portal and central limiting plates appear as trace reminders of the initial midzonal localization of the necrosis.

Microvesicular, Multivacuolar Fatty Change

Microvesicular, multivacuolar fatty change (15) is such a constant finding in yellow fever that experts have argued that the diagnosis should not be made without this feature (76). It is also a feature relatively independent in its extent and distribution from the other two positive findings. Its extent may not parallel that of eosinophilic degeneration or the degree of midzonal necrosis; its distribution may include cells unaffected by eosinophilic change and cells not in the midzonal area. Indeed, the steatosis may helpfully present in the residual row of hepatocytes around central veins, in cases where necrosis throughout the nodule has obscured midzonal localization. Just as the Councilman body of yellow fever can be separated from the Mallory body of alcoholic liver disease on morphologic grounds, so the many small fat vacuoles of yellow fever, which produce a steatosis that does not displace the central location of the hepatocyte's nucleus, can be distinguished from the few (usually one) large intracytoplasmic vacuoles seen in hepatocytes in alcoholic or other "nutritional" liver diseases, which displace the hepatocellular nuclei to the periphery of the steatotic cell (37).

Important Negative Findings

The most important of three negative findings, the absence of reticulin collapse (12), has already been mentioned in the context of midzonal (zone 2) necrosis. This absence is, in turn, associated with a lack of fibroblastic response in the portal zone. The absence of inflammatory white blood cells deserves almost as much emphasis (67). Only occasional macrophages, usually attracted to small foci of necrotic hepatocytes, and even rarer PMNs in the same setting, can be demonstrated. As Strano et al. maintained, "the presence of more than a minimal inflammatory response should raise doubts about the diagnosis of yellow fever" (76). However, the possibility of acute yellow fever superimposed on chronic hepatitis must also be considered in this context. The third useful absence, already mentioned above, is that of striking hepatic parenchymal hemorrhage (48). In marked contrast to the extrahepatic findings in yellow fever, only hepatic sinusoidal dilatation and congestion, without erythrocytes transgressing the hepatocellular plates, is the usual, rather minimal extent of abnormal red blood cell distribution in the liver; however, occasional foci of extravasated erythrocytes outside of the sinusoids should not be taken as obstructing the diagnosis of yellow fever.

The possibility of acute yellow fever superimposed on chronic hepatitis must be considered

While the Councilman body is an important diagnostic finding in yellow fever, two other historical designations, the Torres body and the Villela body, are not (Table 2.4) (76). There are, however, different reasons for this. The Torres body, a homogeneous, amphophilic intranuclear coagulum of host protein, not a viral inclusion, is more frequently demonstrated in simian yellow fever than in human infection (81). This lack of species sensitivity is one reason for its lack of utility. The other consideration is that, although Torres bodies are not an artifact, they are seen more often in Zenker-fixed than in formalin-fixed tissue. Since Zenker's fixative is rarely available, this is a practical disadvantage.

Table 2.4   The "bodies" of yellow fever diagnosis

Name	Location	Composition	Species specificity	Utility
Councilman	Cytoplasmic	Eosinophilic protein	Both human and simian	High
Torres	Nuclear	Amphophilic protein	Simian more than human	Low[a]
Villela	Cytoplasmic	?	?	None

[a]Fixative dependent.

The diagnostic histopathology of yellow fever consists of a variable mix of six characteristic findings

The Villela body is a granular, bright-yellow to ochre, small cytoplasmic structure of uncertain origin (87). It has been variously considered to be a degenerated, bile-pigmented Councilman body or a necrotic, pigment-laden Kupffer cell. (The distinction between these two possibilities may itself be false.) As these suggestions imply, the Villela body appears late in the course of yellow fever, among many more diagnostically useful examples of eosinophilic degeneration and Councilman bodies. In this context, it adds neither sensitivity nor specificity to the other findings present. To this disadvantage is added observer variation in recognizing these structures as specific entities in the spectrum of eosinophilic debris. This makes the Villela body a poorly reproducible, as well as usually insensitive, pathologic finding.

In summary, the diagnostic histopathology of yellow fever consists of a variable mix of six characteristic findings. Three of the findings are positive: (i) eosinophilic degeneration of Kupffer cells and hepatocytes, (ii) a midzonal pattern of hepatocellular necrosis, and (iii) microsteatotic fatty change in the hepatocellular cytoplasm. Three of these characteristics are negative: (i) no stromal collapse, (ii) almost no inflammatory infiltration, and (iii) no hepatic parenchymal hemorrhage.

Histopathologic Differential Diagnosis (76)

In the final topic of yellow fever pathology, the characteristic picture just described is compared with the histopathologic appearances of other conditions that, in various ways, may resemble yellow fever (Table 2.5). Three sorts of pathologic entities make up this differential diagnosis: (i) conditions featuring focal hepatocellular necrosis, (ii) conditions featuring striking (microsteatotic) fatty change, and (iii) conditions featuring a combination of hemorrhagic diathesis and sudden liver failure. The conditions in the first group are mostly infectious; among these, infections due to other viruses predominate, but some due to bacteria and protozoa are also included, as are some toxin-precipitated conditions and other "toxin-like" conditions whose pathologic appearances resemble toxic effects. In the second group, namely, conditions presenting with microsteatotic fatty change, the conditions in the differential diagnostic list tend even more frequently to be toxic or toxic-like. The third group includes especially conditions due to acute vascular obstruction and/or visceral intravascular volume contraction. The segments of the differential spectrum can be organized according to the subgroups of conditions which share salient positive findings with yellow fever.

Table 2.5 Histopathic differential diagnosis of yellow fever

Focal hepatocellular necrosis
    Other flavivirus infections
    Other non-flavivirus hemorrhagic fevers
    Alphabetized (non-flavivirus) agents of viral hepatitis (A, B ± D, E)
    Bacterial infections (typhoid, relapsing, and Q fevers)
    Protozoal infections (malaria, toxoplasmosis)
    Amanita toxin injury, eclampsia
Microsteatotic fatty changes
    Tetracycline-induced steatosis
    Halothane hepatitis
    Aflatoxin injury
    Phosphorus poisoning
    Kwashiorkor
Hemorrhagic diathesis and acute liver failure
    (Hepatic) venous obstruction
    Heat stroke

Focal Hepatocellular Necrosis

Among viral infections, the most difficult to differentiate from yellow fever histopathologically are other flavivirus infections, including not only dengue and other hemorrhagic fever viruses but also hepatitis C virus (72) and non-flavivirus agents of hemorrhagic fevers (27). All these infections cause Kupffer cell hyperplasia (as, indeed, do most of the other viral infections listed below), but more specifically, they cause eosinophilic degeneration, producing Councilman bodies, and variable (macro-microsteatotic) fatty change. In dengue and other flavivirus infections, however, the focal hepatocellular necrosis tends to be paracentral (in zone 3 around the central vein) rather than midlobular. In general, the hepatocellular necrosis in dengue and other flavivirus infections is also less striking than it is in yellow fever. In flavivirus hemorrhagic fever, hepatitis C, and non-flavivirus hemorrhagic fevers, there is, in addition, often a variable lymphocytic infiltrate in the portal zone of the hepatic lobule that is not characteristic of yellow fever (Table 2.6).

The most difficult viral infections to differentiate from yellow fever histopathologically are other flavivirus infections

Table 2.6 Hepatic pathology of yellow fever and other flavivirus infections compared and contrasted

Pathology	Yellow fever	Other flaviviruses
Councilman bodies	Present	Present
Distribution of hepatocellular necrosis	Midzonal	Around central vein
Microsteatotic fatty change	Present	Present
Lymphocytic infiltrate	Absent	Variable/portal
Reticulin collapse	Absent	Absent
Hepatic parenchymal hemorrhage	Absent	Variable

The non-flavivirus, alphabetized agents of endemic acute viral hepatitis are the most common infectious agents in the differential

If other flaviviruses and other non-flavivirus causes of hemorrhagic fever are the most difficult elements in the viropathologic differential diagnosis of yellow fever, the non-flavivirus, alphabetized agents of endemic acute viral hepatitis, which tend to have an abrupt onset of symptomatic infection, are the most common infectious agents in the differential. The enteroviral hepatitis A (78), the hepadnaviral hepatitis B (70)—especially in combination with its coinfecting agent, the plant viroid-like hepatitis D (85)—and the more recently characterized calicivirus hepatitis E (26) can all present with the clinical syndrome of fulminant viral hepatitis, which resembles yellow fever. In this syndrome, however, the gross finding of acute yellow atrophy of the liver and the microscopic finding of submassive hepatocellular necrosis are typical of the rare fatal cases of hepatitis A, the cases of combined hepatitis B and D infection that take a rapid course, and cases of hepatitis E in pregnant women that are fatal. These gross and microscopic findings are not found in yellow fever patients. Indeed, in aggressive infections due to the endemic acute hepatitis agents, the dropout of hepatocytes tends to be uniform rather than localized in rapidly fatal cases; even in fatal yellow fever, by contrast, the dropout tends to be localized to the midzone of the hepatic lobule. Similarly, although fine microsteatotic vacuolar change can be demonstrated in both acute viral hepatitis and yellow fever, in the acute hepatitis presentation the fatty change is less prominent and appears against a background of ballooning viable hepatocytes. In yellow fever, it appears together with hepatocellular necrosis, without ballooning. Four other negative findings can usually exclude yellow fever from the histologic differential diagnosis of acute hepatitis (73): (i) yellow fever's hepatocellular necrosis does not cause reticulin collapse; (ii) yellow fever does not attract a predominantly lymphocytic-plasmacytic inflammatory infiltrate that localizes in the (pericentral and, predominantly, periportal) periphery of the lobule; (iii) yellow fever does not stimulate cholangeal and even portal ductal proliferation at the lobule's biliary pole; (iv) finally, yellow fever is not associated with an endophlebitis of the central vessel at the lobule's venous pole (Table 2.7).

It is important, however, to keep in mind that many yellow fever patients may have been previously and chronically infected with hepatitides B and/or C. A small fraction of patients infected with hepatitis B, but particularly those who were vertically infected in the perinatal period, and a large

Table 2.7 Hepatic histopathology of yellow fever contrasted with acute viral hepatitis

Histopathology	Yellow fever	Viral hepatitis
Hepatocellular "dropout"	Midzonal	Uniform
Cytoplasmic change	Eosinophilic degeneration	Balloon degeneration
Fatty change	Microsteatotic, prominent	Microsteatotic, variable
Reticulin collapse	Absent	Present
Lymphocytic infiltrate	Absent	Present, peripheral
Cholangeal proliferation (portal) fibrosis	Absent	Present
(Central) venous endophlebitis	Absent	Present

fraction of patients infected with hepatitis C, whose initial acquisition is often asymptomatic, may have the histologic findings of chronic hepatitis, including piecemeal necrosis in the periportal zone, reticulin collapse causing bridging fibrosis between portal areas, and a portal plus/minus an intralobular lymphocytic infiltrate, with or without bile duct proliferation (74). It can be challenging to subtract these chronic histopathologic changes from the acute hepatocellular necrosis, etc., that yellow fever superimposes upon them. An historical example of this problem is the Amazonian Labréa hepatitis (24): "dropout" necrosis without zonal distribution, large and small vacuole fatty change, lymphocytic infiltration in portal triads and sinusoids, and absent Kupffer cell hyperplasia, but with "morula" of necrotic cells and a "spider cell" pattern of necrosis. This entity was part of the differential diagnosis of yellow fever in part of the Amazon basin. Without agent-specific immunohistochemical reagents, such complex differential presentations may be impossible to sort out by histopathology alone. (Most cases of Labréa hepatitis are now thought to have been combined hepatitis B and D infections [7].)

The third group of viruses that produce histopathologic injury that must be distinguished from yellow fever's effects are the human *Herpesviridae*. Herpesviruses can all produce foci of hepatocellular necrosis which, especially if widespread, may include eosinophilic degeneration; however, the specific agents in this family produce characteristic histologic changes that separate them from those of yellow fever infection, as follows. (i) Herpes simplex virus and herpes-varicella-zoster virus produce both intranuclear viral inclusions (Cowdry type A intranuclear inclusions) and hemorrhagic necrosis, neither of which is seen in yellow fever (34). (ii) Cytomegalovirus produces both intranuclear (Cowdry type A) and intracytoplasmic inclusions. Neither inclusion type is seen in yellow fever. The necrosis associated with cytomegalovirus infection is indeed often localized, but its focality is rarely limited to the midzone (zone 2) of the hepatic lobule (84). (iii) There is also an inflammatory finding that distinguishes herpesvirus infection from yellow fever. All of the herpesvirus hepatitides listed above stimulate lymphocytic infiltrates, particularly in and around portal areas, but such infiltrates are not seen in yellow fever. These infiltrates are particularly dense, of mixed cytologic composition, and most strikingly widespread and sinusoidal (as "Indian file lymphocytes") in EBV infection. The striking lymphocytic infiltrate in EBV hepatitis is a helpful differential finding, because EBV infection does not produce a histologically apparent intranuclear inclusion as do the other herpesviruses described above (64).

The fourth category of infectious agents that can cause focal hepatocellular necrosis is bacteria, particularly bacterial infection prevalent where yellow fever is endemic. Among these bacterial infections, the following infections all cause focal hepatocellular necrosis: (i) brucellosis (due to *Brucella* spp.) and typhoid fever (invasive *Salmonella typhi* infection), (ii) visceral cat-scratch disease (*Bartonella henselae*) and listeriosis (*Listeria monocytogenes*), (iii) relapsing fever (*Borrelia recurrentis* infection) and leptospirosis (*Leptospira* spp. infection), and (iv) Q fever (*Coxiella burnetii*

The specific agents in the human Herpesviridae produce characteristic histologic changes that separate them from those of yellow fever infection

infection) and other tick-borne infections (*Rickettsia* spp.). As with herpesviruses, the hepatic histopathology of each of these classes of agents has distinctive features that distinguish them from yellow fever. For example, (i) typhoid infection produces a characteristic, striking histiocytic (macrophage) infiltrate surrounding a zone of hepatocellular encrons (a "typhoid nodule") (19); (ii) listeriosis produces microabscesses of PMNs, in which the diagnostic gram-positive bacilli can be seen (76). Furthermore, (iii) leptospirosis also produces a histiocytic infiltrate out of proportion to relatively scant foci of hepatocellular necrosis. In leptospirosis the necrosis is usually limited to the periportal zone; in addition, leptospirosis characteristically produces striking intracanalicular cholestasis, predominantly around the central vein (18). Finally, (iv) mononuclear forms also distinguish Q fever, in which the histiocytic cells actually aggregate into well-formed, sometimes characteristically circular granulomata (65).

The fifth category of infectious agents in the differential diagnosis of yellow fever is protozoa. Two protozoal infections enter into the differential diagnosis of focal hepatocellular necrosis. Malaria is distinguished by the characteristic parasitized red blood cells and characteristic pigment in hepatocytes (22, 63), and *Toxoplasma gondii* infection produces an exuberant lymphocytic infiltrate similar to that seen in EBV infection (90).

The sixth and last category, in this focal hepatocellular necrosis segment of the yellow fever differential list, is a series of toxic or toxic-like disorders that also produce focal hepatocellular necrosis similar to, but—by various characteristics—distinguishable from, the histopathology of yellow fever. The most common of these, alcoholic hepatitis, has already been mentioned above, when the Mallory body of alcoholic hepatocellular necrosis was distinguished from the Councilman body of yellow fever. The centrilobular (zone 3) necrosis and PMN infiltrate of alcoholic hepatitis are distinct from the midzonal (zone 2) necrosis and paucity of inflammatory infiltrate in yellow fever, just as the macrovesicular paucivacuolar fatty change of alcohol toxicity distinguishes it from the microvesicular multivacuolar fatty change of yellow fever. Two other examples can serve to show how necrotizing toxic injury can be separated from yellow fever. First, *Amanita* toxin injury (caused by a mushroom toxin) has, like acute alcohol injury, three features that distinguish it from yellow fever: the hemorrhagic appearance of the necrosis, its central zonal (pericentral vein) distribution, and the PMN infiltrate that it attracts (91). An anesthetic agent, halothane, also produces a hepatocellular necrotizing toxic effect, but its appearances include a diffuse pattern of necrosis and vigorous PMN infiltrate. Both these latter findings help separate it from yellow fever (6). As an example of a "toxin-like" condition, eclampsia of pregnancy is similar to yellow fever in causing a noninflammatory hepatocellular necrosis. It can be distinguished, however, by the striking fibrin deposition in arterioles, sinusoids, and small veins, by sinusoidal hemorrhage, and by the prominence of cholestasis (69).

T wo protozoal infections enter into the differential diagnosis of focal hepatocellular necrosis

Microsteatosis
Other toxin-mediated and toxin-like conditions produce, rather than a characteristic hepatocellular necrosis, a microsteatotic fatty change similar

to that seen in yellow fever. This finding produces another series of differential possibilities. Aflatoxin is another fungal toxin; however, it is associated with mold and fatty change, in contrast to the *Amanita* toxin mentioned above, which is associated with mushrooms and hemorrhagic necrosis. Aflatoxin produces microsteatotic fatty change and focal necrosis, but these findings are distinguished from those in yellow fever by ductal proliferation at the portal end of the lobule and an endophlebitis at the venous end. Tetracycline-induced toxicity produces a pattern of panlobular involvement of microsteatotic fatty change, but this is also associated with central vein endophlebitis, centrilobular necrosis, and PMN infiltrate (16). These findings distinguish this antimicrobial-drug-induced toxic effect from yellow fever's focal, midzonal necrosis with scant infiltrate. Reye's syndrome is a now rare, toxin-like presentation, resembling aflatoxin poisoning, of striking fine vacuolar fatty change and "drop out" necrosis (14). The latter, however, is characteristically focused in the peripheral lobule (zones 1 and 3, rather than the midlobular zone 2) (42). Kwashiorkor, a putative "nutritional" entity of protein starvation first described in the yellow fever zone of West Africa, is also associated with a toxin-like appearance of fatty change in a characteristic distribution, most striking in the periphery of the lobule. Again, fatty change in yellow fever does not have these peripheral zonal predispositions.

Hemorrhagic Diathesis and Acute Liver Failure

In the third and last set of differential diagnoses in the context of yellow fever, the most frequent noninfectious, nontoxic cause of illness is vascular insult to the liver. Infarction due to hepatic venous (outflow) obstruction tends to produce centrilobular coagulative necrosis with a striking PMN infiltrate (33). Both the central (venous pole) distribution of necrosis and the prominence of the PMN infiltrate contrast with the midzonal and pauci-inflammatory findings in yellow fever (45). As mentioned above, in the visceral hypovolemic and coagulopathic syndrome of heat stroke, necrosis may indeed be midzonal (sinusoidal) and bland, but tends to be hemorrhagic.

The most frequent noninfectious, nontoxic cause of illness is vascular insult to the liver

In summary, one needs to bear in mind that other viruses, other nonviral (bacterial and protozoal) infectious agents, and toxic and toxic-like (including "nutritional") conditions can produce either the components of the tripartite pathologic findings (focal hepatocellular necrosis, fatty change, and minimal inflammatory infiltrate) or the fulminant course seen in yellow fever (89). Because yellow fever presents, in its extrahepatic manifestations, as hemorrhagic fever, vascular and circulatory conditions become especially prominent in the latter consideration. The possibility of another flavivirus causing the presentation is the most difficult to eliminate on histopathologic evidence alone. The next most difficult task is to separate yellow fever from non-flavivirus causes of the acute hemorrhagic fever syndrome. The separation of yellow fever from acute fulminant hepatitis A, B ± D, or E is a more straightforward histopathologic challenge. Yellow fever superimposed on chronic hepatitis B ± D or C, however, can require extrahistopathic evidence to sort out the source of the condition. Otherwise, the other infectious, toxic, and toxic-like conditions have findings that render yellow fever unlikely, such as viral inclusions, lymphohistiocytic inflammation, abscess formation, canalicular cholestasis, bile duct proliferation, characteristic portal and/or central patterns of hepatocellular necrosis, similarly specific distributions of fatty change, or hepatic parenchymal hemorrhage.

Treatment and Prevention

No specific antiviral drug has been documented to be useful either in humans or in experimental animals

The treatment of yellow fever is symptomatic, and no specific antiviral drug has been documented to be useful either in humans or in experimental animals (51). Since most patients with yellow fever around the world are diagnosed and treated in remote medical facilities, some simple recommendations should be followed. All acutely ill patients with suspected or confirmed yellow fever should be placed under a bed net to prevent mosquito bites and spread of the infection. Universal precautions should be followed to prevent accidental infection through contaminated needles or blood (8). Acetaminophen may be used to treat headache and fever, but salicylates or aspirin-containing compounds should be avoided. As mentioned above, yellow fever has some features in common with Reye's syndrome and may, like Reye's syndrome, be potentiated by salicylates. Antacids and H_2-blockers to reduce the risk of gastric bleeding, fluid and electrolyte replacement, and oxygen should be used as needed. The use of vitamin K has been advocated but is probably ineffective when there is severe hepatic necrosis. The use of heparin has also been proposed to lessen the severity of the coagulopathy, but most authorities recommend that heparin only be considered when there is strong laboratory evidence of disseminated intravascular coagulation and the patient can be closely monitored (51).

Immunization is the primary means for preventing yellow fever, and an effective vaccine against yellow fever has existed for over 50 years (2). Yellow fever 17D vaccine (a live, attenuated strain of yellow fever virus) is produced from chicken embryos and delivered as a single 0.5-ml subcutaneous dose (13). This vaccine induces long-lasting immunity in greater than 95% of those immunized. In no instance should infants less than 4 months of age receive yellow fever vaccine because of the risk of encephalitis. This human neonatal encephalitis is analogous to a brain inflammation induced in mice in an animal model used in the past to diagnose yellow fever as well as to produce attenuated strains of the virus. Pregnant women theoretically should not be vaccinated, and travel to areas where yellow fever is present should be postponed until after delivery; however, if a pregnant woman must travel, she should be vaccinated. During a massive immunization campaign after an outbreak of yellow fever in Nigeria in 1986–1987 no complications were detected among those women who were vaccinated while pregnant (61). Nevertheless, congenital yellow fever virus infection after immunization during pregnancy has been documented (83). Persons with severe immunosuppression (e.g., AIDS) should also not be vaccinated, nor should persons with severe egg allergy receive vaccine (13).

Yellow fever vaccination is the only practical public health intervention that may control this disease. In endemic countries where yellow fever vaccine has been widely used, the disease has disappeared. For example, during the last yellow fever epidemic in The Gambia in 1978–1979 (56) the government conducted a mass vaccination campaign and since then has added yellow fever vaccine to its Expanded Program on Immunization. Today The Gambia has the highest yellow fever vaccine coverage of children in Africa, and no further outbreaks of the disease have occurred (92). However, of the 33 African countries at risk for yellow fever, only 17 now have a national policy of inclusion of yellow fever vaccine in the childhood immunization program despite such a recommendation in 1988 by a joint WHO/UNICEF Technical Group and the clear cost-effectiveness of such an intervention (58). As of May 1996, coverage data had been reported to WHO by 16 countries, with levels ranging from 1% (Mali) to 87% (The Gambia); only three countries exceeded 50% coverage (92). A new WHO initiative to rapidly expand vaccination coverage for yellow fever in Africa by linking it with mass campaigns against polio and measles is currently under way (93).

The amount of cross-protection between the different flaviviruses is unclear. Prior immunization with dengue caused a significant reduction in viremia of monkeys challenged with yellow fever, and we speculate that this may be why yellow fever is absent in Asia despite the presence in that continent of a competent vector (79). On the other hand, concern has recently been expressed about the possible increased risk of hemorrhagic dengue fever after yellow fever vaccination (36).

Several studies suggest that yellow fever immunity persists for at least 30 to 35 years and probably for life (62), but, for travel certification, revaccination is recommended every 10 years (13). A yellow fever vaccination certificate is now the only certificate required for international travel. Most countries require a valid International Certificate of Vaccination for travelers arriving from infected areas or from countries with infected areas, or who have been in transit through those areas, but some countries require a certificate for all entering travelers. Because requirements change, travelers should consult with public health authorities to determine requirements and regulations for vaccination, but vaccination should be suggested to travelers visiting endemic areas even for short periods (3).

The control of the mosquito vector is also important in the prevention of yellow fever and other diseases transmitted by the same vectors (like dengue fever). In an effort to prevent urban yellow fever, the Pan American Health Organization, led by Dr. Fred Stoper, organized a campaign that eradicated *Aedes aegypti* from most of Central and South American countries in the 1950s and 1960s (35, 82). The *Aedes aegypti* eradication program in the United States was officially discontinued in 1970, and such programs gradually eroded elsewhere in the Americas. In 1995, *Aedes aegypti* was again widely distributed in the Americas. Today, the disease continues to be a major health problem in much of the world (68).

Yellow fever vaccination is the only practical public health intervention that may control this disease

Figure 2.1 Low-power view of midzonal necrosis. Note central vein on the left-hand side of the frame and portal triad on the right-hand side. Hematoxylin and eolin (H&E) stain, ×90.

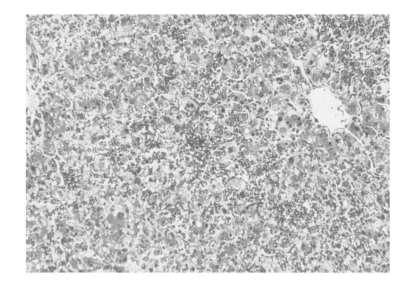

Figure 2.2 Mid-power view of a central vein in yellow fever midzonal necrosis. Note the preservation of a row of hepatocytes around the central vein against a background of hepatocellular necrosis. H&E, ×195.

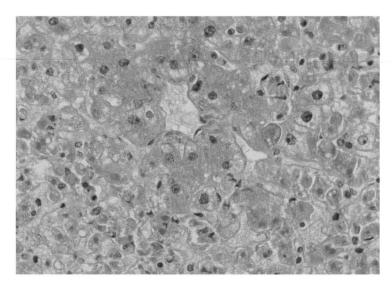

Figure 2.3 Mid-power view of a portal triad in yellow fever midzonal necrosis. Note the preservation of a row of hepatocytes around the portal and the paucity of inflammatory infiltrate in that area. H&E, ×180.

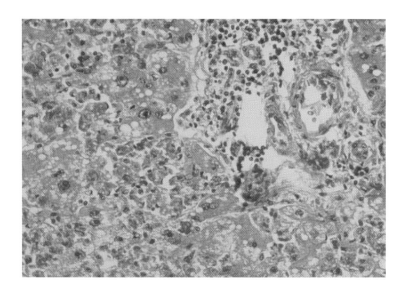

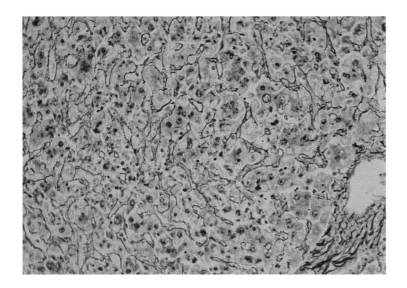

Figure 2.4 Mid-power reticulum stain of mid-zonal necrosis in yellow fever. Note the *absence* of reticulum collapse (that is, the absence of groups of fibers with little or no space between them). Wilder's reticulum stain, ×115.

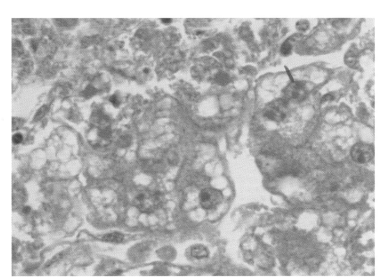

Figure 2.5 High-power view of microsteatotic fatty change in yellow fever. Note the multiple intracellular vesicles and the central location of nuclei. H&E, ×485.

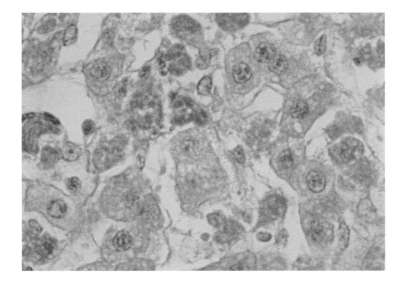

Figure 2.6 High-power view of multiple Councilman bodies in yellow fever. Note their cytoplasmic cytologic localization and their sinusoidal histologic localization. H&E, ×485.

Figure 2.7 High-power view of typical pauci-cellular inflammatory response in yellow fever. Note the Councilman bodies. H&E, ×350.

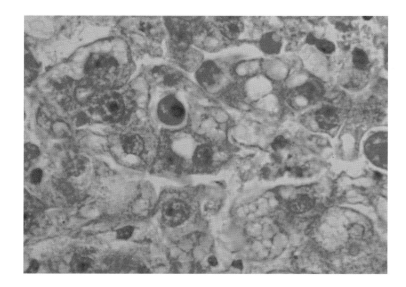

Figure 2.8 Low-power view of midzonal local-ization of necrosis in yellow fever. This slide repre-sents the deceptively subtle usual lower-power appearance of the liver in yellow fever. H&E, ×120.

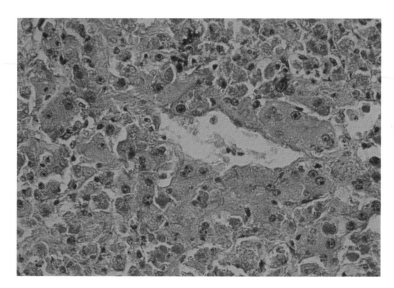

Figure 2.9 High-power view of marked fatty change with microsteatosis. Oil Red O stain, ×485.

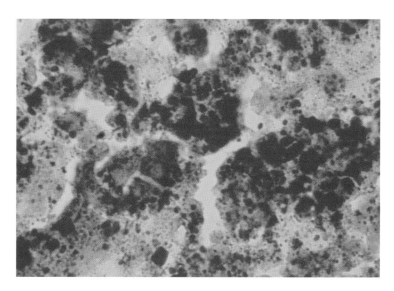

References

1. **Anonymous.** 1968. Present status of yellow fever: memorandum from a PAHO meeting. *Bull. W.H.O.* **64:**511–524.

2. **Barrett, A. D.** 1997. Yellow fever vaccines. *Biologicals* **25:**17–25.

3. **Barros, M. L., and G. Boeken.** 1996. Jungle yellow fever in the Central Amazon. *Lancet* **348**(9032):969–970. (Letter.)

4. **Bearcroft, W. G. C.** 1957. The histopathology of the liver of yellow fever infected Rhesus monkeys. *J. Pathol. Bacteriol.* **74:**295–303.

5. **Bearcroft, W. G. C.** 1960. Cytological and cytochemical studies on the liver cells of yellow fever infected Rhesus monkeys. *J. Pathol. Bacteriol.* **80:**19–31.

6. **Benjamin, S. E., Z. D. Goodman, K. G. Ishak, H. J. Zimmerman, and N. W. Irey.** 1981. The morphologic spectrum of halothane-induced hepatic injury: analysis of 77 cases. *Hepatology* **1:**255–263.

7. **Bensabath, G., S. C. Hadler, M. C. Pereira Soares, H. Fields, L. B. Dias, H. Popper, and J. E. Maynard.** 1987. Hepatitis delta virus infection and Labréa hepatitis. *JAMA* **258:**479–483.

8. **Berry, G. P., and S. F. Kitchen.** 1931. Yellow fever accidentally contracted in the laboratory: a study of seven cases. *Am. J. Trop. Med. Hyg.* **11:**365–434.

9. **Bhamorapravate, N., P. Tuchinda, and V. Boonyapaknoruk.** 1967. Pathology of Thailand hemorrhagic fever: a study of 100 autopsy cases. *Ann. Trop. Med. Parasitol.* **61:**500–510.

10. **Bianchi, L., H. Ohnacker, K. Beck, and M. Zimmerli-Ning.** 1972. Liver damage in heat stroke and its regression: a biopsy study. *Hum. Pathol.* **3:**237–248.

11. **Bugher, J. C.** 1951. The pathology of yellow fever, p. 139–163. *In* G. K. Strode (ed.), *Yellow Fever*. McGraw-Hill, New York.

12. **Camain, R., and D. Lambert.** 1967. Histopathologie des fois amarils prelevés post mortem et par ponction biopsie hépatique. *Bull. W.H.O.* **36:**129–136.

13. **Centers for Disease Control and Prevention.** 1990. Yellow fever vaccine. Recommendations of the immunization practices advisory committee (ACIP). *Morbid. Mortal. Weekly Rep.* **39**(RR-6):1–6.

14. **Chavez-Carballo, E., R. D. Ellefson, and M. R. Gomez.** 1976. An aflatoxin in the liver of a patient with Reye-Johnson syndrome. *Mayo Clin. Proc.* **51:**50–68.

15. **Child, P. L., R. B. MacKenzie, L. R. Valverde, and K. M. Johnson.** 1967. Bolivian hemorrhagic fever: a pathologic description. *Arch. Pathol.* **83:**434–445.

16. **Combes, B., P. J. Whalley, and R. H. Adams.** 1972. Tetracycline and the liver. *Progr. Liver Dis.* **4:**589.

17. **David-West, T. S., N. A. Labzoffsky, and J. J. Hamvas.** 1972. Morphogenesis of yellow fever virus in mouse brain. *Arch. Ges. Virusforsch.* **36:**372–379.

18. **DeBrito, T., M. M. Machado, S. D. Montans, S. Hoshino, and E. Freymuller.** 1967. Liver biopsy in human leptospirosis: a light and electron microscopic study. *Virchow's Arch.* (A) **342:**61–69.

19. **DeBrito, T., W. Trench Vierra, and M. D'Agostino Dias.** 1977. Jaundice in typhoid hepatitis: a light and electron microscopic study based on liver biopsies. *Acta Hepato-Gastroenterol.* **24:**426–433.

20. **DeCock, K. M., T. P. Monath, A. Nasidi, P. M. Tukei, J. Enriquez, P. Lichfield, R. B. Craven, A. Fabiyi, B. C. Okafor, C. Ravaonjanahary, and A. Sorungbe.** 1988. Epidemic yellow fever in Eastern Nigeria, 1986. *Lancet* **i:**630–633.

21. **Delaponte, F.** 1941. *The History of Yellow Fever: an Essay on the Birth of Tropical Medicine.* MIT Press, Cambridge, Mass.

22. **Deller, J. J., P. S. Ciforelli, S. Berque, and R. Buchanan.** 1967. Malaria hepatitis. *Milit. Med.* **132:**614–620.

23. **Dennis, H., B. E. Reisberg, J. Crosbie, D. Crozier, and M. E. Conrad.** 1969. The original hemorrhagic fever: yellow fever. *Br. J. Haematol.* **17:**455–462.

24. **DePaola, D., A. J. Strano, and H. C. Hopps.** 1968. Labréa hepatitis (black fever): a problem in geographic pathology. *Int. Pathol. Bull.* **9:**43–48.

25. **Deubel, V., V. Mouly, J.-J. Salaun, C. Adam, M. M. Diop, and J. P. Digoutte.** 1983. Comparison of the enzyme-linked immunosorbent assay (ELISA) with standard tests used to detect yellow fever virus antibodies. *Am. J. Trop. Med. Hyg.* **32:**565–568.

26. **Dienes, H. P., T. Hütterroth, L. Bianchi, M. Grün, and W. Thoenes.** 1986. Hepatitis A-like non-A, non-B hepatitis: light and electron microscopic observations of three cases. *Virchow's Arch.* (A) **409:**657–667.

27. **Elisaf, M., S. Stefanaki, M. Repante, H. Korakis, E. Tsianos, and K. C. Sianopoulos.** 1993. Liver involvement in hemorrhagic fever with renal syndrome. *J. Clin. Gastroenterol.* **17:**33–37.

28. **Elton, N. W.** 1950. Pathologic features of yellow fever in Panama. *U.S. Armed Forces Med. J.* **1:**596–601.

29. **Engelthaler, D. M., M. Fink, C. E. Levy, and M. J. Leslie.** 1997. The reemergence of *Aedes aegypti* in Arizona. *Emerg. Infect. Dis.* **3**(2):241–242.

30. **Francis, T. I., D. L. Moore, G. M. Edington, and J. A. Smith.** 1972. A clinicopathological study of human yellow fever. *Bull. W.H.O.* **46:**659–667.

31. **French, S. W.** 1983. Present understanding of the development of Mallory's body. *Arch. Pathol. Lab. Med.* **107:**445–450.

32. **French, S. W., J. Nash, P. Shitabata, K. Kachi, C. Hara, A. Chedid, and C. L. Mendenhall.** 1993. Pathology of alcoholic liver disease. *Semin. Liver Dis.* **13:**154–169.

33. **Gitlin, N., and K. M. Serio.** 1992. Ischemic hepatitis: widening horizons. *Am. J. Gastroenterol.* **87:**831–836.

34. **Goodman, Z. D., K. G. Ishak, and I. A. Sesterhenn.** 1986. Herpes simplex hepatitis in apparently immunocompetent adults. *Am. J. Clin. Pathol.* **85:**694–699.

35. **Gubler, D. J., and G. G. Clark.** 1995. Dengue/dengue hemorrhagic fever: the emergence of a global health problem. *Emerg. Infect. Dis.* **1**(2):55–57.

36. **Guzman, J. R., and M. A. Kron.** 1997. Threat of dengue hemorrhagic fever after yellow fever vaccination. *Lancet* **349**(9068):1841. (Letter.)

37. **Hoyumpa, A. M., H. L. Greene, G. D. Dunn, and S. S. Schenker.** 1975. Fatty liver: biochemical and clinical considerations. *Dig. Dis.* **20:**1142–1170.

38. **Ishak, K. G., D. H. Walker, J. A. W. Coetzer, J. J. Gardner, and L. Gorelkin.** 1982. Viral hemorrhagic fevers with hepatic involvement: pathologic aspects with clinical correlations. *Prog. Liver Dis.* **7:**495–515.

39. **Jones, E. M. M., and D. C. Wilson.** 1972. Clinical features of yellow fever cases at Vom Christian Hospital during the 1969 epidemic on the Jos Plateau, Nigeria. *Bull. W.H.O.* **46:**653–657.

40. **Kerr, J. A.** 1951. The clinical aspects and diagnosis of yellow fever, p. 387–425. *In* G. K. Strode (ed.), *Yellow Fever.* McGraw-Hill, New York.

41. **Kilpatrick, Z. M.** 1966. Structural and functional abnormalities of liver in infectious mononucleosis. *Arch. Intern. Med.* **117:**47–53.

42. **Kimura, S., T. Kobayashi, Y. Tanaka, and Y. Sasaki.** 1991. Liver histopathology in clinical Reye syndrome. *Brain Dev.* **13:**95–100.

43. **Klotz, O., and T. H. Belt.** 1930. The pathology of the liver in yellow fever. *Am. J. Pathol.* **6:**663–688.

44. **Kuo, C. H., D.-I. Tai, C.-S. Chang-Chien, C.-K. Lan, S.-S. Chiou, and Y.-F. Liaw.** 1992. Liver biochemical tests and dengue fever. *Am. J. Trop. Med. Hyg.* **47:**265–270.

45. **Lefkowitch, J. H., and L. Mendez.** 1986. Morphologic features of hepatic injury in cardiac disease and shock. *J. Hepatol.* **2:**313–327.

46. **Lefkowitch, J. H., E. R. Schiff, G. L. Davis, R. P. Perrillo, K. Kindsay, H. C. Bodenheimer, Jr., L. A. Balart, T. J. Ortego, J. Payne, J. L. Dienstag, A. Gibas, I. M. Jacobson, C. H. Tamburro, W. Carey, C. O'Brien, R. Sampliner, D. H. Van Thiel, D. Feit, J. Albrecht, C. Meschievitz, B. Samghui, R. D. Vaughan, and the Hepatitis International Therapy Group.** 1993. Pathological diagnosis of chronic hepatitis C: a multicenter comparative study with chronic hepatitis B. *Gastroenterology* **104:**595–603.

47. **MacGavran, M. H., and J. D. White.** 1964. Electron microscopic and immunofluorescent observations on monkey liver and tissue culture cells infected with the Asibi strain of yellow fever virus. *Am. J. Pathol.* **45:**501–517.

48. **MacNamara, F. N.** 1957. A clinicopathological study of yellow fever in Nigeria. *West Afr. Med. J.* **6:**137–146.

49. **McFarland, J. M., L. M. Baddur, J. E. Nelson, S. K. Elkins, R. B. Craven, B. C. Cropp, G. J. Chang, A. D. Grindstaff, A. S. Craig, and R. J. Smith.** 1997. Imported yellow fever in a United States citizen. *Rev. Infect. Dis.* **25:**1143–1147.

50. **Miyake, M.** 1964. The pathology of Japanese encephalitis. *Bull. W.H.O.* **30:** 153–160.

51. **Monath, T. P.** 1987. Yellow fever: a medically neglected disease. Report on a seminar. *Rev. Infect. Dis.* **9:**165–175.

52. **Monath, T. P.** 1990. Yellow fever, p. 661–674. *In* K. S. Warren and A. A. F. Mahmoud (ed.), *Tropical and Geographical Medicine*, 2nd ed. McGraw-Hill, Inc., New York.

53. **Monath, T. P.** 1991. Yellow fever: Victor, Victoria? Conqueror, conquest? Epidemics and research in the last forty years and prospects for the future. *Am. J. Trop. Med. Hyg.* **45:**1–43.

54. **Monath, T. P.** 1995. Flaviviruses (yellow fever, dengue, dengue hemorrhagic fever, Japanese encephalitis, tick-borne encephalitis), p. 1465–1474. *In* G. L. Mandell, J. E. Bennett, and R. Dolin (ed.), *Principles and Practice of Infectious Diseases*, 4th ed. Churchill Livingstone, New York.

55. **Monath, T. P., K. R. Brinker, F. W. Chandler, G. E. Kemp, and C. B. Crupp.** 1981. Pathophysiologic correlations in a rhesus monkey model of yellow fever. *Am. J. Trop. Med. Hyg.* **30:**431–443.

56. **Monath, T. P., R. B. Craven, A. Adjukiewicz, M. Germain, D. B. Francy, L. Ferrara, E. M. O. Samba, H. N'jie, K. Cham, S. A. Fitzgerald, P. H. Crippen, D. I. H. Simpson, E. T. W. Bowen, A. Fabiyi, and J. J. Salaun.** 1980. Yellow fever in the Gambia 1978–79: epidemiologic aspects. *Am. J. Trop. Med. Hyg.* **29:**912–928.

57. **Monath, T. P., L. J. Hill, N. V. Brown, C. B. Cropp, J. J. Schlesinger, J. F. Saluzzo, and J. R. Wands.** 1986. Sensitive and specific monoclonal immunoassay for detecting yellow fever virus in laboratory and clinical specimens. *J. Clin. Microbiol.* **23:**129–134.

58. **Monath, T. P., and A. Nasidi.** 1993. Should yellow fever vaccine be included in the expanded program of immunization in Africa? A cost-effectiveness analysis for Nigeria. *Am. J. Trop. Med. Hyg.* **48:**274–299.

59. **Monath, T. P., and R. R. Nystrom.** 1984. Detection of yellow fever virus in serum by enzyme immunoassay. *Am. J. Trop. Med. Hyg.* **33:**151–157.

60. **Montenegro, J.** 1937. Diagnostico anatomopathologico du febre amarella. *Arq. Hig. Saude Publica* **3:**109–119.

61. **Nasidi, A., T. P. Monath, J. Vandenberg, O. Tomori, C. H. Calisher, X. Hurtgen, G. R. R. Munube, A. O. O. Sorugbe, G. C. Okafor, and S. Wali.** 1993. Yellow fever vaccination in pregnancy: a four-year prospective study. *Trans. R. Soc. Trop. Med. Hyg.* **87:**337–339.

62. **Poland, J. D., C. H. Calisher, T. P. Monath, W. G. Downs, and K. Murphy.** 1981. Persistence of neutralizing antibody 30–35 years after immunization with 17D yellow fever vaccine. *Bull. W.H.O.* **59:**895–900.

63. **Pounder, D. J.** 1983. Malarial pigment and hepatic anthracosis. *Am. J. Surg. Pathol.* **7:**501–502.

64. **Purtilo, D. T., and K. Sakamoto.** 1981. Epstein-Barr virus and human disease: immune response determines the clinical and pathologic expression. *Hum. Pathol.* **12:**677–679.

65. **Qizilbash, A. H.** 1983. The pathology of Q fever as seen on liver biopsy. *Arch. Pathol. Lab. Med.* **107:**364–367.

66. **Rice, C. M., E. M. Lenches, S. R. Eddy, S. J. Shir, R. L. Sheets, and J. H. Struss.** 1985. Nucleotide sequence of yellow fever virus: implications for flavivirus gene expression and evolution. *Science* **229:**726–733.

67. **Ricosse, J. H., R. Loubierre, J. P. Albert, M. Elte, and F. Roux.** 1972. La diagnostic anatomo-pathologique de la fievre jaune à-propos de l'épidemie survenue en Haute-Volta en 1969. *Ann. Anat. Pathol.* (Paris) **17:**21–38.

68. **Robertson, S. E., B. P. Hull, O. Tomori, O. Bele, J. W. LeDuc, and K. Esteves.** 1996. Yellow fever: a decade of reemergence. *JAMA* **276:**1157–1162.

69. **Rolfes, D. B., and K. G. Ishak.** 1986. Liver disease in toxemia of pregnancy. *Am. J. Gastroenterol.* **81:**1138–1144.

70. **Rugge, M., M.-J. Vanstapel, V. Ninfo, G. Realdi, F. Tremolada, P. G. Montanari, B. van Damme, J. Fevery, J. de Groote, and V. J. Desmet.** 1983. Comparative histology of acute hepatitis B and non-A, non-B in Leuven and Padova. *Virchow's Arch.* (A) **401:**275–288.

71. **Sanders, E. J., P. Borus, G. Ademba, G. Kuria, P. M. Tukei, and J. W. LeDuc.** 1996. Sentinel surveillance for yellow fever in Kenya, 1993 to 1995. *Emerg. Infect. Dis.* **2**(3):236–238.

72. **Scheuer, P. J., P. Ashrafzadeh, S. Sherlock, D. Brown, and G. M. Dushieko.** 1992. The pathology of hepatitis C. *Hepatology* **15:**567–571.

73. **Scheuer, P. J., and J. H. Lefkowitch.** 1994. Acute hepatitis, p. 62–80. *In* P. J. Scheuer and J. H. Lefkowitch (ed.), *Liver Biopsy Interpretation*, 5th ed. Saunders, London.

74. **Scheuer, P. J., and J. H. Lefkowitch.** 1994. Chronic hepatitis, p. 117–134. *In* P. J. Scheuer and J. H. Lefkowitch (ed.), *Liver Biopsy Interpretation*, 5th ed. Saunders, London.

75. **Stocker, J. T., and K. G. Ishak.** 1975. *Syllabus: Morphologic Changes in Viral Hepatitis*, p. 14–16. Armed Forces Institute of Pathology, Washington, D.C.

76. **Strano, A. J., J. R. Dooley, and K. G. Ishak.** 1974. *Syllabus: Yellow Fever and Its Histopathologic Differential Diagnosis*, p. 1–54. Armed Forces Institute of Pathology, Washington, D.C.

77. **Strode, G. K. (ed.).** 1951. *Yellow Fever*. McGraw-Hill, New York.

78. **Teixeira, Jr., M. R., D. Weller IV, A. M. Murray, M. Bamber, H. C. Thomas, S. Sherlock, and P. J. Scheuer.** 1982. The pathology of hepatitis A in man. *Liver* **2:**53–60.

79. **Theiler, M., and C. R. Anderson.** 1975. The relative resistance of dengue-immune monkeys to yellow fever virus. *Am. J. Trop. Med. Hyg.* **24:**115–117.

80. **Theiler, M., and J. Casals.** 1958. The serological reactions in yellow fever. *Am. J. Trop. Med. Hyg.* **7:**585–594.

81. **Torres, C. M.** 1928. Inclusions nucléaires acidophiles (degeneresence oxychromatique) dans le foie de *Macacus rhesus* inoculé avec le virus Bresilien. *C. R. Soc. Biol.* (Paris) **99:**1344–1345.

82. **Trapido, H., and D. Galindo.** 1956. The epidemiology of yellow fever in Middle America. *Exp. Parasitol.* **5:**285–323.

83. **Tsai, T. F., R. Paul, M. C. Lynberg, and G. W. Letson.** 1993. Congenital yellow fever virus infection after immunization in pregnancy. *J. Infect. Dis.* **168:**1520–1523.

84. **Vanstapel, M. J., and V. J. Desmet.** 1983. Cytomegalovirus hepatitis: a histological and immunohistochemical study. *Appl. Pathol.* **1:**41–49.

85. **Verme, G., P. Amoroso, G. Lettieri, P. Pierri, E. David, F. Sessa, R. Rizzi, F. Bonino, S. Recchai, and M. Rizzetto.** 1986. A histological study of hepatitis delta virus liver disease. *Hepatology* **6:**640–644.

86. **Vieira, W. T., L. C. Gayotto, C. P. deLima, and T. deBrito.** 1983. Histopathology of the human liver in yellow fever with special emphasis on the diagnostic role of the Councilman body. *Histopathology* **7:**195–208.

87. **Villela, E.** 1941. Histology of human yellow fever when death is delayed. *Arch. Pathol.* **31:**665–669.

88. **Walker, D. H., J. B. McCormick, K. M. Johnson, P. A. Webb, G. Komba-Kono, L. H. Elliott, and J. J. Gardner.** 1982. Pathologic and virologic study of fatal Lassa fever in man. *Am. J. Pathol.* **107:**349–356.

89. **Webber, B. L., and I. Freiman.** 1974. The liver in Kwashiorkor: a clinical and electron microscopical study. *Arch. Pathol.* **98:**400–408.

90. **Weitberg, A. B., J. C. Alper, I. Diamond, and Z. Fligiel.** 1979. Acute granulomatous hepatitis in the course of acquired toxoplasmosis. *N. Engl. J. Med.* **300:**1093–1096.

91. **Welper, W., and K. Opitz.** 1972. Histologic changes in the liver biopsy in *Amanita phalloides* intoxication. *Hum. Pathol.* **3:**249–254.

92. **World Health Organization.** 1996. Yellow fever. *W.H.O. Weekly Epidemiol. Record* **42:**313–318.

93. **World Health Organization.** 1996. WHO appeals for action to combat "dramatic resurgence" of yellow fever in Africa. Press release WHO/67. World Health Organization, Geneva.

chapter 3

Dengue and Other Viral Hemorrhagic Fevers

Duane J. Gubler and Sherif R. Zaki

Dengue and dengue hemorrhagic fever (DHF) are important resurgent tropical diseases caused by infection with dengue viruses. Hemorrhagic fever (HF) of infectious origin is a clinical syndrome caused by a group of infectious agents including viruses, chlamydiae, rickettsiae, bacteria, fungi, spirochetes, and protozoa. However, the term "hemorrhagic fever viruses" is withheld for a special group of viruses transmitted to humans by arthropods and rodents (Table 3.1). These viruses persist in nature through zoonotic cycles, although in the case of dengue and sometimes yellow fever viruses, human-to-human transmission through the bite of a mosquito vector is an important factor in disease maintenance. Because these viruses are often extremely virulent and associated with disease outbreaks with high mortality rates, they have gained considerable public notoriety and are considered among the most threatening examples of what are commonly called emerging pathogens.

Duane J. Gubler, Division of Vector-Borne Infectious Diseases, Centers for Disease Control and Prevention, P.O. Box 2087 (Foothills Campus), Fort Collins, CO 80520. **Sherif R. Zaki,** Infectious Disease Pathology Activity, Division of Viral and Rickettsial Diseases, National Center for Infectious Diseases, Centers for Disease Control and Prevention, Mailstop G-32, 1600 Clifton Road, Atlanta, GA 30333

Pathology of Emerging Infections 2
Edited by Ann Marie Nelson and C. Robert Horsburgh, Jr.
© 1998 American Society for Microbiology, Washington, D.C.

Table 3.1 HF viruses[a]

Virus	Disease name	Case fatality (%)	Vertebrate host	Arthropod vector
Arenaviruses				
Junin	Argentine HF	15–30	Rodents (*Calomys musculinus*)	None
Machupo	Bolivian HF	15–30	Rodents (*Calomys callosus*)	
Guanarito	Venezualen HF	15–30	Rodents (*Zygodontomys brevicauda*)	None
Sabia	Brazilian HF	15–30	Presumably an unidentified rodent	None
Lassa	Lassa fever	~15	Rodents (*Mastomys*)	None
Bunyaviridae				
Rift Valley fever	Rift Valley fever	~50	Vertebrates (sheep, cattle)	Mosquito, *Aedes* and others
Crimean-Congo HF	Crimean-Congo HF	15–30	Vertebrates (birds, hares, large ungulates)	Ticks, especially *Hyalomma*
Hantaan, Seoul, Puumala, and others	Hemorrhagic fever with renal syndrome (HFRS)	1–15	Rodents	None
Sin Nombre, Black Creek Canal, and others	Hantavirus pulmonary syndrome (HPS)	50	Rodents	None
Filoviridae				
Marburg	Marburg HF	25	Unknown	Unknown
Ebola	Ebola HF	50–90	Unknown	Unknown
Flaviviridae				
Yellow fever	Yellow fever	20	Primates	Mosquito, especially *Aedes*
Dengue 1, 2, 3, 4	DHF/DSS	5	Primates, humans	Mosquito, especially *Aedes aegypti*
Kyasanur Forest disease	Kyasanur Forest disease	0.5–9	Rodents	Ticks
Omsk HF	Omsk HF	0.5–9	Rodents	Ticks

[a]Adapted from reference 106.

Natural History

Dengue and DHF are caused by infection with dengue viruses. There are four dengue serotypes, dengue 1, 2, 3, and 4. These viruses are closely related to each other antigenically, and as a result, serologic tests reflect extensive cross-reactivity; however, infection with any one serotype does not provide cross-protective immunity against the others. Persons living in an endemic area can be infected with each of the four dengue serotypes during their lifetime.

Infection with dengue viruses is transmitted through the bite of an infective *Aedes aegypti* mosquito (30). *A. aegypti* is a small, black-and-white,

> *Infection with any one dengue serotype does not provide cross-protective immunity against the others*

highly domesticated mosquito that prefers to lay its eggs in artificial containers commonly found in and around homes in the tropics, for example, containers used for water storage, flower vases, old automobile tires, and buckets, that collect rainwater. The adult mosquitoes prefer to rest indoors, are unobtrusive, and prefer to feed on humans during daylight hours. As a result, inhabitants are rarely aware of the presence of this mosquito, making its control difficult.

After a person is bitten by an infective mosquito, the virus undergoes an incubation period of 3 to 14 days (average, 4 to 7 days), after which the person may experience acute onset of fever accompanied by a variety of nonspecific signs and symptoms. During this acute febrile period, which may be as short as 2 days and as long as 10 days, dengue viruses may circulate in the infected person's peripheral blood. If other A. *aegypti* mosquitoes bite the ill person during this febrile viremic stage, those mosquitoes may become infected and subsequently transmit the virus to other uninfected persons after an extrinsic incubation period of 8 to 12 days.

Epidemiology

Dengue viruses and A. *aegypti* mosquitoes are distributed throughout the tropical areas of the world (Fig. 3.1); over 2.5 billion people live in dengue-endemic areas (37, 41, 75). Currently, dengue fever causes more illness and death than any other arboviral disease acquired by humans. Each year, an estimated 50 to 100 million cases of dengue fever and several hundred thousand cases of DHF occur, depending on epidemic activity (34, 64). The severe and fatal form of the disease, DHF, is a leading cause of hospitalization and death among children in many Southeast Asian countries (2). Epidemics of DHF first occurred in the Southeast Asian region in the 1950s, spread to the South Pacific islands in the 1970s, and reached the Caribbean Basin in the 1980s (2, 5, 34, 37, 38). Current evidence suggests that the pattern of severe hemorrhagic disease is evolving in the American region in a manner similar to the way it did in Southeast Asia in the 1960s (32).

Dengue fever has been known in the medical literature for over 200 years but was characterized by relatively infrequent epidemics until the 1950s. The disease pattern associated with dengue changed with the ecologic disruption in Southeast Asia during and following World War II, which created ideal conditions for increased transmission of mosquito-borne diseases in urban areas. In this setting, a global pandemic of dengue began, epidemic transmission increased, hyperendemicity (the co-circulation of multiple dengue virus serotypes) developed in Southeast Asian cities, and DHF, a newly described disease, emerged (34, 37, 42). The first known epidemic of DHF occurred in Manila in 1953–54, but within 20 years it had spread throughout Southeast Asia; by the mid-1970s, DHF had become a leading cause of hospitalization and death among children in the region (2). In the 1980s and 1990s, dengue transmission in Asia further intensified, with increased incidence and geographic expansion of epidemic DHF west into India, Pakistan, Sri Lanka, and the Maldive Islands, and east into China (34, 37, 42). At the same time, the

Currently, dengue fever causes more illness and death than any other arboviral disease acquired by humans

geographic distribution of epidemic DHF was expanding into new regions: the Pacific Islands in the 1970s and 1980s and the American tropics in the 1980s and 1990s (5, 32, 34, 37, 38, 42, 72, 75).

Epidemiologic changes in the Americas have been the most dramatic. In the 1960s and most of the 1970s, epidemic dengue was rare in the American region because the principal mosquito vector, A. aegypti, had been eradicated from most of Central and South America (31, 37). The eradication program was discontinued in the early 1970s, and this species then began to reinvade those countries where it had been eradicated. By the 1990s, A. aegypti had regained the geographic distribution it had before "eradication" (Fig. 3.2). Epidemic dengue invariably followed after reinfestation of a country by A. aegypti. By the 1980s, the American region was experiencing major epidemics of dengue in countries that had been free of the disease for 35 to 130 years (32, 37, 72). With increased epidemic activity came the development of hyperendemicity and the emergence of epidemic DHF much as had occurred in Southeast Asia 25 years earlier (32). From 1981 to 1997, 23 American countries reported laboratory-confirmed DHF (Fig. 3.3) (34, 37, 72).

While Africa has not yet had a major epidemic of DHF, sporadic cases have occurred as epidemic dengue fever has increased markedly in the past 17 years. Before the 1980s, little was known of the distribution of dengue viruses in Africa. Since then, however, major epidemics caused by all four serotypes have occurred in both East and West Africa. Outbreaks have been more common in East Africa in the 1990s, with major epidemics in Djibouti in 1991 and in Jeddah, Saudi Arabia, in 1994; both were the first outbreaks in those countries in over 50 years (34, 37).

The emergence of epidemic dengue/DHF as a global public health problem in the past 17 years is closely associated with demographic and societal changes that have occurred over the past 50 years (34, 37). A major factor has been unprecedented population growth and, with that, unplanned and uncontrolled urbanization, especially in tropical developing countries. The substandard housing and the deterioration in water, sewer, and waste management systems associated with unplanned urbanization have created ideal conditions for increased transmission of mosquito-borne diseases in tropical urban centers.

Increased air travel provides the ideal mechanism for the transport of dengue and other urban pathogens between population centers of the world

Another major factor in the global emergence of dengue/DHF is the jet airplane and increased air travel, which provides the ideal mechanism for the transport of dengue and other urban pathogens between population centers of the world. For instance, in 1994, an estimated 40 million persons departed the United States by air, 51% of whom traveled for business or holiday to tropical dengue-endemic countries (33). Many travelers become infected while visiting tropical areas, but become ill after returning home, resulting in a constant movement of dengue viruses in infected humans to all areas of the world and ensuring repeated introductions of new dengue virus strains and serotypes into areas where the mosquito vectors occur. The result is increased epidemic activity, the development of hyperendemicity, and the emergence of epidemic DHF.

The United States is not immune to the introduction of dengue viruses. Each year for the past 20 years, imported dengue cases have been documented by the Centers for Disease Control and Prevention (CDC) (33, 73). These cases represent introductions of all four virus serotypes from all tropical regions of the world. Most dengue introductions into the United States come from the American and Asian tropics and reflect the increased number of Americans traveling to those areas. Overall, from 1976 to 1994, 2,265 suspected cases of imported dengue have been reported to the CDC (33, 73). Although adequate blood samples were received from only a portion of these patients, 498 (22%) have been confirmed as dengue.

These cases represent only the "tip of the iceberg" because most physicians in the United States have a low index of suspicion for dengue, which they often do not include in their differential diagnosis, even if the patient recently traveled to a tropical country. As a result, many imported dengue cases are never reported. It is important to increase awareness of dengue/DHF among physicians in temperate areas, however, because the disease can be life-threatening. For example, two cases of the severe form of DHF, dengue shock syndrome (DSS), were recently described in Swedish tourists returning from holiday in Asia (98). In the United States, imported cases appear to be increasingly severe (14). Thus, from 1986 to 1993, there were 13 hospitalized patients among 166 laboratory-confirmed cases (8%). In 1994, however, 6/46 (13%) of confirmed imported cases required hospitalization. Moreover, three of those patients (7%) had severe hemorrhagic disease (14). Thus, it is important that physicians in the United States consider dengue in the differential diagnosis of viral syndrome in all patients with a travel history to any tropical area.

There is a potential for epidemic dengue transmission in the United States. On four occasions in the past 17 years, autochthonous transmission, secondary to importation of the virus in humans, has occurred in Texas (1980, 1986, 1995, and 1997). Although the outbreaks were small, they underscore the potential for dengue transmission in the United States, where two competent mosquito vectors occur. A. *aegypti*, the most important and efficient epidemic vector of dengue viruses, has been in the country for over 200 years and has been responsible for transmitting major epidemics in the past (22). Currently, this species is found only in the Gulf Coast states from Texas to Florida. *Aedes albopictus* was introduced to the continental United States in the early 1980s and has since become widespread in the eastern half of the country. It currently occurs in counties in 25 of the continental states; this species has also been found in Hawaii for over 90 years. Both A. *aegypti* and A. *albopictus* can transmit dengue viruses to humans, and their presence in an area increases the risk of autochthonous dengue transmission, secondary to imported cases (30).

There is a potential for epidemic dengue transmission in the United States

Clinical Manifestations

Dengue virus infection in humans causes a spectrum of illness ranging from inapparent or mild febrile illness to severe and fatal hemorrhagic disease. In dengue-endemic areas, many dengue infections are clinically nonspecific, especially in children, with symptoms of a viral syndrome that has a variety

The same viruses can cause dengue fever and DHF, and severe hemorrhagic disease can be caused by all four dengue serotypes

of local names. Important risk factors influencing the proportion of patients who have severe disease during epidemic transmission include the strain and serotype of the infecting virus, the immune status of the individual, the age of the patient, and the genetic background of the human host (2, 5, 30, 38, 40, 41, 75). The same viruses can thus cause dengue fever and DHF, and severe hemorrhagic disease can be caused by all four dengue serotypes.

Classic dengue fever is primarily a disease of older children and adults. It is characterized by sudden onset of fever and a variety of nonspecific signs and symptoms, including frontal headache, retro-orbital pain, body aches, nausea and vomiting, joint pains, weakness, and rash (94). Patients may be anorexic and have altered taste sensation and mild sore throat. Lymphadenopathy is common. Dengue fever is generally self-limiting and rarely fatal. The acute phase of illness lasts for 3 to 7 days, but the convalescent phase may be prolonged and may be associated with weakness and depression. No permanent sequelae are known to be associated with dengue infection.

DHF, on the other hand, is primarily a disease of children under the age of 15 years, although it may also occur in adults (2). It too is characterized by sudden onset of fever, usually of 2 to 7 days duration, and a variety of nonspecific signs and symptoms. During the acute phase of illness, it is difficult to distinguish DHF from dengue fever and other illnesses found in tropical areas (Table 3.2). The differential diagnosis should include measles, rubella, influenza, typhoid, leptospirosis, malaria, other viral HFs (VHFs), and any other disease that may present in the acute phase as a nonspecific viral syn-

Table 3.2 Signs and symptoms associated with confirmed DHF, Jakarta, Indonesia, 1975–1977

Sign or symptom	No.	% Positive
Hepatomegaly	297/601[a]	49
Abdominal pain	281/619	45
Vomiting	279/619	45
Cough	142/619	23
Constipation	101/619	16
Nausea	90/618[a]	15
Headache	82/619	13
Sore throat	53/619	9
Rhinitis	50/619	8
Diarrhea	50/619	8
Chills	30/619	5
Myalgia	24/619	4
Joint pain	15/619	2
Stiff neck	15/619	2
Backache	12/619	2
Conjunctivitis	6/619	1
Pruritus	4/619	1
Paresthesia	1/619	1

[a]Data not available on all patients.

drome. Children frequently have concurrent infections with other viruses and bacteria causing upper respiratory symptoms. There is no pathognomonic sign or symptom for DHF (Table 3.2).

The critical stage in DHF occurs most frequently from about 24 h before to 24 h after the temperature falls to normal or below. During this time, hemorrhagic manifestations and, more importantly, signs of circulatory failure usually occur. Blood tests during this period will usually show that the patient has thrombocytopenia (platelet count of <100,000/µl) and evidence of a vascular leak syndrome.

Common hemorrhagic manifestations include skin hemorrhages such as petechiae, purpuric lesions, and ecchymoses. Epistaxis, bleeding gums, gastrointestinal (GI) hemorrhage, and hematuria occur less frequently. The tourniquet test may be diagnostically helpful to the physician. This is done by inflating the blood pressure cuff to the midpoint between the systolic and diastolic pressures for 5 min and then releasing the pressure. In persons with increased capillary fragility, a "shower" of petechiae will appear below the cuff. The test is positive if 20 or more petechiae per square inch are observed. Some noninfected persons may have a positive tourniquet test, however, so it does not mean that a person has DHF when the test is positive, only that he or she has increased capillary fragility and that the physician should be concerned and do further tests.

Common hemorrhagic manifestations include skin hemorrhages such as petechiae, purpuric lesions, and ecchymoses

Scattered petechiae are the most common hemorrhagic manifestation observed; they appear most often on the extremities, but also on the trunk and other parts of the body. Purpuric lesions may appear on various parts of the body but are most common at the site of venipuncture. In some patients, large ecchymotic lesions develop on the trunk and extremities, and other patients bleed actively at the site of venipuncture, some profusely. More severely ill patients have GI hemorrhage, which is manifested by hematemesis or melena. Classic hematemesis and melena usually occur after prolonged shock, but patients may develop massive, frank upper GI hemorrhage as well. Without early diagnosis and proper management, some patients experience shock due to blood loss, which may be mild or severe (25, 85, 86). More commonly, shock is caused by plasma leakage; it may be mild and transient or progress to profound shock with undetectable pulse and blood pressure (2). Children with profound shock often are somnolent, exhibit petechiae on the face, and have perioral cyanosis.

It is convenient for both clinicians and epidemiologists to classify DHF into four grades of illness based on severity (Table 3.3) (2). Grade I is mild DHF; the only hemorrhagic manifestation is scattered petechiae and/or a positive tourniquet test. Grade II DHF is more severe, with one or more overt hemorrhagic manifestations such as those mentioned above. Grades III and IV represent a more severe form of disease called DSS (dengue shock syndrome). Grade III illness is characterized by mild shock with signs of circulatory failure; the patient may be lethargic or restless and have cold extremities, clammy skin, a rapid but weak pulse, narrowing of pulse pressure to 20 mm Hg or less, and/or hypotension. Grade IV, the most severe form of DHF/DSS, is characterized by profound shock with undetectable pulse and blood pressure.

Table 3.3 World Health Organization Classification of DHF[a]

Grade I	Fever accompanied by nonspecific constitutional symptoms, with a positive tourniquet test or sporadic petechiae as the only hemorrhagic manifestation
Grade II	The same as grade I, but with spontaneous hemorrhagic manifestations
Grade III	Circulatory failure manifested by rapid, weak pulse, narrowing of pulse pressure (20 mm Hg or less), or hypotension
Grade IV	Profound shock with undetectable pulse and blood pressure

[a]Adapted from reference 2.

In severe cases of DSS, fever of a few days duration is followed by the sudden deterioration of the patient's condition. At the time of (or shortly after) the fall in temperature, the patient's skin may become cool, blotchy, and congested; circumoral cyanosis is frequently observed, and the pulse becomes rapid and weak. Although some patients appear lethargic at first, they become restless and then rapidly pass into a critical stage of shock. They frequently experience acute abdominal pain shortly before the onset of shock (2).

In mild cases of DHF, all signs and symptoms abate after fever subsides. Lysis of fever, however, may be accompanied by profuse sweating and mild changes in pulse rate and blood pressure, together with coolness of extremities and skin congestion. These changes reflect mild and transient circulatory disturbances as a result of plasma leakage. Patients usually recover spontaneously or after fluid and electrolyte therapy (2). Patients in shock are in danger of dying without appropriate management. The duration of shock is usually short; the patient may die within 12 to 24 h or recover rapidly following antishock therapy. Convalescence for those with DHF, with or without shock, is usually short and uneventful. Even in patients with undetectable pulse and blood pressure, once the shock is overcome, the surviving patients recover within 2 to 3 days.

Thrombocytopenia and hemoconcentration are constant findings in DHF/DSS. A platelet count of less than 100,000/μl is usually found between days 3 and 8 of illness. Hemoconcentration, indicating plasma leakage, is almost always present in classic DHF but is more severe in patients with shock. Hepatomegaly is a common but not a constant finding (25, 85, 86). In some countries, most patients with confirmed DHF/DSS have been found to have an enlarged liver. In other countries, however, hepatomegaly varies from one epidemic to another, suggesting that the strain and/or serotype of virus may influence liver involvement (25).

Diagnosis

A definitive diagnosis of dengue infection can only be made in the laboratory

A definitive diagnosis of dengue infection can only be made in the laboratory and depends on either isolating the virus or detecting specific antibodies in the patient's serum (36). An acute-phase blood sample should always be taken as soon as possible after onset of illness, and a convalescent-phase sample should be taken 2 to 3 weeks after onset. Because it is frequently difficult to obtain convalescent-phase samples, however, a second sample should always be taken from hospitalized patients on the day of discharge from hospital.

Virus can often be isolated from acute-phase blood samples taken in the first 5 days of illness (36). Two serologic tests are used to detect antibodies. The immunoglobulin M (IgM) capture enzyme-linked immunosorbent assay (ELISA) detects IgM antibody, which usually appears by day 5 after onset and persists for 2 to 3 months (36, 53). The hemagglutination-inhibition test and an IgG ELISA detect IgG antibody, which appears simultaneously or shortly after IgM but persists for life. For this reason, diagnosis using IgG requires paired acute- and convalescent-phase blood samples to demonstrate a fourfold or greater rise in specific antibody (36).

It should be emphasized that DHF is new to the Americas (32). Epidemics that occur in areas where the medical community is unaware of this disease and its pathophysiology may have high fatality rates (20 to 40%) because diagnosis of DHF/DSS is made too late or not at all. Moreover, cases of dengue infection are being more frequently imported into temperate regions such as the United States and Europe (33, 73, 98). It is important, therefore, that physicians everywhere learn to recognize and properly manage DHF/DSS.

Pathology and Pathogenesis

The primary pathophysiologic abnormality seen in DHF/DSS is an acute increase in vascular permeability that leads to leakage of plasma into the extravascular compartment, resulting in hemoconcentration and decreased blood pressure (2). Plasma volume studies have shown a reduction of more than 20% in severe cases. Supporting evidence of plasma leakage includes serous effusion found postmortem, pleural effusion on X-ray, hemoconcentration, and hypoproteinemia. There are no apparent destructive vascular lesions, suggesting that the transient functional vascular changes are due to a short-acting pharmacologic mediator (2).

Hemostatic changes in DHF involve three factors: vascular changes, thrombocytopenia, and coagulation disorders (2). Almost all DHF patients have increased vascular fragility and thrombocytopenia, and many have abnormal coagulograms, suggesting disseminated intravascular coagulation, which is also evidenced by concomitant thrombocytopenia, prolonged partial thromboplastin time, decreased fibrinogen level, and increased fibrinogen degradation products. GI hemorrhage is found at autopsy in the majority of patients who die.

Hemostatic changes in DHF involve three factors: vascular changes, thrombocytopenia, and coagulation disorders

Some cases of severe hemorrhagic disease do not fit the above classification and may have a different pathogenesis (86). These patients generally present with similar signs and symptoms during the acute phase of illness, but develop frank upper GI bleeding without any evidence of plasma leakage (hemoconcentration) or circulatory failure as seen in patients with classical DSS. Generally, the upper GI bleeding occurs 3 to 5 days after onset of illness and is often the reason the patient is brought to the hospital. All such patients have significant thrombocytopenia. In many cases, bleeding may be severe enough to cause shock due to blood loss rather than plasma leakage. In one study in Indonesia, 30% of patients with virologically confirmed fatal DHF had this type of severe upper GI hemorrhaging (86). Blood transfusions are always indicated for these patients, whose disease is generally more difficult to manage than classic DSS (86).

Finally, some patients with dengue infection may present with neurologic disorders such as convulsions, spastic paresis, and change in consciousness, with or without hemorrhagic manifestations (35). These patients, who may be admitted to the neurologic ward with a diagnosis of viral encephalitis, may subsequently develop hemorrhagic manifestations and shock. Their cerebrospinal fluid findings are normal, and most evidence suggests that the virus does not cross the blood-brain barrier, although recent studies suggest that this may occur in some patients (57, 76, 77). Further studies are necessary to identify what factors contribute to these unusual manifestations.

Generally speaking, the gross pathologic findings in DHF are similar to those seen in many other VHFs. Autopsy findings in fatal cases of dengue include widespread petechial hemorrhages and ecchymoses involving skin, mucous membranes, and internal organs. Hemorrhages are especially prominent around needle puncture sites. While hemorrhage can be striking in some cases, the amount of bleeding is usually minimal and sometimes absent. Hemorrhagic effusions can be seen in rare cases; however, serous effusions are more common, with accumulation of a high protein fluid in pleural, peritoneal, and pericardial cavities. Necrosis and major organ damage are not usually observed at the gross level in most cases. However, in some cases with a prolonged hypovolemia, widespread, focal, and sometimes massive necrosis can be observed in multiple organ systems and is usually ischemic in nature.

None of the histopathologic features seen in DHF is considered to be pathognomonic. In general, the histopathology of the disease is similar to that seen in many other VHFs (107) (Fig. 3.4–3.13). Some of the characteristic features that may support the histopathologic diagnosis of DHF and other VHFs are summarized in Table 3.4. Variable degrees of generalized congestion are usually seen in fatal cases of DHF; however, morphological changes of vascular wall and endothelium are exceedingly uncommon. Occasionally, the endothelial cells lining capillaries and venules are prominent and swollen. Microscopic perivascular hemorrhages can occasionally be seen in various organs, and ischemic necrotic lesions, except those attributed to shock, are not common. Microvascular thrombosis can be seen in tissues of a small proportion of patients with severe hemorrhage.

The most consistent microscopic findings in DHF are seen in the liver and consist of hepatocellular necrosis, Councilman bodies, and microvesicular fatty change (Fig. 3.4). These hepatic histopathologic features (4, 9–12, 27) are somewhat similar to those seen in fatal yellow fever (83, 89) (Fig. 3.9). The acidophil or Councilman body, once considered to be diagnostic for yellow fever (18), is not pathognomonic of the disease and can be seen in DHF and other VHFs, as well as other hepatic diseases. In yellow fever the hepatic necrosis is extensive and midzonal in distribution, while in fatal

The gross pathologic findings in DHF are similar to those seen in many other VHFs

Table 3.4 Pathologic features in VHF[a]

Disease	References	Pathologic features[b]
Argentine HF Bolivian HF Venezuelan HF Lassa fever	17, 24, 29, 58 15, 62, 63, 87 79 21, 48, 60, 80, 91, 92, 96, 97	Multifocal hepatocellular necrosis with minimal inflammatory response, interstitial pneumonitis, myocarditis, and lymphoid depletion. Extensive parenchymal cell and reticuloendothelial infection, more than morphologic lesions would suggest.
Rift Valley fever	1, 61, 88, 90	Widespread hepatocellular necrosis and hemorrhage, sometimes with midzonal distribution, minimal inflammatory response, DIC, lymphoid depletion, and encephalitis. Rift Valley fever antigens in very few individual hepatocytes.
Crimean Congo HF	8, 13, 49, 84	Widespread hepatocellular necrosis and hemorrhage with minimal or no inflammatory cell response and lymphoid depletion. Hepatic and endothelial cell infection and damage.
Hemorrhagic fever with renal syndrome (HFRS)	16, 43, 50, 51, 54–56, 82, 100	Retroperitoneal edema in severe HFRS; mild to severe renal pathologic changes. Congestion and hemorrhagic necrosis of renal medulla, right atrium of the heart, and anterior pituitary. Extensive endothelial infection mainly in renal and cardiac microvasculature.
Hantavirus pulmonary syndrome (HPS)	20, 70, 93, 100, 102, 105	Large bilateral pleural effusions and heavy edematous lungs, mild to moderate interstitial pneumonitis, immunoblasts and atypical lymphocytes in lymphoid tissues and peripheral blood. Extensive infections of endothelial cells in pulmonary microvasculature.
Ebola HF	6, 7, 19, 23, 26, 28, 44, 47, 65, 69, 78, 101, 103, 104, 106	Extensive and disseminated infection and necrosis in major organs such as liver, spleen, lung, kidney, skin, and gonads. Extensive hepatocellular necrosis associated with formation of characteristic intracytoplasmic viral inclusions. Lymphoid depletion, microvascular infection and injury.
Marburg HF	52, 66, 67, 74, 101	Similar to Ebola HF.
Yellow fever	39, 81, 83, 89	Midzonal hepatocellular necrosis; minimal inflammatory response. Councilman bodies and microvesicular fatty change. Hepatocellular and Kupffer cell infection.
Dengue HF/DSS	4, 9–12, 27, 81	Centrilobular and midzonal hepatocellular necrosis with minimal inflammatory response; Councilman bodies and microvesicular fatty change. Hyperplasia of mononuclear phagocytic cells in lymphoid tissues and atypical lymphocytes in peripheral blood. Widespread infection of mononuclear phagocytic and endothelial cells.
Kyasanur Forest disease (KFD)	45, 46, 95	Focal hepatocellular degeneration, fatty change, and necrosis. Pulmonary hemorrhage, depletion of malpighian follicles, sinus histiocytosis, erythrophagocytosis, mild myocarditis, and encephalitis.
Omsk HF	59	Little known; scattered focal hemorrhage, interstitial pneumonia, and normal lymphoid tissues.

[a]Adapted from reference 107.

[b]These features represent the more characteristic pathologic findings in the different VHFs. More general findings seen to variable degrees in all HF are not listed in this table (see text).

DHF/DSS it is less severe and tends to be centrilobular or midzonal. In severe cases of both diseases the necrosis may extend beyond the midzone, resulting in almost complete necrosis of the lobule; however, a rim of intact hepatocytes usually remains around the portal tracts and central veins. Immunohistochemistry is extremely valuable in providing a definitive diagnosis and differentiating these infections from other VHFs and diseases with similar histopathologic features such as viral hepatitis and leptospirosis (39, 81, 99) (Fig. 3.4–3.13).

In lymphoid tissues of fatal DHF, there is usually a marked proliferation of lymphocytes with an increase in the number of plasma cells and immunoblasts (Fig. 3.5). These proliferative changes are somewhat similar to those seen in hantavirus-related illnesses. This is in contrast to most other VHFs, where lymphoid necrosis and depletion are the general rule. Commonly observed histopathologic findings in the lungs include variable degrees of congestion, interstitial pneumonitis, and diffuse alveolar damage (Fig. 3.8). In the heart, histopathologic findings are nonspecific and consist of hypoxic changes and edema (Fig. 3.6).

The histopathologic features in arenaviral infections are strikingly similar

The histopathologic features in arenaviral infections such as Lassa fever (21, 48, 60, 80, 91, 92, 96, 97), Argentine HF (17, 24, 29, 58), Bolivian HF (15, 62, 63, 87), and Venezuelan HF (79) are strikingly similar (Fig. 3.10). The histopathologic features in the liver are very similar to those in DHF and consist of multifocal hepatocellular necrosis with cytoplasmic eosinophilia, Councilman body formation, nuclear pyknosis, and cytolysis. Inflammatory cell infiltrates and necrotic areas are usually mild and, when present, consist of neutrophils and mononuclear cells. In contrast to DHF, immunohistochemical studies demonstrate hepatocellular infection in association with focal areas of necrosis (Fig. 3.10). Extensive infection of macrophages and mesothelial cells lining several serosal surfaces is characteristic of arenavirus infections and helps explain serous effusions commonly seen in patients with these infections (Fig. 3.10) (71, 80).

The pathologic features of hantavirus-associated diseases, namely hantavirus fever with renal syndrome (HFRS) (16, 43, 50, 51, 54, 55, 56, 82) and hantavirus pulmonary syndrome (HPS) (20, 68, 100, 102, 105), are shown in Fig. 3.11 (100). In contrast to DHF, histopathologic changes in the liver of fatal cases of HFRS and HPS are minimal and nonspecific in nature. Histopathologic changes of HPS are mainly seen in the lungs and spleen. Microscopic examination of the lungs, in most cases, reveals a mild to moderate interstitial pneumonitis with variable degrees of congestion, edema, and mononuclear cell infiltration. The cellular infiltrate is composed of a mixture of small and enlarged mononuclear cells with the appearance of immunoblasts. Focal hyaline membranes, as well as extensive intra-alveolar edema, fibrin, and variable numbers of inflammatory cells, are observed. In typical cases, neutrophils are scanty and the respiratory epithelium is intact with no evidence of cellular debris, nuclear fragmentation, or type II pneumocyte hyperplasia. Other characteristic histopathologic findings in HPS cases include the presence of variable numbers of immunoblasts within the red pulp and periarteriolar sheaths of the spleen and paracortex, within sinuses of lymph nodes, and in the peripheral blood. The most dramatic and characteristic microscopic lesions seen in HFRS involve the kidney. The mildest changes are seen in nephropathia epidemica and include slight tubular dilatation, interstitial edema, diffuse but sparse interstitial inflammatory infiltrate, interstitial medullary hemorrhage, and mild hypercellularity of the glomeruli. In Hantaan virus-associated HFRS, the renal pathologic changes are more severe; in addition to the characteristic medullary hemorrhage and edema, tubular lesions including dilatation, degeneration, necrosis, and sloughing of the tubular epithelium are more prominent.

In Crimean-Congo HF (8, 49, 84) and Rift Valley fever (1, 61, 88), the main histopathologic lesions are seen in the liver, spleen, and lung (Fig. 3.12). The changes in the liver are similar to those seen in DHF and consist of widespread hepatocellular necrosis, usually midzonal in the case of Rift Valley fever, associated with variable degrees of hemorrhage and Councilman body formation. As in the case of Lassa HF, the inflammatory cellular response in necrotic areas is minimal or absent, and only a mild periportal mononuclear infiltrate is sometimes seen. Immunostaining reveals only focal infection of hepatocytes, Kupffer cells, and sinusoidal lining cells (3, 13). The essential histopathologic features in lymphoid tissue include sinusoidal dilatation and generalized lymphoid depletion.

Compared to DHF and other VHFs, the filoviruses cause the most widespread destructive tissue lesions (Fig. 3.13). The pathologic changes are similar in Marburg virus (52, 66, 67, 74) and Ebola virus (6, 7, 19, 23, 26, 28, 44, 47, 65, 69, 78, 103, 104) infections, although the latter tends to be more severe (71, 101, 106, 107). Necrosis is seen in many organs and is maximal in liver, spleen, kidney, and gonads. The necrosis is both related to cytopathic effect of the virus and ischemic in nature. As with DHF, the most characteristic histologic features are seen in the liver with widespread hepatocellular necrosis, Councilman bodies, microvesicular fatty change, and Kupffer cell hyperplasia. The portal tracts usually exhibit extensive karyorrhectic debris and a mononuclear inflammatory infiltrate. The most pathognomonic finding is the presence of characteristic intracytoplasmic viral inclusions within hepatocytes (Fig. 3.13). These are usually numerous, eosinophilic, and oval or filamentous in shape. Ultrastructurally, the inclusions are seen to be composed of aggregates of viral nucleocapsids. The viral inclusions and distribution of antigens can be confirmed and studied by immunohistochemistry (Fig. 3.13) (47, 103, 104). Lymphoid tissues show extensive follicular necrosis and necrotic debris. Similar to DHF, myocardial edema is seen but is not associated with any appreciable inflammatory infiltrates. The lungs are usually hemorrhagic and show features of diffuse alveolar damage.

In summary, the diagnosis of DHF and other VHFs suspected by history and clinical manifestations can also be supported histopathologically, and the overall pattern of histopathologic lesions may suggest a specific diagnosis. However, because of similar pathologic features seen in VHF and a variety of other viral, rickettsial, and bacterial infections, unequivocal diagnosis can only be made by laboratory tests such as immunohistochemistry and

Compared to DHF and other VHFs, the filoviruses cause the most widespread destructive tissue lesions

serology. The main pathological differential diagnosis should include viral hepatitis, leptospirosis, malaria, and rickettsial diseases.

Treatment of DHF

With adequate fluid administration, DSS is rapidly reversible

Early and effective fluid replacement of lost plasma with electrolyte solutions, plasma, or plasma expanders usually results in a favorable outcome. With adequate fluid administration, DSS is rapidly reversible. Rapid replacement of fluid will usually prevent disseminated intravascular coagulation. Prognosis depends on early recognition of shock, based on careful monitoring.

In dengue-endemic areas, it is often not possible and not necessary to hospitalize all patients with suspected DHF/DSS, since shock may develop in only about one-third of the patients (2). The rather constant finding that a decrease in platelet count usually precedes the rise in hematocrit is of great diagnostic and prognostic value. In order to be able to recognize the early signs of shock and thus take preventive action, parents or family members should be advised to bring the patient back for repeat platelet and hematocrit determinations every 24 h. They should also be instructed to keep a careful watch for any signs of clinical deterioration or warning signs of shock such as restlessness and/or lethargy, acute abdominal pain, cold extremities, skin congestion, or oliguria, usually on or after day 3 of illness. Patients with mild DHF can usually be rehydrated orally and an antipyretic drug may be all that is needed. Salicylates should be avoided.

Patients should be hospitalized and treated immediately if they have any signs or symptoms of shock such as restlessness/lethargy, cold extremities, circumoral cyanosis, rapid, weak pulse, narrowing of pulse pressure to 20 mm Hg or less, hypotension, a sudden rise in hematocrit, or continuously elevated hematocrit despite the administration of intravenous fluids (2). Frequent recording of vital signs, hematocrit determinations, and urine output monitoring are important in evaluating the results of treatment. Blood transfusions are contraindicated in patients with severe plasma leakage in the absence of hemorrhage; if given, they may cause pulmonary edema. Blood transfusions may be indicated for patients with significant clinical bleeding. It may be difficult to recognize internal bleeding in the presence of hemoconcentration. A drop in hematocrit of 10% with no clinical improvement, despite adequate fluid administration, indicates significant internal hemorrhage (2). Transfusion of fresh whole blood is preferable; fresh frozen plasma and/or concentrated platelets may be indicated in some cases when consumptive coagulopathy causes massive bleeding.

There is some controversy surrounding the use of steroids, but the general consensus is that they have no beneficial effect in management of severe DHF/DSS. Although some physicians still use them in treatment of shock cases, two double-blind studies, in Thailand and Indonesia, have shown no increase in survival rates of patients with grade IV DSS who were administered steroids (2).

Prevention

Although progress in developing a vaccine against dengue viruses shows promise, there is currently none available. Prevention and control depend on controlling the mosquito vector, A. aegypti, in and around the home where most transmission occurs. Space sprays with insecticides to kill adult mosquitoes are usually ineffective. The most effective way to control the mosquitoes that transmit dengue is larval source reduction, i.e., to eliminate or clean water-holding containers that serve as the breeding sites for A. aegypti in the domestic environment (31).

There is no completely effective method of preventing dengue infection in travelers to tropical areas. The risk of infection can be significantly decreased, however, by understanding the basic behavior and habits of the mosquito vector and by taking a few simple precautions, such as using aerosol bomb insecticides to kill adult mosquitoes indoors, using a repellent containing N,N-diethyl-m-toluamide (DEET) on exposed skin and clothing, and wearing protective clothing. The risk of exposure may be lower in modern, air-conditioned hotels with well-kept grounds and in rural areas.

There is no completely effective method of preventing dengue infection in travelers to tropical areas

Physicians in the United States who see patients with suspected dengue should monitor the temperature, blood pressure, pulse, hematocrit, and platelets. Thrombocytopenia (<100,000/μl), any evidence of vascular leakage or circulatory failure, and hemorrhagic manifestations are indications of severe dengue disease. Acetaminophen products are recommended for management of fever because of the anticoagulant properties of aspirin. All suspected cases should be reported to respective state health departments. Paired acute- and convalescent-phase blood samples should be obtained and sent for laboratory confirmation through the state health department laboratory to CDC's Dengue Branch, Division of Vector-Borne Infectious Diseases, National Center for Infectious Diseases, Calle Casia 2, San Juan, Puerto Rico 00921, telephone (787) 766-5181.

Figure 3.1 Global distribution of dengue fever and the principal mosquito vector, A. *aegypti*.

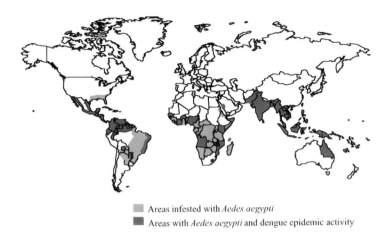

Areas infested with *Aedes aegypti*
Areas with *Aedes aegypti* and dengue epidemic activity

Figure 3.2 Distribution of A. *aegypti* in the Americas (shaded) in the 1930s, 1970, and 1997.

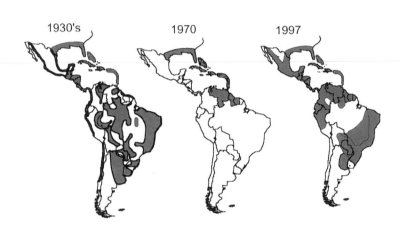

1930's   1970   1997

Figure 3.3 American countries reporting laboratory-confirmed DHF (shaded) prior to 1981 and from 1981 to 1997.

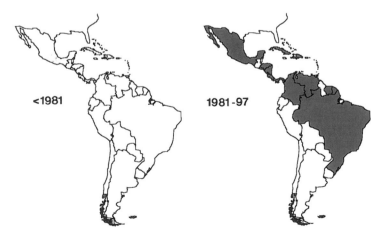

<1981   1981-97

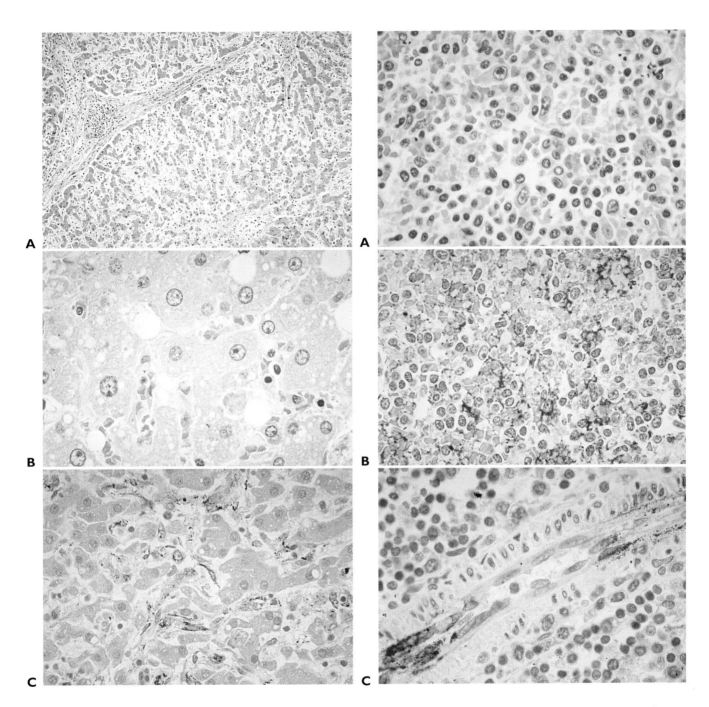

Figure 3.4   DHF. (A) Paracentral hepatic necrosis and sinusoidal congestion. Note rim of intact hepatocytes surrounding central vein. (B) Higher-power detail showing microvesicular fatty change and focal hepatocellular necrosis. (C) Immunostaining of liver showing viral antigens predominantly within sinusoidal Kupffer cells. Note absence of staining of hepatocytes. Original magnifications: A, ×25; B, ×158; C, ×100. Stains: A and B, hematoxylin and eosin (H&E); C, immunoalkaline phosphatase, Naphthol fast red substrate with light hematoxylin counterstain.

Figure 3.5   DHF. (A) Numerous reactive mononuclear cells with prominent nucleoli are seen in section of spleen. (B) Delicate reticular pattern of immunostaining of dengue virus antigens in lymphoid follicle of spleen. (C) Immunostaining of dengue antigens within vascular endothelial cells of spleen. Original magnifications: A–C, ×158. Stains: A, H&E; B and C, immunoalkaline phosphatase staining, Naphthol fast red substrate with light hematoxylin counterstain.

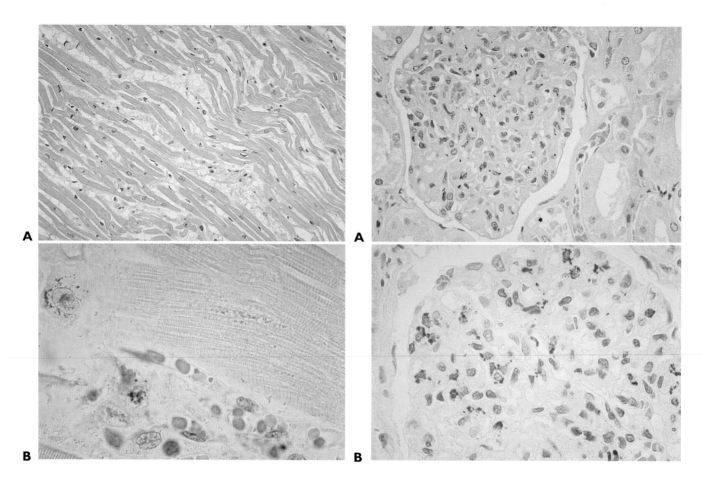

Figure 3.6 DHF. (A) Myocardium showing interstitial edema and fibrosis. (B) Immunostaining of dengue antigens within interstitial macrophages in the myocardium. Original magnifications: A, ×50; B, ×250. Stains: A, H&E; B, immunoalkaline phosphatase staining, Naphthol fast red substrate with light hematoxylin counterstain.

Figure 3.7 DHF. (A) Photomicrograph of kidney showing slight proliferation of glomerular mesangial cells. (B) Immunostaining of dengue viral antigens in mesangial and endothelial cells in a glomerulus. Original magnifications: A, ×100; B, ×158. Stains: A, H&E; B, immunoalkaline phosphatase staining, Naphthol fast red substrate with light hematoxylin counterstain.

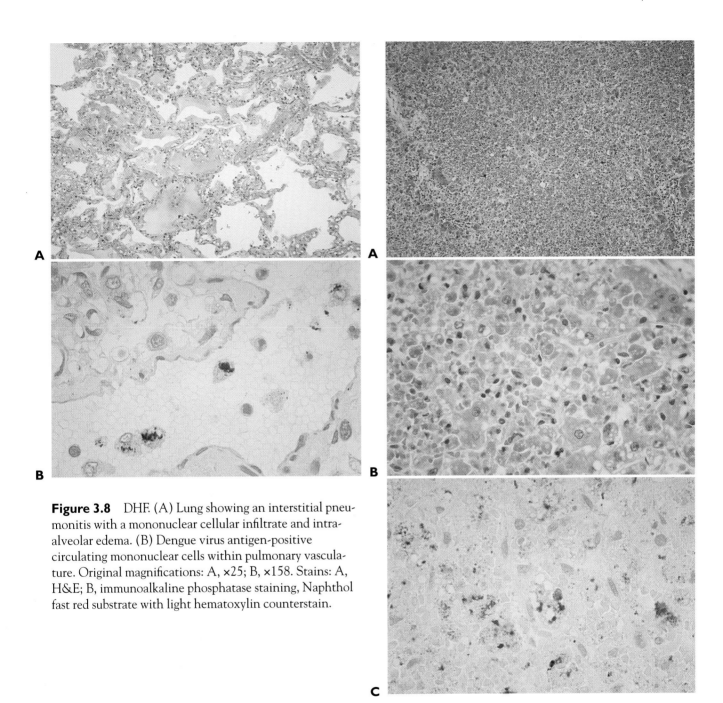

Figure 3.8 DHF. (A) Lung showing an interstitial pneumonitis with a mononuclear cellular infiltrate and intra-alveolar edema. (B) Dengue virus antigen-positive circulating mononuclear cells within pulmonary vasculature. Original magnifications: A, ×25; B, ×158. Stains: A, H&E; B, immunoalkaline phosphatase staining, Naphthol fast red substrate with light hematoxylin counterstain.

Figure 3.9 Yellow fever. (A) Extensive midzonal hepatic necrosis and mild mononuclear portal infiltrates. (B) High-power magnification showing acidophilic necrosis with Councilman bodies and microvesicular fatty change. (C) Abundant immunostaining of yellow fever viral antigens is seen within hepatocytes and Kupffer cells primarily within midzonal area of hepatic lobule. Original magnifications: A, ×25; B, ×100; C, ×158. Stains: A and B, H&E; C, immunoalkaline phosphatase staining, Naphthol fast red substrate with light hematoxylin counterstain.

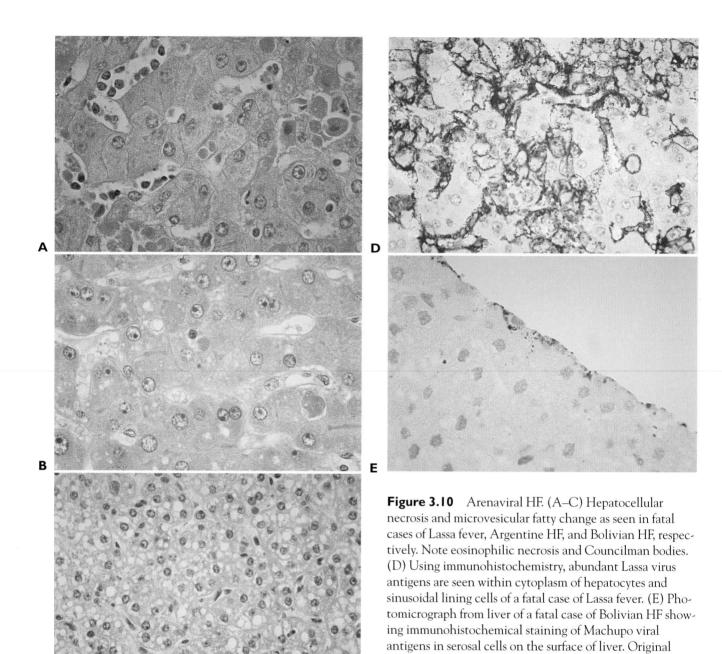

Figure 3.10   Arenaviral HF. (A–C) Hepatocellular
necrosis and microvesicular fatty change as seen in fatal
cases of Lassa fever, Argentine HF, and Bolivian HF, respectively. Note eosinophilic necrosis and Councilman bodies.
(D) Using immunohistochemistry, abundant Lassa virus
antigens are seen within cytoplasm of hepatocytes and
sinusoidal lining cells of a fatal case of Lassa fever. (E) Photomicrograph from liver of a fatal case of Bolivian HF showing immunohistochemical staining of Machupo viral
antigens in serosal cells on the surface of liver. Original
magnifications: A and B, ×158; C and D, ×100; E, ×158.
Stains: A–C, H&E; D and E, immunoalkaline phosphatase
staining, Naphthol fast red substrate with light
hematoxylin counterstain.

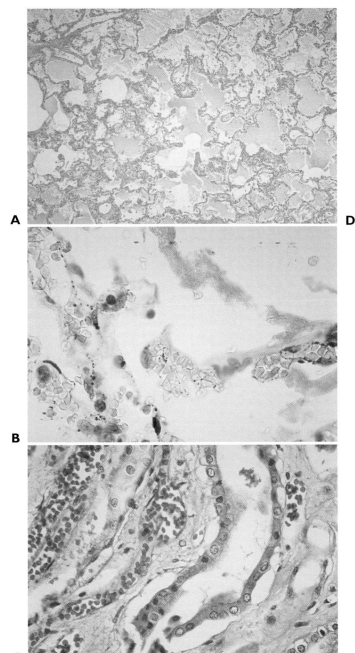

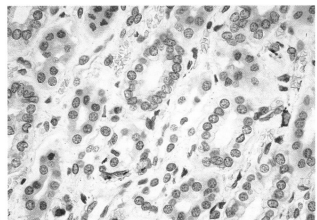

Figure 3.11 Hantavirus-associated diseases (HPS and HFRS). (A) Photomicrographs showing typical interstitial pneumonitis and intra-alveolar edema in lung of a fatal case of HPS. (B) Hantaviral antigens in lung of the same HPS patient, as determined by immunohistochemistry. Note prominent immunostaining in pulmonary microvasculature. (C) Capillary congestion, patchy dilatation of tubules, and slight interstitial edema in renal medulla of an HFRS patient. Note variation in size, intensity of staining, and location of nuclei within tubules. (D) Hantaan antigen-positive endothelial cells in an interstitial vessel in renal medulla. Original magnifications: A, ×12.5; B, ×158; C and D, ×100. Stains: A and C, H&E; B and D, immunoalkaline phosphatase staining, Naphthol fast red substrate with light hematoxylin counterstain.

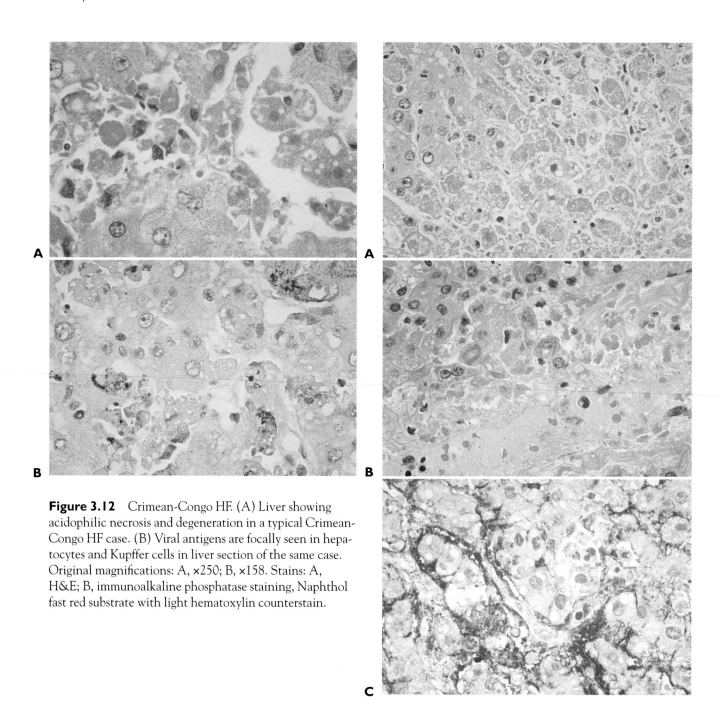

Figure 3.12 Crimean-Congo HF. (A) Liver showing acidophilic necrosis and degeneration in a typical Crimean-Congo HF case. (B) Viral antigens are focally seen in hepatocytes and Kupffer cells in liver section of the same case. Original magnifications: A, ×250; B, ×158. Stains: A, H&E; B, immunoalkaline phosphatase staining, Naphthol fast red substrate with light hematoxylin counterstain.

Figure 3.13 Filovirus HF. (A) Section of liver from a fatal case of Marburg HF showing extensive hepatocellular necrosis as well as sinusoidal dilatation and congestion. (B) Section of liver from a fatal case of Ebola HF showing necrotic debris and hepatocytes containing typical intracytoplasmic, eosinophilic Ebola viral inclusions. (C) Large amounts of viral antigens are seen in hepatocytes and sinusoidal lining cells in section of liver from a case of Ebola HF. Original magnifications: A, ×100; B and C, ×158. Stains: A and B, H&E; C, immunoalkaline phosphatase staining, Naphthol fast red substrate with light hematoxylin counterstain.

References

1. **Abdel-Wahab, K. S. E., L. M. El Baz, E. M. El Tayeb, and M. A. M. Ossman.** 1978. Rift Valley fever virus infections in Egypt: pathological and virological findings in man. *Trans. R. Soc. Trop. Med. Hyg.* **72:**392–396.

2. **Anonymous.** 1986. *Dengue Haemorrhagic Fever, Diagnosis, Treatment and Control,* p. 58. World Health Organization, Geneva.

3. **Arborio, M., and W. C. Hall.** 1989. Diagnosis of a human case of Rift Valley fever by immunoperoxidase demonstration of antigen in fixed liver tissue. *Res. Virol.* **140:**165–168.

4. **Aung-Khin, M., M. M. Khin, M. Thant-Zin, and M. Tin-U.** 1975. Changes in the tissues of the immune system in dengue haemorrhagic fever. *J. Trop. Med. Hyg.* **78:**256–261.

5. **Barnes, W. J. S., and L. Rosen.** 1974. Fatal hemorrhagic disease and shock associated with primary dengue infection on a Pacific island. *Am. J. Trop. Med. Hyg.* **23:**495–506.

6. **Baskerville, A., E. T. W. Bowen, G. S. Platt, L. B. McArdell, and D. I. H. Simpson.** 1978. The pathology of experimental Ebola virus infection in monkeys. *J. Pathol.* **125:**131–138.

7. **Baskerville, A., S. P. Fisher-Hoch, G. H. Neild, and A. B. Dowsett.** 1985. Ultrastructural pathology of experimental Ebola haemorrhagic fever virus infection. *J. Pathol.* **147:**199–209.

8. **Baskerville, A., A. G. O. Satti, F. A. Murphy, and D. I. H. Simpson.** 1981. Congo-Crimean haemorrhagic fever in Dubai: histopathological studies. *J. Clin. Pathol.* **34:**871–874.

9. **Bhamarapravati, N., P. Tuchinda, and V. Boonpucknavig.** 1967. Pathology of Thailand haemorrhagic fever: a study of 100 autopsy cases. *Ann. Trop. Med. Parasitol.* **61:**500–510.

10. **Boonpucknavig, S., V. Boonpucknavig, N. Bhamarapravati, and S. Nimmannitya.** 1979. Immunofluorescence study of skin rash in patients with dengue hemorrhagic fever. *Arch. Pathol. Lab. Med.* **103:**463–466.

11. **Boonpucknavig, V., N. Bhamarapravati, S. Boonpucknavig, P. Futrakul, and P. Tanpaichitr.** 1976. Glomerular changes in dengue hemorrhagic fever. *Arch. Pathol. Lab. Med.* **100:**206–212.

12. **Burke, T.** 1968. Dengue haemorrhagic fever: a pathological study. *Trans. R. Soc. Trop. Med. Hyg.* **62:**682–691.

13. **Burt, F. J., R. Swanepoel, W.-J. Shieh, J. F. Smith, P. A. Leman, P. W. Greer, L. M. Coffield, P. E. Rollin, T. G. Ksiazek, C. J. Peters, and S. R. Zaki.** 1997. Immunohistochemical and in situ localization of Crimean-Congo hemorrhagic fever (CCHF) virus in human tissues and implications for CCHF pathogenesis. *Arch. Pathol. Lab. Med.* **121:**839–846.

14. **Centers for Disease Control and Prevention.** 1995. Imported dengue—United States, 1993 and 1994. *Morbid. Mortal. Weekly Rep.* **44:**353–356.

15. **Child, P. L., R. B. MacKenzie, L. R. Valverde, and K. M. Johnson.** 1967. Bolivian hemorrhagic fever. A pathologic description. *Arch. Pathol.* **83:**434–445.

16. **Collan, Y., M. Mihatsch, J. Lahdevirta, E. Jokinen, T. Romppanen, and E. Janunen.** 1991. Nephropathia epidemica: mild variant of hemorrhagic fever with renal syndrome. *Kidney Int.* **40:**S62–S71.

17. **Cossio, P., R. Laguens, R. Arana, A. Segal, and J. Maiztegui.** 1975. Ultrastructural and immunohistochemical study of the human kidney in Argentine hemorrhagic fever. *Virchows Arch. A Pathol. Anat. Histol.* **368:**1–9.

18. **Councilman, W. T.** 1980. Report of Dr. William T. Councilman, p. 151–159. *In* G. M. Sternberg (ed.), *Report on Etiology and Prevention of Yellow Fever.* U. S. Marine Hospital Service Public Report Bulletin no. 2.

19. **Dietrich, M., H. H. Schumacher, D. Peters, and J. Knobloch.** 1978. Human pathology of Ebola (Maridi) virus infection in the Sudan, p. 37–41. *In* S. R. Pattyn (ed.), *Ebola Virus Haemorrhagic Fever.* Elsevier/North-Holland Biomedical Press, Amsterdam.

20. **Duchin, J. S., F. T. Koster, C. J. Peters, G. L. Simpson, B. Tempest, S. R. Zaki, P. E. Rollin, S. Nichol, E. T. Umland, R. L. Moolenaar, S. E. Reef, K. B. Nolte, M. M. Gallagher, J. C. Butler, R. F. Breiman, and Hantavirus Study Group.** 1994. Hantavirus pulmonary syndrome: a clinical description of 17 patients with a newly recognized disease. *N. Engl. J. Med.* **330:**949–955.

21. **Edington, G. M., and H. A. White.** 1972. The pathology of Lassa fever. *Trans. R. Soc. Trop. Med. Hyg.* **66:**381–389.

22. **Ehrankramz, N. J., A. K. Ventura, R. R. Cuadrado, W. L. Pond, and J. E. Porter.** 1971. Pandemic dengue in Caribbean countries and the southern United States—past, present and potential problems. *N. Engl. J. Med.* **285:**1460–1469.

23. **Ellis, D. S., D. I. H. Simpson, D. P. Francis, J. Knobloch, E. T. W. Bowen, P. Lolik, and I. M. Deng.** 1978. Ultrastructure of Ebola virus particles in human liver. *J. Clin. Pathol.* **31:**201–208.

24. **Elsner, B., E. Schwarz, O. C. Mando, J. Maiztegui, and A. Vilches.** 1973. Pathology of 12 fatal cases of Argentine hemorrhagic fever. *Am. J. Trop. Med. Hyg.* **22:**229–236.

25. **Eram, S., Y. Setyabudi, T. I. Sadono, D. S. Sutrisno, D. J. Gubler, and J. Sulianti Saroso.** 1979. Epidemic dengue hemorrhagic fever in rural Indonesia. II. Clinical studies. *Am. J. Trop. Med. Hyg.* **28:**711–716.

26. **Fisher-Hoch, S. P., T. L. Brammer, S. G. Trappier, L. C. Hutwagner, B. B. Farrar, S. L. Ruo, B. G. Brown, L. M. Hermann, G. I. Perez-Oronoz, C. S. Goldsmith, M. A. Hanes, and J. B. McCormick.** 1992. Pathogenic potential of filoviruses: role of geographic origin of primate host and virus strain. *J. Infect. Dis.* **166:**753–763.

27. **Fresh, J. W., V. Reyes, E. J. Clarke, and C. V. Uylangco.** 1969. Philippine hemorrhagic fever: a clinical, laboratory, and necropsy. *J. Lab. Clin. Med.* **73:**451–458.

28. **Geisbert, T. W., P. B. Jahrling, M. A. Hanes, and P. M. Zack.** 1992. Association of Ebola-related Reston virus particles and antigen with tissue lesions of monkeys imported to the United States. *J. Comp. Pathol.* **106:**137–152.

29. **Gonzalez, P. H., P. M. Cossio, R. M. Arana, J. I. Maiztegui, and R. P. Laguens.** 1980. Lymphatic tissue in Argentine hemorrhagic fever: pathologic features. *Arch. Pathol. Lab. Med.* **104:**250–254.

30. **Gubler, D. J.** 1988. Dengue, p. 223–260. *In* T. P. Monath (ed.), *Epidemiology of Arthropod-Borne Viral Diseases.* CRC Press Inc., Boca Raton, Fla.

31. **Gubler, D. J.** 1989. *Aedes aegypti* and *Aedes aegypti*-borne disease control in the 1990s: top down or bottom up. *Am. J. Trop. Med. Hyg.* **40:**571–578.

32. **Gubler, D. J.** 1993. Dengue and dengue hemorrhagic fever in the Americas, p. 9–22. *In* P. Thongcharoen (ed.), *Monograph on Dengue/Dengue Hemorrhagic Fever*. Regional Publication, SEARO No. 22, New Delhi, India.

33. **Gubler, D. J.** 1996. Arboviruses as imported disease agents: the need for increased awareness. *Arch. Virol.*, 11(Suppl.):21–32.

34. **Gubler, D. J., and G. G. Clark.** 1995. Dengue/dengue hemorrhagic fever: the emergence of a global health problem. *Emerg. Infect. Dis.* **1:**55–57.

35. **Gubler D. J., G. Kuno, and S. H. Waterman.** 1983. Neurologic disorders associated with dengue infection, p. 290–306. *In* T. Pan and R. Pathmanathan (ed.), *Proceedings of the International Conference on Dengue/DHF*. University Malaysia Press, Kuala Lumpur, Malaysia.

36. **Gubler, D. J., and G. E. Sather.** 1990. Laboratory diagnosis of dengue and dengue hemorrhagic fever, p. 291–322. *In Proceedings of the International Symposium on Yellow Fever and Dengue*. Rio de Janeiro, Brazil.

37. **Gubler, D. J., and D. W. Trent.** 1994. Emergence of epidemic dengue/dengue hemorrhagic fever as a public health problem in the Americas. *Infect. Agents Dis.* **2:**383–393.

38. **Guzman, M. G., G. P. Kouri, J. Bravo, M. Soler, S. Vasquez, M. Santos, R. Villaescusa, P. Basanta, G. Indan, and J. M. Ballester.** 1984. Dengue haemorrhagic fever in Cuba. II. Clinical investigations. *Trans. R. Soc. Trop. Med. Hyg.* **78:**239–241.

39. **Hall, W. C., T. P. Crowell, D. M. Watts, V. L. R. Baoors, H. Kruger, F. Pinheiro, and C. J. Peters.** 1991. Demonstration of yellow fever and dengue antigens in formalin-fixed paraffin-embedded human liver by immunohistochemical analysis. *Am. J. Trop. Med. Hyg.* **45:**408–417.

40. **Halstead, S. B.** 1970. Observations related to pathogenesis of dengue hemorrhagic fever. VI. Hypotheses and discussion. *Yale J. Biol. Med.* **42:**350–362.

41. **Halstead, S. B.** 1980. Dengue hemorrhagic fever—public health problem and a field for research. *Bull. W.H.O.* **58:**1–21.

42. **Halstead, S. B.** 1992. The XXth Century dengue pandemic: need for surveillance and research. *World Health Stat. Q.* **45:**292–298.

43. **Hullinghorst, R. L., and A. Steer.** 1953. Pathology of epidemic hemorrhagic fever. *Ann. Intern. Med.* **38:**77–101.

44. **International Study Team.** 1978. Ebola haemorrhagic fever in Sudan, 1976. *Bull. W.H.O.* **56:**247–270.

45. **Iyer, C. G. S., R. Laxmana, T. H. Work, and D. P. N. Murthy.** 1959. Kyasanur Forest disease. VI. Pathological findings in three fatal human cases of Kyasanur Forest disease. *Indian J. Med. Sci.* **13:**1011–1022.

46. **Iyer, C. G. S., T. H. Work, D. P. N. Murthy, H. Trapido, and P. K. Rajagopalan.** 1960. Kyasanur Forest disease. VII. Pathological findings in monkeys, *Presbytis entellus* and *Macaca radiata*, found dead in the forest. *Indian J. Med. Res.* **48:**276–286.

47. **Jaax, N. J., K. J. Davis, T. J. Geisbert, P. Vogel, G. P. Jaax, M. Topper, and P. B. Jahrling.** 1996. Lethal experimental infection of rhesus monkeys with Ebola-Zaire (Mayinga) virus by the oral and conjunctival route of exposure. *Arch. Pathol. Lab. Med.* **120:**140–155.

48. **Jahrling, P. B., R. A. Hesse, G. A. Eddy, K. M. Johnson, R. T. Callis, and E. L. Stephen.** 1980. Lassa virus infection of rhesus monkeys: pathogenesis and treatment with ribavirin. *J. Infect. Dis.* **141:**580–589.

49. **Joubert, J. R., J. B. King, D. J. Rossouw, and R. Cooper.** 1985. A nosocomial outbreak of Crimean-Congo haemorrhagic fever at Tygerberg hospital. Part III. Clinical pathology and pathogenesis. *South Afr. Med. J.* **68:**722–728.

50. **Kessler, W. H.** 1953. Gross anatomic features found in 27 autopsies of epidemic hemorrhagic fever. *Ann. Intern. Med.* **38:**73–76.

51. **Kikuchi, K., M. Imamura, H. Ueno, T. Takami, H. Koshiba, K. Ogawa, K. Dempo, M. Mori, T. Minase, Y. Yoshida, and K. Muroya.** 1982. An autopsy case of epidemic hemorrhagic fever (Korean hemorrhagic fever). *Sapporo Med. J.* **51:**K17–K31.

52. **Kissling, R. E., F. A. Murphy, and B. E. Henderson.** 1970. Marburg virus. *Ann. N. Y. Acad. Sci.* **174:**932–945.

53. **Kuno, G., I. Gomez, and D. J. Gubler.** 1991. An ELISA procedure for the diagnosis of dengue infections. *J. Virol. Methods* **33:**101–113.

54. **Lahdevirta, J.** 1971. Nephropathia epidemica in Finland. A clinical, histological, and epidemiological study. *Ann. Clin. Res.* **3:**1–154.

55. **Lahdevirta, J., Y. Collan, E. J. Jokinen, and R. Hiltunen.** 1978. Renal sequelae to nephropathia epidemica. *Acta Pathol. Microbiol. Scand.* **86:**265–271.

56. **Lukes, R. J.** 1954. The pathology of thirty-nine fatal cases of epidemic hemorrhagic fever. *Am. J. Med.* **16:**639–650.

57. **Lum, L. C., S. K. Lam, Y. S. Choy, R. George, and F. Harun.** 1996. Dengue encephalitis: a true entity? *Am. J. Trop. Med. Hyg.* **54:**256–259.

58. **Maiztegui, J. I., R. P. Laguens, P. M. Cossio, M. B. Casanova, M. T. de la Vega, V. Ritacco, A. Segal, N. J. Fernandez, and R. M. Arana.** 1975. Ultrastructural and immunohistochemical studies in five cases of Argentine hemorrhagic fever. *J. Infect. Dis.* **132:**35–43.

59. **McCormick, J. B., and K. M. Johnson.** 1984. Viral hemorrhagic fevers, p. 676–697. *In* K. S. Warren and A. A. F. Mahmoud (ed.), *Tropical and Geographical Medicine.* McGraw-Hill, New York.

60. **McCormick, J. B., D. H. Walker, I. J. King, P. A. Webb, L. H. Elliott, S. G. Whitfield, and K. M. Johnson.** 1986. Lassa virus hepatitis: a study of fatal Lassa fever in humans. *Am. J. Trop. Med. Hyg.* **35:**401–407.

61. **McGavran, M. H., and B. C. Easterday.** 1963. Rift Valley fever virus hepatitis. Light and electron microscopic studies in the mouse. *Am. J. Pathol.* **42:**587–607.

62. **McLeod, C. G., J. L. Stookey, G. A. Eddy, and S. K. Scott.** 1976. Pathology of chronic Bolivian hemorrhagic fever in the rhesus monkey. *Am. J. Pathol.* **84:**211–224.

63. **McLeod, C. G., J. L. Stookey, J. D. White, G. A. Eddy, and G. A. Fry.** 1978. Pathology of Bolivian hemorrhagic fever in the African green monkey. *Am. J. Trop. Med. Hyg.* **27:**822–826.

64. **Monath, T. P.** 1994. Dengue: the risk to developed and developing countries. *Proc. Natl. Acad. Sci. USA* **91:**2395–2400.

65. **Murphy, F. A.** 1978. Pathology of Ebola virus infection, p. 43–59. *In* S. R. Pattyn (ed.), *Ebola Virus Haemorrhagic Fever.* Elsevier/North-Holland Biomedical Press, Amsterdam.

66. **Murphy, F. A., D. I. H. Simpson, S. G. Whitfield, I. Zlotnik, and G. B. Carter.** 1971. Marburg virus infection in monkeys. Ultrastructural studies. *Lab. Invest.* **24:**279–291.

67. **Murphy, F. A., D. I. H. Simpson, S. G. Whitfield, I. Zlotnik, and G. B. Carter.** 1972. Marburg virus infection in monkeys. Ultrastructural studies. *Med. Chir. Dig.* **1:**325–332.

68. **Nolte, K. B., R. M. Feddersen, K. Foucar, S. R. Zaki, F. T. Koster, D. Madar, T. L. Merlin, E. T. Umland, P. J. McFeeley, and R. E. Zumwalt.** 1995. Hantavirus pulmonary syndrome in the United States: pathologic description of a disease caused by a new agent. *Hum. Pathol.* **26:**110–120.

69. **Pereboeva, L. A., V. K. Tkachev, L. V. Kolesnikova, L. Y. Krendeleva, E. I. Ryabchikova, and M. P. Smolina.** 1993. Ultrastructural changes of guinea pig organs in sequential passages of Ebola virus. *Voprosy Virusolog.* **4:**179–182.

70. **Peters, C. J., and S. R. Zaki.** 1997. Hantavirus pulmonary syndrome, p. 95–106. *In* C. R. Horsburgh, Jr., and A. M. Nelson (ed.), *Pathology of Emerging Infections.* ASM Press, Washington, D.C.

71. **Peters, C. J., S. R. Zaki, and P. E. Rollin.** 1997. Viral hemorrhagic fevers, p. 10.1–10.26. *In* G. L. Mandell (ed.), *Atlas of Infectious Diseases.* Churchill Livingstone, Philadelphia.

72. **Pinheiro, F. P.** 1989. Dengue in the Americas, 1980–1987. *Epi. Bull. Pan Am. Health Org.* **10:**1–8.

73. **Rigau-Perez, J. G., D. J. Gubler, and A. V. Vorndam.** 1994. Dengue surveillance—United States. *Morbid. Mortal. Weekly Rep.* **43:**7–19.

74. **Rippey, J. J., N. J. Schepers, and J. H. S. Gear.** 1984. The pathology of Marburg virus disease. *South Afr. Med. J.* **66:**50–54.

75. **Rosen, L.** 1982. Dengue—an overview, p. 484-493. *In* J. S. Mackenzie (ed.), *Viral Diseases in Southeast Asia and the Western Pacific.* Academic Press, Sydney, Australia.

76. **Rosen, L., M. M. Khin, and U. Tin.** 1989. Recovery of virus from the liver of children with fatal dengue: reflections on the pathogenesis of the disease and its possible analogy with that of yellow fever. *Res. Virol.* **140:**351–360.

77. **Row, D., P. Weinstein, and S. Murray-Smith.** 1996. Dengue fever with encephalopathy in Australia. *Am. J. Trop. Med. Hyg.* **54:**253–255.

78. **Ryabchikova, E. I., S. G. Baranova, V. K. Tkachev, and A. A. Grazhdantseva.** 1993. Morphological changes in Ebola virus infection in guinea pigs. *Voprosy Virusolog.* **4:**176–179.

79. **Salas, R., N. de Manzione, R. B. Tesh, R. Rich-Hesse, R. E. Shope, A. Betancourt, O. Godoy, R. Bruzual, M. E. Pacheco, B. Ramos, M. E. Taibo, J. G. Tamayo, E. Jaimes, C. Vasquez, F. Araoz, and J. Querales.** 1991. Venezuelan haemorrhagic fever. *Lancet* **338:**1033–1036.

80. **Shieh, W.-J., P. W. Greer, S. L. Ruo, T. G. Ksiazek, C. J. Peters, and S. R. Zaki.** 1997. Lassa fever: immunohistochemical analysis of human tissues and pathogenetic implications. *Lab. Invest.* **76:**141A.

81. **Shieh, W.-J., T. G. Ksiazek, F. R. Bethke, P. W. Greer, and S. R. Zaki.** 1996. Immunohistochemical diagnosis of flavivirus infection in paraffin-embedded human tissues. *Lab. Invest.* **74:**131A.

82. **Steer, A.** 1955. Pathology of hemorrhagic fever: a comparison of the findings—1951 and 1952. *Am. J. Pathol.* **31:**201–221.

83. **Strano, A. J.** 1976. Yellow fever, p. 1–4. *In* C. H. Binford and D. H. Connor (ed.), *Pathology of Tropical and Extraordinary Diseases.* Armed Forces Institute of Pathology, Washington, D.C.

84. **Suleiman, M. N. E. H., J. M. Muscat-Baron, J. R. Harries, and A. G. O. Satti.** 1980. Congo/Crimean haemorrhagic fever in Dubai. *Lancet* **ii:**939–941.

85. **Sumarmo, S. P. S.** 1983. Demam berdarah dengue pada anak di Jakarta, p. 236. Thesis/Dissertation. University of Indonesia, Jakarta.

86. **Sumarmo, S. P. S., H. Wulur, E. Jahja, D. J. Gubler, W. Suharyono, and K. Sorensen.** 1983. Clinical observations on virologically confirmed fatal dengue infections in Jakarta, Indonesia. *Bull. W.H.O.* **61:**693–701.

87. **Terrell, T. G., J. L. Stookey, G. A. Eddy, and M. D. Kastello.** 1973. Pathology of Bolivian hemorrhagic fever in the rhesus monkey. *Am. J. Pathol.* **73:**477–494.

88. **van Velden, D. J. J., J. D. Meyer, J. Olivier, J. H. S. Gear, and B. McIntosh.** 1977. Rift Valley fever affecting humans in South Africa. A clinicopathological study. *South Afr. Med. J.* **51:**867–871.

89. **Vieira, W. T., L. C. Hayotto, C. P. de Lima, and T. de Brito.** 1983. Histopathology of the human liver in yellow fever with special emphasis on the diagnostic role of the Councilman body. *Histopathology* **7:**195–208.

90. **Walker, D. H.** 1988. The pathogenesis and pathology of the hemorrhagic state in viral and rickettsial infections, p. 9–45. *In* J. H. S. Gear (ed.), *CRC Handbook of Viral and Rickettsial Hemorrhagic Fevers.* CRC Press, Inc., Boca Raton, Fla.

91. **Walker, D. H., K. M. Johnson, J. V. Lange, J. J. Gardner, M. P. Kiley, and J. B. McCormick.** 1982. Experimental infection of rhesus monkeys with Lassa virus and a closely related arenavirus, Mozambique virus. *J. Infect. Dis.* **146:**360–368.

92. **Walker, D. H., J. B. McCormick, K. M. Johnson, P. A. Webb, G. Komba-Kono, L. H. Elliott, and J. J. Gardner.** 1982. Pathologic and virologic study of fatal Lassa fever in man. *Am. J. Pathol.* **107:**349–356.

93. **Walker, D. H., and F. A. Murphy.** 1987. Pathology and pathogenesis of arenavirus infections. *Curr. Top. Microbiol. Immunol.* **133:**89–113.

94. **Waterman, S. H., and D. J. Gubler.** 1989. Dengue fever. *Clin. Dermatol.* **7:**117–123.

95. **Webb, H. E., and J. Burston.** 1966. Clinical and pathological observations with special reference to the nervous system in *Macaca radiata* infected with Kyasanur Forest disease virus. *Trans. R. Soc. Trop. Med. Hyg.* **60:**325–331.

96. **Winn, W. C., T. P. Monath, F. A. Murphy, and S. G. Whitfield.** 1975. Lassa virus hepatitis. Observations on a fatal case from the 1972 Sierra Leone epidemic. *Arch. Pathol.* **99:**599–604.

97. **Winn, W. C., and D. H. Walker.** 1975. The pathology of human Lassa fever. *Bull. W.H.O.* **52:**535–545.

98. **Wittesjo, B., R. Eitrem, and B. Niklasson.** 1993. Dengue fever among Swedish tourists. *Scand. J. Infect. Dis.* **25:**699–704.

99. **Zaki, S. R.** 1996. Leptospirosis associated with outbreak of acute febrile illness and pulmonary haemorrhage, Nicaragua, 1995. *Lancet* **347:**535–536.

100. **Zaki, S. R.** 1997. Hantavirus-associated diseases, p. 125–136. *In* D. H. Connor, F. W. Chandler, D. A. Schwartz, H. J. Manz, and E. E. Lack (ed.), *Diagnostic Pathology of Infectious Diseases.* Appleton and Lange, Stamford, Conn.

101. **Zaki, S. R., and C. S. Goldsmith.** 1998. Human pathology of filovirus infections. *Curr. Top. Microbiol. Immunol.* p. 95–114.

102. **Zaki, S. R., P. W. Greer, L. M. Coffield, C. S. Goldsmith, K. B. Nolte, K. Foucar, R. M. Feddersen, R. E. Zumwalt, G. L. Miller, A. S. Khan, P. E. Rollin, T. G. Ksiazek, S. T. Nichol, B. W. J. Mahy, and C. J. Peters.** 1995. Hantavirus pulmonary syndrome: pathogenesis of an emerging infectious disease. *Am. J. Pathol.* **146:**552–579.

103. **Zaki, S. R., P. W. Greer, L. M. Coffield, C. S. Goldsmith, P. E. Rollin, P. Callain, A. S. Khan, T. G. Ksiazek, and C. J. Peters.** Outbreak of Ebola virus hemorrhagic fever, Kikwit, Zaire, 1995: pathologic, immunopathologic, and ultrastructural study. In preparation.

104. **Zaki, S. R., P. W. Greer, C. S. Goldsmith, L. M. Coffield, P. E. Rollin, P. Callain, A. S. Khan, T. G. Ksiazek, and C. J. Peters.** 1996. Ebola virus hemorrhagic fever: pathologic, immunopathologic, and ultrastructural study. *Lab. Invest.* **74:**133A.

105. **Zaki, S. R., A. S. Khan, R. A. Goodman, L. R. Armstrong, P. W. Greer, L. M. Coffield, T. G. Ksiazek, P. E. Rollin, C. J. Peters, and R. F. Khabbaz.** 1996. Retrospective diagnosis of hantavirus pulmonary syndrome, 1978–1993: implications for emerging infectious disease. *Arch. Pathol. Lab. Med.* **120:**134–139.

106. **Zaki, S. R., and P. H. Kilmarx.** 1997. Ebola virus hemorrhagic fever, p. 299–312. *In* C. R. Horsburgh, Jr., and A. M. Nelson (ed.), *Pathology of Emerging Infections.* ASM Press, Washington, D.C.

107. **Zaki, S. R., and C. J. Peters.** 1997. Viral hemorrhagic fevers, p. 347–364. *In* D. H. Connor, F. W. Chandler, D. A. Schwartz, H. J. Manz, and E. E. Lack (ed.), *Diagnostic Pathology of Infectious Diseases.* Appleton and Lange, Stamford, Conn.

chapter 4

Leptospirosis

Sherif R. Zaki and Richard A. Spiegel

eptospirosis is a zoonosis of worldwide distribution with many wild and domestic animal reservoirs. Human infection typically results from exposure to infected animal urine, by either direct contact or indirect exposure through water or soil. The early clinical presentation is often nonspecific, with fever, headache, chills, myalgia, and abdominal pain. Two classic forms of leptospirosis are described: the anicteric (most common) and the icteric (Weil's syndrome), which causes severe renal, hepatic, and vascular dysfunction. Mild pulmonary involvement has been reported in 20 to 70% of leptospirosis patients, but it is often overshadowed by manifestations of other organ system involvement.

Sherif R. Zaki, Infectious Disease Pathology Activity, Division of Viral and Rickettsial Diseases, National Center for Infectious Diseases, Centers for Disease Control and Prevention, Mailstop G-32, 1600 Clifton Road, Atlanta, GA 30333. **Richard A. Spiegel,** Division of Bacterial and Mycotic Diseases, National Center for Infectious Diseases, Centers for Disease Control and Prevention, Mailstop C-23, 1600 Clifton Road, Atlanta, GA 30333.

Pathology of Emerging Infections 2
Edited by Ann Marie Nelson and C. Robert Horsburgh, Jr.
© 1998 American Society for Microbiology, Washington, D.C.

The genus Leptospira contains both pathogenic and nonpathogenic strains

Morphology and Taxonomy

Leptospires (from Greek *leptos*, meaning "fine," and *speira*, meaning "a coil") are thin, finely coiled, filamentous spirochetes measuring 6 to 20 μm in length and 0.1 μm in width, with characteristic curved or hooked ends. The genus *Leptospira* contains both pathogenic and nonpathogenic strains. Traditionally, pathogenic leptospires have been included in the species *L. interrogans*, which contains more than 300 antigenically distinct variants known as serovars (39, 86). Recently, taxonomic classifications of pathogenic leptospires using genomic schemes based on DNA relatedness have been proposed (93). Genetic classification divides the genus *Leptospira* into seven pathogenic species, viz., *L. interrogans*, *L. borgpeterseni*, *L. inadai*, *L. noguchii*, *L. santarosai*, *L. weillii*, and *L. kirschneri*. Identification and classification of species of *Leptospira* are important since different serovars cause different clinical diseases and have different host preferences.

Epidemiology

Leptospirosis is an infectious disease of worldwide distribution. Because it is most prevalent in areas where diagnostic capabilities are limited, and because its clinical presentation is variable, there are few reliable data on its global incidence. The disease has been reported to be the most common zoonosis affecting many species of wild and domestic animals such as rodents, livestock, wild mammals, dogs, and cats (86). Human infection can occur either through direct contact with infected animals or, more commonly, through indirect contact with water or soil contaminated by the urine of infected animals (37). Person-to-person transmission is considered to be extremely rare since humans are a dead-end host for leptospiral dissemination (38). In contrast, leptospires can survive for a long time in the renal tubules of infected animals (maintenance hosts) without causing illness. Most human infections occur in young adult men and children and are often related to occupational or environmental exposure (37). Epidemiologic studies indicate that infection is commonly associated with certain occupational groups such as farmers, sewage workers, veterinarians, and animal handlers. Leptospirosis can also be transmitted through recreational activities such as hiking, swimming, and canoeing (5, 20, 40).

Leptospires can survive in unchlorinated water for months or years but cannot survive desiccation or saltwater (37). Only sporadic cases of leptospirosis are seen in arid climates and deserts. In comparison, the disease is endemic in tropical and temperate areas, areas with heavy precipitation, and areas with high levels of subsurface water. Hence, China, Southeast Asia, Africa, and South and Central America have vast areas endemic for leptospirosis. Leptospirosis occurs sporadically in these areas, with a peak seasonal incidence in summer; large epidemics have been reported following periods of unusually heavy rainfall and monsoons.

In this section, we describe a number of epidemiologic settings in which leptospirosis has been an active problem in the 1990s. The settings are (i) a large epidemic of leptospirosis in Nicaragua in 1995; (ii) an outbreak of leptospirosis in United States travelers to Costa Rica in 1996; (iii) hyperendemic leptospirosis in Brazil; (iv) a report of significant numbers of leptospirosis cases presenting to the Puerto Rico dengue surveillance system; and (v) a large outbreak of uveitis associated with leptospirosis in India.

In October 1995, Nicaraguan health authorities identified an epidemic of "hemorrhagic fever" initially thought to be dengue in the rural towns of Achuapa and El Sauce (population 37,030) following a period of heavy rainfall and flooding (60) (Fig. 4.1). No jaundice or renal manifestations were reported. An investigation, including laboratory studies and a case-control study, was conducted to describe the epidemic, identify case-patient risk factors, and confirm the etiology. During October and November, 2,259 Achuapa and El Sauce residents were identified with non-malarial febrile illnesses meeting the clinical case definition for leptospirosis (Fig. 4.2). In the study area 6.1% were found to have leptospirosis, and 15 patients (0.7%) died with pulmonary hemorrhage. Case patients were more likely than controls to report walking in creeks or seeing rodents in household food storage areas, or to own dogs with positive titers against *Leptospira* spp. *L. interrogans* serovar canicola was isolated from six dogs, two humans, and one rodent; serogroup pyrogenes was isolated from two humans; and serovar pomona was isolated from one pig. In this outbreak, the epidemic likely resulted from floodwaters contaminated by infected animal urine. Dogs most likely played a role in the peridomestic amplification and transmission of leptospirosis.

A multi-state investigation of leptospirosis among 26 male whitewater rafters who ran a river in Costa Rica during September 27–28, 1996, was reported (20). Nine (34.6%) patients were identified with leptospires, and two were hospitalized. Ingesting river water and having one's head under water after falling into the river were significantly associated with illness. Serologic, epidemiologic, and clinical findings implicated leptospirosis in causing illness among the rafters. River water was the probable source of illness. This outbreak was significant in highlighting the occurrence of leptospirosis in the tropics with identification of the cases in the United States, where there is a decreased awareness of leptospirosis.

Ingesting river water and having one's head under water after falling into the river were significantly associated with illness

In Brazil, epidemics of acute renal failure, hepatitis, and pulmonary hemorrhage are reported annually in urban centers of Brazil (55). Although these epidemics are attributed to leptospirosis, the lack of local surveillance by diagnostic laboratories prevents case confirmation and determination of the impact of these epidemics. The annual incidence for clinical cases of severe leptospirosis is 10.5/100,000 population. Of the cases for which paired sera were submitted, 90% (117/130) had a confirmed or probable diagnosis by the microagglutination test. *L. interrogans* serogroup icterohaemorrhagiae was identified as the etiologic agent in 10 of 12 serotyped patient isolates. Major clinical complications included renal failure requiring intraperitoneal dialysis (27%), hemorrhagic manifestations (25%), and arrhythmia as documented by irregular pulse (13%). The case fatality rate was 16% (43/276), and 56% (34/43) of the deaths occurred in the first 48 h after admission to a health care facility. Because of a concurrent dengue epidemic, 64% of these patients were diagnosed with dengue during their initial visit. The Brazilian researchers stressed the need for early case detection and development of rapid diagnostic methods so that antibiotic therapy may be initiated promptly and medical complications prevented.

Leptospirosis is rarely reported in Puerto Rico, but after a hurricane and widespread floods in September 1996, a study was carried out to determine the increase of leptospirosis (76). Of the patient specimens submitted to the dengue laboratory and found to be seronegative for dengue, 5 (6.9%) of 72 patients tested before the hurricane, and 19 (26.8%) of 71 tested afterward, were found positive for leptospirosis by rapid diagnostic tests (43). Eighteen (85.7%) of 21 confirmed cases were male, including 2 fatal cases. The case fatality rate for leptospirosis patients was 9.5%.

Researchers in Tamil Nadu State of India reported clinical features of 73 consecutive cases of uveitis linked clinically to an outbreak of leptospirosis in the region. In these 73 patients, the pattern of ocular involvement was unilateral in 35 and bilateral in 38. Panuveitis, retinal periphlebitis, hypopyon, and cataracts were widely reported in leptospirosis-associated cases. The researchers concluded that uveitis associated with leptospirosis may be a significant contributor to uveitis in the region and pointed out the need to define the nature and magnitude of this serious public health problem in India (73).

Uveitis associated with leptospirosis may be a significant contributor to uveitis in the region

Clinical Aspects

The incubation period of leptospirosis ranges from 2 to 26 (usually 7 to 12) days. In general, leptospirosis can be divided into two distinct clinical syndromes: 90% of patients present with a mild anicteric febrile illness, and 10% are severely ill with jaundice and other manifestations (Weil's syndrome). Both anicteric and icteric leptospirosis may follow a biphasic course. In the initial or septicemic phase, patients usually present with an abrupt onset of fever, chills, headache, myalgias, skin rashes, nausea, vomiting, conjunctivitis, and prostration. The fever may be high, reaching a peak of 40°C before defervescence. Conjunctival suffusion is characteristic and usually appears on day 3 or 4. Myalgias typically involve the muscles in the calf, abdomen, and paraspinous region and can be very severe. When present in the neck they may cause nuchal rigidity resembling meningitis. In the abdomen, myalgias may mimic acute abdomen, leading to confusion with surgical intra-abdominal emergencies (14). The skin manifestations seen in mild leptospirosis include transient urticaria and macular or maculopapular, erythematous, or purpuric rash (41). The first phase of illness lasts 3 to 9 days, followed by 2 or 3 days of defervescence; the disease then enters the second or "immune" phase.

The immune phase is characterized by leptospiruria and coincides with the initial appearance of immunoglobulin M (IgM) antibodies in the serum. Fever and earlier constitutional symptoms recur in some patients, and signs of meningitis such as headache, photophobia, and nuchal rigidity may develop. Central nervous system involvement in leptospirosis most commonly occurs as aseptic meningitis (34, 45, 82). Complications such as optic neuritis, uveitis (12), iridocyclitis, chorioretinitis (46), and peripheral neuropathy occur more commonly in the immune phase (33). Prolonged or recurrent uveitis was demonstrated in 2% of patients, with onset several months after initial symptoms of clinical leptospirosis (1) (Fig. 4.3).

The icteric, or more severe, form of leptospirosis is usually associated with hepatic dysfunction, renal insufficiency, hemorrhage, myocarditis (24, 52), and high mortality. Hemorrhage may present as petechiae, purpura, conjunctival hemorrhage, gastrointestinal hemorrhage, and/or pulmonary hemorrhage. Severe pulmonary hemorrhage has been described in China (6), Korea (66), and recently in Nicaragua (94), where patients died from pulmonary hemorrhage with no significant renal dysfunction or jaundice. Other less common manifestations of leptospirosis are generalized lymphadenopathy (89), pharyngitis, cholecystitis (59), and adult respiratory distress syndrome (27).

Most routine laboratory tests show nonspecific findings. The white blood cell count can be low, normal, or elevated, but usually demonstrates a left shift. Mild anemia and thrombocytopenia are common; hemolytic anemia and disseminated intravascular coagulation have been described in severe cases (26, 70). Thrombocytopenia is found in over 50% of patients and is significantly associated with renal failure (30, 32). Liver involvement may be mild or severe, with bilirubin levels reaching 60 to 80 mg/dl in extreme cases (72). Hepatomegaly is more common in icteric disease but occurs in up to 15% of anicteric cases. Proteinuria, pyuria, hematuria, and hyaline or granular casts are common findings on urinalysis, even in the absence of renal dysfunction (42). Renal function impairment is primarily the result of tubular damage; however, hypovolemia may play a critical role in the subsequent development of renal insufficiency (8, 54). In the cerebrospinal fluid (CSF), neutrophils usually predominate in the early course of meningitis but are surpassed by lymphocytes after day 7. The CSF protein may be normal or elevated up to 300 mg/dl, while the glucose concentration is normal. Although abnormal CSF findings are reported in up to 80% of leptospirosis cases, only half of these are symptomatic.

Chest X-ray abnormalities are common in patients with leptospirosis (70, 71). Arrhythmias or significant cardiac irritability were documented in 35% of patients who were subjected to continuous cardiac monitoring for 24 h (33). Arrhythmias include atrial fibrillation, flutter, and tachycardia. Premature ventricular contractions are common and can progress to subsequent ventricular fibrillation. Echocardiograms on 88 patients in one study revealed pericarditis and small pericardial effusions in 6% of patients (33). The chest X-ray abnormalities can include pulmonary edema, diffuse pneumonitis, nonsegmental or basal linear opacities, and pleural effusions (48, 90) (Fig. 4.4).

The differential diagnosis of leptospirosis depends on the epidemiology of acute febrile illnesses in the particular area. A high index of suspicion is needed in endemic areas, and leptospirosis must be considered when a patient presents with acute onset of fever, headache, and myalgia. However, in locations where dengue fever or malaria is also present, the differentiation may be very difficult since these diseases usually have similar

The icteric, or more severe, form of leptospirosis is usually associated with hepatic dysfunction, renal insufficiency, hemorrhage, myocarditis, and high mortality

clinical manifestations. Laboratory confirmation is crucial, especially when these diseases are occurring simultaneously during the same rainy season. Other conditions to be considered in the differential diagnosis include influenza, meningitis or encephalitis, viral hepatitis, rickettsioses, typhoid fever, Kawasaki syndrome, septicemia, toxoplasmosis, brucellosis, yellow fever, hantavirus infection, and Legionnaires disease. When the patient presents with jaundice during or after an acute febrile illness, leptospirosis must be differentiated from other causes of jaundice. A good history should help to differentiate patients with alcoholic hepatitis.

The prognosis of leptospirosis depends on the severity of the disease and associated complications. Anicteric leptospirosis usually carries a good prognosis, although fatal pulmonary hemorrhage and myocarditis have been reported in anicteric cases (94). The mortality rate of Weil's syndrome is 15 to 40%, and the rate is higher in patients >60 years old (19). In a recent study in the French West Indies during the period 1989–1993, five factors were independently associated with mortality due to leptospirosis: dyspnea, oliguria, white blood cell count of >12,900, electrocardiogram abnormalities, and alveolar infiltrates on chest X-ray (29).

Pathology and Pathogenesis

Leptospires can penetrate abraded skin or intact mucous membranes, after which they enter the circulation and rapidly disseminate to various tissues (39). Penetration and invasion of tissues is presumably accomplished through a burrowing motion produced by a pair of axial filaments and release of hyaluronidase (58). The dissemination and proliferation of the spirochetes in various tissues results in a systemic illness with a broad spectrum of clinical manifestations including fever, headache, chills, myalgia, abdominal pain, and conjunctival suffusion; more severe manifestations include renal failure, jaundice, meningitis, hypotension, hemorrhage, and hemorrhagic pneumonitis.

In fatal cases various degrees of jaundice are usually present (9). Generalized petechiae or ecchymosis in the skin and most internal organs is also commonly seen. Microscopically, a systemic vasculitis with endothelial injury is seen. The damaged endothelial cells usually show different degrees of swelling, denudation, and necrosis. The main histopathological findings are usually found in liver, kidney, heart, and lungs (9, 28, 69, 80). Hepatic changes include mild degenerative changes in hepatocytes, prominent hypertrophy and hyperplasia of Kupffer cells, erythrophagocytosis, and cholestasis (23) (Fig. 4.5). Focal necrosis with occasional acidophilic bodies may be seen; however, there is no particular zonal distribution associated with the necrosis. Mild to moderate mononuclear cell infiltrates in portal tracts are also present. In the kidney, the main histopathologic feature is a diffuse tubulointerstitial inflammation characterized by a mixed inflammatory cell infiltrate of lymphocytes, plasma cells, macrophages, and polymorphonuclear leukocytes (Fig. 4.6). Tubular necrosis is also a common finding. Glomeruli show mild hyperplasia of mesangial cells and occasional infiltra-

Penetration and invasion of tissues is presumably accomplished through a burrowing motion produced by a pair of axial filaments and release of hyaluronidase

tion with inflammatory cells (67). Grossly, the lungs are heavy and severely congested, with focal areas of hemorrhage. Microscopically, the lungs show congestion with foci of intra-alveolar hemorrhage (95) (Fig. 4.7). In some cases, pulmonary features include diffuse alveolar damage and variable degrees of severe air space disorganization.

The pathogenesis of leptospirosis is not fully understood; there is a marked disparity between the profound clinical illness and the paucity of histologic lesions. In the septicemic (first) phase of human infections and experimental animal models, vascular injury is seen in various organs (2, 3, 8, 10, 22, 25). Spirochetes can be found in the walls of capillaries and medium- and large-sized vessels (94). The exact mechanism of vascular damage is not clear. A direct toxic effect of the leptospires has been proposed to cause the vascular injury, but no bacterial endotoxin has been demonstrated. In the immune (second) phase of illness, the host immune response including immune complex deposition may play a role in endothelial injury (24, 32).

Diagnosis

The definitive diagnosis of leptospirosis depends on laboratory findings. There are several different methods for the laboratory diagnosis of leptospirosis, including microbiological, immunological, pathological, and molecular biological methods. Current laboratory criteria of leptospirosis at the Centers for Disease Control and Prevention (CDC) are: (i) isolation of leptospires from a clinical specimen; (ii) fourfold or greater increase in agglutination titer between acute- and convalescent-phase sera obtained at least 2 weeks apart and studied at the same laboratory; and (iii) demonstration of leptospires in a clinical specimen by immunohistochemistry or immunofluorescence.

The definitive diagnosis of leptospirosis depends on laboratory findings

The most commonly used microbiological methods are isolation and animal inoculation. Leptospires are fastidious organisms that do not grow in ordinary blood culture broth or on routine agar plates (21). Isolation generally requires special semisolid, protein-supplemented media, such as Fletcher, Stuart, Ellinghausen, or Tween 80-albumin media (35, 53). Organisms can be cultured from blood, CSF, kidney, or brain in the first 1 to 2 weeks after onset. Urine provides the highest yield of positive cultures after 1 to 2 weeks of illness. Preferably, cultures should be obtained before antibiotic therapy is initiated. No more than 2 to 3 drops of the specimen should be used per 4 ml of culture medium, since excess tissue in the tube is harmful to the microorganisms and usually will result in isolation failures. Samples for leptospiral isolation should be kept at room temperature before incubation, and then incubated at 28 to 30°C in the dark and aerobic conditions for at least 6 weeks before being discarded.

Animal inoculation methods are particularly useful for isolating leptospires from contaminated material. The best laboratory animals for this purpose are weaning hamsters and young guinea pigs that are free from natural infections. Material for diagnosis is inoculated intraperitoneally or

The most commonly used immunological method is the microscopic agglutination test for detecting specific antileptospiral antibodies

subcutaneously in at least three animals. Whenever signs of disease are present in these animals, heart blood for culture and microscopic examination is obtained, and the kidneys are harvested.

The most commonly used immunological method is the microscopic agglutination test (MAT) for detecting specific antileptospiral antibodies (18). It is highly sensitive and highly serovar specific (75). The test evaluates the acute-phase (within the first week) and convalescent-phase (2 to 3 weeks after onset) serum specimens. MAT confirms the diagnosis of leptospirosis with a fourfold rise in titer and is suggestive of leptospirosis with a titer greater than or equal to 1:400. It is noteworthy that delayed seroconversion (a month or more after onset) may occur. The serum specimens are tested against a battery of live or formalin-treated leptospiral antigens (64), and the antigen battery should preferably include serovars that are most frequently isolated locally as well as one or more saprophytic types. These saprophytic types can sometimes cross-react with pathogenic serovars and cause a confusing "paradoxical reaction" that represents an early postinfection sample with a high agglutination titer against one or more serovars unrelated to the causative one (77). Therefore, the antigen battery should be selected with caution because the use of inappropriate antigens can potentially fail to diagnose clinical cases of human and animal leptospirosis.

Other immunological methods include macroscopic agglutination, enzyme-linked immunosorbent assay (ELISA), immunofluorescent antibody (7, 88), indirect hemagglutination (63, 83), hemolytic tests (13), and complement fixation (44). The macroscopic agglutination test is less labor-intensive than the MAT but is also less sensitive and specific (81). The test uses a battery of single or pooled formalin-fixed antigens that are mixed with the sera to be tested on a slide or plate; the antigens and sera are allowed to react and are then examined by the naked eye for presence of agglutination. The test can be used as a quick and inexpensive screening method for the diagnosis of acute leptospirosis, but is not recommended for use in routine laboratories as a confirmatory test.

The ELISA is available for the diagnosis of human and animal leptospirosis. It can detect specific antibodies earlier than the MAT (91). This technique also allows an assessment of the presence of specific IgM and IgG, thereby providing insight on the phase of infection. In addition, it is useful for the preliminary laboratory diagnosis of leptospirosis during acute phase without a paired serology. A dot ELISA which uses a proteinase K-resistant antigen (PK-Dot-ELISA) has been described as a sensitive and economical test for the detection of leptospiral antibodies (65, 74). Although the ELISA is gaining general acceptance, it still has technical pitfalls and should only be used as a preliminary test at present. Further confirmation by the classic MAT or other specific methods such as dipstick test is always recommended (43). Immunofluorescent antibody, indirect hemagglutination, hemolytic tests, and complement fixation have all been used as alternative methods; however, they are not as sensitive or specific as MAT and therefore are not recommended as confirmatory tests.

Pathological methods of diagnosis include examination of tissue samples using dark-field microscopy, special stains, immunohistochemical staining, and in situ hybridization methods. Direct dark-field microscopy of urine, CSF, or bronchoalveolar lavage specimens can sometimes be valuable in the preliminary diagnosis of leptospirosis; however, this requires expertise in differentiating the spirochetes from background material. The Dieterle, Steiner's, and Warthin-Starry silver impregnation stains can demonstrate leptospires in tissues and body fluids. These silver stains also need special expertise in interpretation since confusion with nerve fibers, cell membrane fragments, and fibrin filaments can occur. Immunohistochemical techniques using immunoalkaline phosphatase (94, 95) or immunoperoxidase (4, 84) staining methods can readily demonstrate leptospiral antigens and intact leptospira in various tissues (Fig. 4.8). Examination of post-mortem human tissues such as kidney, liver, lymph node, and lung by the immunoalkaline phosphatase method has proved to be a valuable method in the investigation of leptospirosis outbreaks (94). In situ hybridization using biotin-labeled leptospiral DNA is a simple method for rapid diagnosis of leptospirosis (36, 85). The technique combines the advantage of visualization of the leptospiral morphology with the specificity of the hybridization reaction and is very practical for detection of leptospires in blood, urine, and tissues.

PCR (polymerase chain reaction) is a rapid and sensitive molecular method for the diagnosis of leptospiral infection, especially during the first few days of the disease before serologic conversion (17). It is a valuable diagnostic tool when the clinical manifestation of the disease is confusing and when early diagnosis is required for patient management (57). PCR with leptospiral DNA probes which identify specific sequences can also be used to examine genetic variability among different strains. PCR using primers to amplify a specific 5′ region of 16S rDNA can detect as little as 10^{-1} pg of purified leptospiral DNA and as few as 10 leptospires (47). Leptospiral DNA can be detected in blood, serum, CSF, urine, and aqueous humor (49). The combination of PCR and restriction enzyme analysis of the amplified products has been suggested as a simple method for rapid detection of leptospires as well as for large-scale epidemiological studies (78).

PCR is a rapid and sensitive molecular method for the diagnosis of leptospiral infection

Treatment

Death seldom occurs in anicteric leptospirosis, and treatment with antibiotics within the first 4 days of illness will reduce the duration of illness and alleviate the symptoms. Oral doxycycline at 100 mg twice daily for 7 days, or penicillin at 2.4 million to 3.6 million U/day in divided doses for 7 days, are both effective in shortening the clinical course (51, 56). An in vitro study has suggested that cefotaxime has better MIC levels than penicillin and may serve as an alternative choice. Jarisch-Herxheimer type reactions can be seen after initiation of antibiotic treatment (85). Unless there is a high index of suspicion, most cases are not confirmed at an early stage. Treatment therefore has to be early and empirical when the diagnosis is considered in the appropriate setting.

Patients presenting with severe disease are usually jaundiced or have renal insufficiency as part of Weil's disease. They should be treated with meticulous attention to electrolyte balance and rehydration in order to prevent anuric renal failure. If there are early signs of renal failure or pre-renal azotemia, aggressive rehydration over 48 to 72 h with intensive monitoring of the outcome may be beneficial to the patient (61). If the diagnosis of acute renal failure is established, peritoneal dialysis is the treatment of choice. The jaundice requires no treatment. Patients should have serial electrocardiograms performed, and if any abnormality is detected, they should be placed under continuous electrocardiographic monitoring. Arrhythmias in patients with myocarditis should be evaluated and treatment should be instituted to decrease mortality. Aggressive specific therapy for presenting symptoms such as hemorrhage, hypotension, respiratory failure, or changes in levels of consciousness is warranted. Controversy still exists in the literature as to whether antibiotics are of any value in Weil's disease. From several clinical studies, it was concluded that penicillin has little effect on the clinical outcome of severe leptospirosis except for leptospiruria (31, 62, 92). It was also suggested that all patients with anicteric leptospirosis should be treated irrespective of the time of illness. Further studies need to be done with more clearly defined criteria for severe disease and patient exclusion in order to answer the question as to the efficacy of antibiotics in Weil's disease.

Prevention and Control

Prevention and control of leptospirosis mainly require reducing direct contact with infected animals and contaminated water or soil

Prevention and control of leptospirosis mainly require reducing direct contact with infected animals and contaminated water or soil (37). The risk of contact with infected animals may be reduced by sanitation measures among veterinarians, farmers, and other animal handlers. Since rodents are important natural reservoirs for leptospires, reduction of rodent population can decrease incidence of human leptospirosis in endemic areas. It should be noted that in the Nicaragua leptospirosis outbreaks both dogs and rodents appeared to play a role in leptospirosis transmission; thus, rodent control alone is expected to have only partial benefit. In addition, in places with poverty and poor sanitation, reduction of exposure to rodents may be difficult. Indirect exposure, or exposure to contaminated water or soil, is a particular problem, but a common recommendation is to wear rubber boots and protective clothing and, where possible, to reduce exposure to contaminated rivers, streams, still water, and mud. In actual field settings, this recommendation may be extremely difficult to implement.

Prevention programs for domestic animals have long included the use of *Leptospira* vaccines (11, 15, 16, 50). Effective vaccines have been available for cattle, swine, and dogs. The vaccine for cattle generally includes serovar hardjo, that for pigs includes serovar pomona, and the vaccine for dogs includes serovars canicola and icterhemorrhagiae. Vaccinated dogs are protected against clinical leptospirosis but continue to shed live leptospires. In addition, it should be noted that the animal vaccines have only a limited serovar selection and cannot be expected to prevent transmission of other serovars which the animal may acquire in the field. The current canine vaccine in use in the United States does not include serovar grippo-typhosa, although this serovar is being increasingly recognized in dogs in the United States due to increased contact with raccoons, which tend to carry this serovar. Immunization of humans is not a common practice, but trials of human vaccines to specific serovars have been attempted success-fully in mines in Japan and rice fields in Italy and Spain. Vaccine trials are now under way in China, Korea, and Cuba. The major problem with vacci-nation of humans is that immunity is serovar specific and it is very difficult to select serovars to include in the vaccines (68, 79, 87). To be effective, the serovar(s) included must be responsible for the majority of infections in the community. In addition, the incidence should be high enough to justify immunization of persons considered to be at high risk of developing leptospirosis.

The major problem with vacci-nation of humans is that immu-nity is serovar specific and it is very difficult to select serovars to include in the vaccines

Figure 4.1 Typical scene in epidemic area of Achuapa, Nicaragua, 1995.

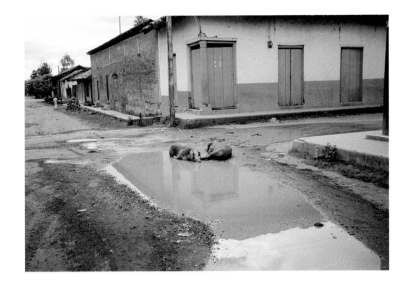

Figure 4.2 Epidemic curve of Nicaraguan leptospirosis outbreak, 1995.

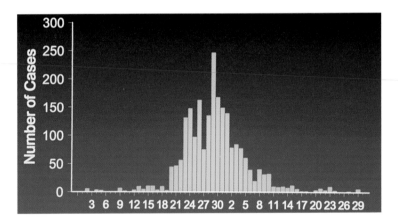

Figure 4.3 Photo of leptospiral uveitis patient, Madurai, Tamil Nadu State, India. (Courtesy of S. R. Rathinam, Aravind Eye Hospital, Madurai, India.)

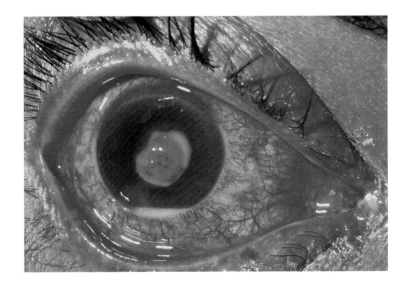

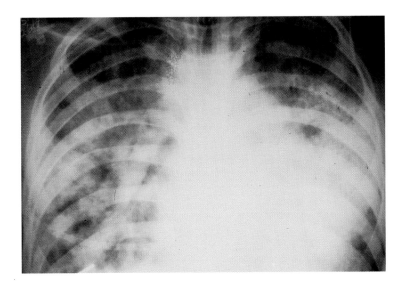

Figure 4.4 X-ray of patient presenting with pulmonary hemorrhage.

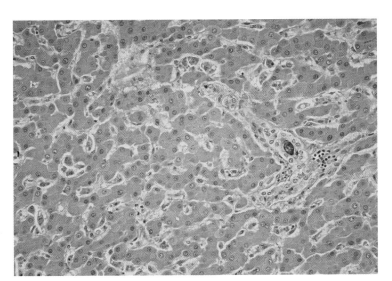

Figure 4.5 Low-power magnification of liver that shows a portal area infiltrated with a moderate number of lymphocytes. Note prominent canalicular plugs and hypertrophic Kupffer cells containing phagocytosed erythrocytes. Hematoxylin and eosin (H&E) stain; ×50.

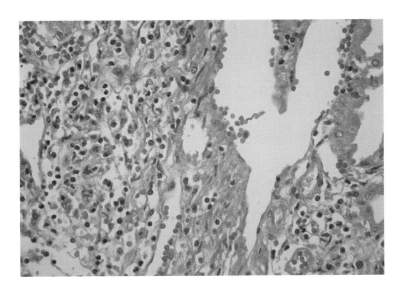

Figure 4.6 Photomicrograph of kidney showing a moderate interstitial mononuclear infiltrate. H&E stain; ×250.

Figure 4.7 Lung showing extensive intra-alveolar hemorrhage in fatal case. Note mild interstitial inflammatory response. H&E stain; ×25.

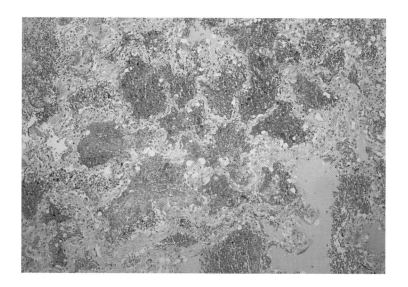

Figure 4.8 Immunostaining of leptospires in kidney. Note intact forms with typical terminal hooks, and granular forms of the bacterium. Immunoalkaline phosphatase stain; ×250.

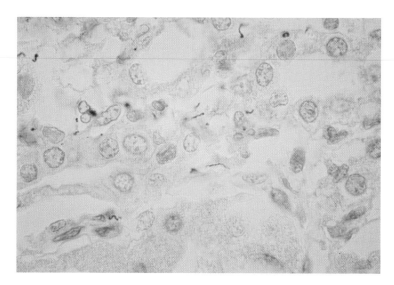

References

1. **Alexander, A., A. Baer, J. R. Fair, W. S. Gochenour, Jr., J. H. King, Jr., and R. H. Yager.** 1952. Leptospiral uveitis: report of bacteriologically verified case. *A. M. A. Arch. Ophthalmol.* **48:**292–297.

2. **Alves, V. A. F., L. C. Gayotto, T. De Brito, R. T. Santos, A. Wakamatsu, M. R. Vianna, and E. E. Sakata.** 1992. Leptospiral antigens in the liver of experimentally infected guinea pig and their relation to the morphogenesis of liver damage. *Exp. Toxic. Pathol.* **44:**425–434.

3. **Alves, V. A. F., L. C. C. Gayotto, P. H. Yasuda, A. Wakamatsu, C. T. Kanamura, and T. De Brito.** 1991. Leptospiral antigens (*L. interrogans* serogroup *ictero-haemorrhagiae*) in the kidney of experimental infected guinea pigs and their relation to the pathogenesis of the renal injury. *Exp. Pathol.* **42:**81–93.

4. **Alves, V. A. F., P. H. Yasuda, E. H. Yamashiro, R. T. Santos, L. U. Yamamoto, and T. De Brito.** 1986. An immunohistochemic assay to localize leptospires in tissue specimens. *Rev. Inst. Med. Trop. Sao Paulo* **28:**170–173.

5. **Anderson, D. C., D. S. Folland, M. D. Fox, C. M. Patton, and A. F. Kaufmann.** 1978. Leptospirosis: a common-source outbreak due to leptospires of the grippotyphosa serogroup. *Am. J. Epidemiol.* **107:**538–544.

6. **Anonymous.** 1973. Emergency treatment and pathogenesis of leptospirosis with massive pulmonary hemorrhage. Chung-Hua i Hsueh Tsa Chih. *Chinese Med. J.* **5:**279–282. (In Chinese.)

7. **Appassakij, H., K. Silpapojakul, R. Wansit, and J. Woodtayakorn.** 1995. Evaluation of the immunofluorescent antibody test for the diagnosis of human leptospirosis. *Am. J. Trop. Med. Hyg.* **52:**340–343.

8. **Arean, V. M.** 1962. Studies on the pathogenesis of leptospirosis. II. A clinicopathologic evaluation of hepatic and renal function in experimental leptospiral infections. *Lab. Invest.* **11:**273–288.

9. **Arean, V. M.** 1962. The pathologic anatomy and pathogenesis of fatal human leptospirosis (Weil's Disease). *Am. J. Pathol.* **40:**393–423.

10. **Arean, V. M., and J. B. Henry.** 1964. Studies on the pathogenesis of leptospirosis. IV. The behavior of transaminases and oxidative enzymes in experimental leptospirosis: a histochemical and biochemical assay. *Am. J. Trop. Med. Hyg.* **13:**430–442.

11. **Banker, D. D.** 1968. Modern practice in immunization. 11. Other bacterial and miscellaneous vaccines. *Indian J. Med. Sci.* **22:**743–751.

12. **Barkay, S., and H. Garzozi.** 1984. Leptospirosis and uveitis. *Ann. Ophthalmol.* **16:**164–168.

13. **Bazovska, S., E. Kmety, and J. Rak.** 1997. Differentiation of pathogenic and saprophytic leptospira strains. *Zentralbl. Bakteriol. Mikrobiol. Hyg. Reihe A* **257(4):**126–141.

14. **Berman, S. J., C. C. Tsat, K. Holmes, J. W. Fresh, and R. H. Watten.** 1973. Sporadic anicteric leptospirosis in South Vietnam: a study of 150 patients. *Ann. Intern. Med.* **79:**167–173.

15. **Bey, R. F., and R. C. Johnson.** 1982. Leptospiral vaccines in dogs: immunogenicity of whole cell and outer envelope vaccines prepared in protein-free medium. *Am. J. Vet. Res.* **43:**831–834.

16. **Bolin, C. A., J. A. Cassells, R. L. Zuerner, and G. Trueba.** 1991. Effect of vaccination with a monovalent Leptospira interrogans serovar hardjo type hardjo-bovis vaccine on type hardjo-bovis infection of cattle. *Am. J. Vet. Res.* **52:**1639–1643.

17. **Brown, P. D., C. Gravekamp, D. G. Carrington, H. Van de Kemp, R. A. Hartskeerl, C. N. Edwards, C. O. Everard, W. J. Terpstra, and P. N. Levett.** 1995. Evaluation of the polymerase chain reaction for early diagnosis of leptospirosis. *J. Med. Microbiol.* **43:**110–114.

18. **Carter, P. L., and T. J. Ryan.** 1975. New microtechnique for the leptospiral microscopic agglutination test. *J. Clin. Microbiol.* **2:**474–477.

19. **Centers for Disease Control and Prevention.** 1986. Centers for Disease Control and Prevention: leptospirosis—cases, by year, United States, 1955–1984. MMWR Annual Summary 1984. *Morbid. Mortal. Weekly Rep.* **33:**31.

20. **Centers for Disease Control and Prevention.** 1997. Outbreak of leptospirosis among white-water rafters—Costa Rica, 1996. *Morbid. Mortal. Weekly Rep.* **46:**577–579.

21. **Cole, J. R., Jr., H. C. Ellinghausen, and H. L. Rubin.** 1979. Laboratory diagnosis of leptospirosis of domestic animals, p. 189–199. *In Proceedings of the 83rd Annual Meeting of the United States Animal Health Association.* United States Animal Health Association.

22. **De Brito, T., G. M. Bohm, and P. H. Yasuda.** 1979. Vascular damage in acute experimental leptospirosis of the guinea-pig. *J. Pathol.* **128:**177–182.

23. **De Brito, T., M. M. Machado, S. D. Montans, S. Hoshino, and E. Freymuller.** 1967. Liver biopsy in human leptospirosis: a light and electron microscopy study. *Virchows Arch. Pathol. Anat. Physiol. Klin. Med.* **342:**61–69.

24. **De Brito, T., C. F. Morais, P. H. Yasuda, C. P. Lancellotti, S. Hoshino-Shimizu, E. Yamashiro, and V. A. Ferreira Alves.** 1987. Cardiovascular involvement in human and experimental leptospirosis: pathologic findings and immunohistochemical detection of leptospiral antigen. *Ann. Trop. Med. Parasitol.* **81:**207–214.

25. **De Brito, T., M. J. B. A. Prado, V. A. C. Negreiros, A. L. Nicastri, E. E. Sakata, P. H. Yasuda, R. T. Santos, and V. A. F. Alves.** 1992. Detection of leptospiral antigen (*L. interrogans* serovar *copenhageni* serogroup Icterohaemorrhagiae) by immunoelectron microscopy in the liver and kidney of experimentally infected guinea-pigs. *Int. J. Exp. Pathol.* **73:**633–642.

26. **de Carvalho, J. E., S. dos Marchiore, E. Guedes, J. B. Silva, B. A. Netto, W. Tavares, and A. V. de Paula.** 1992. Pulmonary compromise in leptospirosis. *Rev. Soc. Brasileira Med. Trop.* **25:**21–30. (In Portuguese.)

27. **de Koning, J., J. G. van der Hoeven, and A. E. Meinders.** 1995. Respiratory failure in leptospirosis (Weil's disease). *Netherlands J. Med.* **47:**224–229.

28. **Dooley, J. R., and K. G. Ishak.** 1976. Leptospirosis, p. 101–106. *In* C. H. Binford and D. H. Connor (ed.), *Pathology of Tropical and Extraordinary Diseases.* Armed Forces Institute of Pathology, Washington, D.C.

29. **Dupont, H., D. Dupont-Perdrizet, J. L. Perie, S. Zehner-Hansen, B. Jarriger, and J. B. Daijardin.** 1997. Leptospirosis: prognostic factors associated with mortality. *Clin. Infect. Dis.* **25:**720–724.

30. **Edwards, C. N., G. D. Nicholson, and C. O. Everard.** 1982. Thrombocytopenia in leptospirosis. *Am. J. Trop. Med. Hyg.* **31:**827–829.

31. **Edwards, C. N., G. D. Nicholson, and T. A. Hassell.** 1988. Penicillin therapy in icteric leptospirosis. *Am. J. Trop. Med. Hyg.* **39:**388–390.

32. **Edwards, C. N., G. D. Nicholson, T. A. Hassell, C. O. Everard, and J. Callender.** 1986. Thrombocytopenia in leptospirosis: the absence of evidence for disseminated intravascular coagulation. *Am. J. Trop. Med. Hyg.* **35:**352–354.

33. **Edwards, C. N., G. D. Nicholson, T. A. Hassell, C. O. Everard, and J. Callender.** 1990. Leptospirosis in Barbados: a clinical study. *W. Indian Med. J.* **39:**27–34.

34. **Edwards, G. A., and B. M. Domm.** 1960. Human leptospirosis. *Medicine* **39:**117–156.

35. **Ellinghausen, H. C., Jr.** 1997. Variable factors influencing the isolation of leptospires involving culture ingredients and testing. *Proc. Annu. Meet. U.S. Animal Health Assoc.* **79:**126–141.

36. **Fach, P., D. Trap, and J. P. Guillou.** 1991. Biotinylated probes to detect Leptospira interrogans on dot blot hybridization or by in situ hybridization. *Lett. Appl. Microbiol.* **12**(5)**:**171–176.

37. **Faine, S.** 1982. Guidelines for the control of leptospirosis. Offset publication no. 67. World Health Organization, Geneva.

38. **Faine, S.** 1993. Brief history of leptospirosis, p. 1–13. *In Leptospira and Leptospirosis.* CRC Press, Boca Raton, Fla.

39. **Farrar, W. E.** 1995. Leptospira species (leptospirosis), p. 2137–2141. *In* J. E. Bennett, G. L. Mandell, and R. Dolin (ed.), *Principles and Practice of Infectious Diseases,* 4th ed. Churchill Livingstone, New York.

40. **Feigin, R. D., and D. C. Anderson.** 1975. Human leptospirosis. *Crit. Rev. Clin. Lab. Sci.* **5:**413–467.

41. **Fraser, D. W., J. W. Glosser, D. P. Francis, C. J. Phillips, J. C. Feeley, and C. R. Sulzer.** 1973. Leptospirosis caused by serotype Fort-Bragg. A suburban outbreak. *Ann. Intern. Med.* **79:**786–789.

42. **Gendron, Y., J. Prieur, X. Gaufroy, and C. Gras.** 1992. [Leptospirosis in French Polynesia: 120 case reports.] *Med. Trop.* **52:**21–27. (In French.)

43. **Gussenhoven, G. C., M. A. van der Hoorn, M. G. Goris, W. J. Terpstra, R. A. Hartskeerl, B. W. Mol, and C. W. van Igen.** 1997. Lepto dipstick, a dipstick assay for detection of *Leptospira*-specific immunoglobulin M antibodies in human sera. *J. Clin. Microbiol.* **35:**92–97.

44. **Hagiwara, M. K., C. A. Santa Rosa, and A. A. Pinto.** 1980. Comparative study between microscopic agglutination and complement fixation tests in experimental canine leptospirosis. *Int. J. Zoonoses* **7:**150–157.

45. **Heath, C. W., Jr., A. D. Alexander, and M. M. Galton.** 1965. Leptospirosis in the United States, analysis of 483 cases in man, 1949–1961. *N. Engl. J. Med.* **273:**857–864.

46. **Hines, M. T.** 1984. Immunologically mediated ocular disease in the horse. *Vet. Clin. North Am. Large Animal Pract.* **6:**501–512.

47. **Hookey, J. V.** 1992. Detection of Leptospiraceae by amplification of 16S ribosomal DNA. *FEMS Microbiol. Lett.* **69:**267–274.

48. **Im, J. G., K. M. Yeon, M. C. Han, C. W. Kim, W. R. Webb, J. S. Lee, Y. C. Han, W. H. Chang, and J. G. Chi.** 1989. Leptospirosis of the lung: radiographic findings in 58 patients. *Am. J. Roentgenol.* **152:**955–959.

49. **Kee, S. H., I. S. Kim, M. S. Choi, and W. H. Chang.** 1994. Detection of leptospiral DNA by PCR. *J. Clin. Microbiol.* **32:**1035–1039.

50. **Kerr, D. D., and V. Marshall.** 1974. Protection against the renal carrier state by a canine leptospirosis vaccine. *Vet. Med. Small Animal Clinician* **69:**1157–1160.

51. **Kocen, R. S.** 1962. Leptospirosis: a comparison of symptomatic and penicillin therapy. *Br. Med. J.* **1:**1181.

52. **Lee, M. G., G. Char, S. Dianzumba, and P. Prussia.** 1986. Cardiac involvement in severe leptospirosis. *W. Indian Med. J.* **35:**295–300.

53. **Lindenbaum, I., E. Eylan, and E. Raanani.** 1975. Enhancement of growth of Leptospira icterohaemorrhagiae by tissue cell cultures. *J. Gen. Microbiol.* **86:**62.

54. **Magaldi, A. J., P. N. Yasuda, L. H. Kudo, A. C. Seguro, and A. S. Rocha.** 1992. Renal involvement in leptospirosis: a pathophysiologic study. *Nephron* **62:**332–339.

55. **Marotto, P. C., M. S. Marotto, D. L. Santos, T. N. Souza, and A. C. Seguro.** 1997. Outcome of leptospirosis in children. *Am. J. Trop. Med. Hyg.* **56:**307–310.

56. **McClain, J. B., W. R. Ballou, and S. M. Harrison.** 1984. Doxycycline therapy for leptospirosis. *Ann. Intern. Med.* **100:**696–698.

57. **Merien, F., G. Baranton, and P. Perolat.** 1995. Comparison of polymerase chain reaction with microagglutination test and culture for diagnosis of leptospirosis. *J. Infect. Dis.* **172:**281–285.

58. **Miller, N. G., R. C. Froehling, and R. J. White.** 1970. Activity of leptospires and their products on L cell monolayers. *Am. J. Vet. Res.* **31:**371–377.

59. **Monno, S., and Y. Mizushima.** 1993. Leptospirosis with acute acalculous cholecystitis and pancreatitis. *J. Clin. Gastroenterol.* **16:**52–54.

60. **Munoz, F., C. Jarquin, A. Gonzalez, J. Amador, J. de los Reyes, R. Jimenez, F. Lamy, N. Jiron, and F. Pinheiro.** 1995. Outbreak of acute febrile illness and pulmonary hemorrhage—Nicaragua, 1995. *Morbid. Mortal. Weekly Rep.* **44:**841–842.

61. **Nicholson, G. D., C. N. Edwards, and T. A. Hassell.** 1989. Urinary diagnostic indices in the management of leptospirosis: selection of patients for dialysis therapy. *W. Indian Med. J.* **33:**33.

62. **Oie, S., K. Hironaga, A. Koshiro, H. Konishi, and Z. Yoshii.** 1983. In vitro susceptibilities of five leptospira strains to 16 antimicrobial agents. *Antimicrob. Agents Chemother.* **24:**905–908.

63. **Palit, A., and G. L. Sharma.** 1971. Comparison of microscopic agglutination, indirect haemagglutination and complement-fixation tests in rabbit and buffalo-calf hyperimmune sera for detection of leptospiral antibodies. *Brit. Vet. J.* **127:**154–162.

64. **Palmer, M. F., S. A. Waitkins, and S. W. Wanyangu.** 1987. A comparison of live and formalised leptospiral microscopic agglutination test. *Zentralbl. Bakteriol. Mikrobiol. Hyg. Reihe A* **265:**151–159.

65. **Pappas, M. G., W. R. Ballou, M. R. Gray, E. T. Takafuji, R. N. Miller, and W. T. Hockmeyer.** 1985. Rapid serodiagnosis of leptospirosis using the IgM-specific Dot-ELISA: comparison with the microscopic agglutination test. *Am. J. Trop. Med. Hyg.* **34:**346–354.

66. **Park, S.-K., S.-H. Lee, Y.-K. Rhee, S.-K. Kang, K.-J. Kim, M.-C. Kim, K.-W. Kim, and W.-H. Chang.** 1989. Leptospirosis in Chonbuk Province of Korea in 1987: a study of 93 patients. *Am. J. Trop. Med. Hyg.* **41:**345–351.

67. **Penna, D., T. De Brito, A. A. Pupo, M. M. Machado, P. A. A. Galvao, and S. S. de Almeida.** 1963. Kidney biopsy in human leptospirosis. *Am. J. Trop. Med. Hyg.* **12:**896–901.

68. **Philip, N. A., and R. B. Tennent.** 1966. Leptospirosis: a report from one practice on the use of a leptospiral vaccine for a period of three years. *New Zealand Med. J.* **65**(Suppl. 15)**:**13–19.

69. **Pierce, P. F., J. P. Utz, and E. E. Lack.** 1997. Leptospirosis, p. 615–620. *In* D. H. Conner and F. W. Chandler (ed.), *Pathology of Infectious Diseases.* Appleton & Lange, Stamford, Conn.

70. **Ragnaud, J. M., M. Dupon, E. Echinard, D. Teboulle, and C. Wone.** 1987. Pulmonary manifestations in severe ictero-hemorrhagic leptospirosis. *Ann. Med. Intern.* **138:**282–286. (In French.)

71. **Ramachandran, S.** 1975. Electrocardiographic abnormalities in leptospirosis. *J. Trop. Med. Hyg.* **78:**210–213.

72. **Ramos-Morales, F., R. S. Diaz-Rivera, A. A. Cintron-Rivera, J. A. Rullan, A. S. Beneson, and A. Acosta-Matienzo.** 1959. The pathogenesis of leptospiral jaundice. *Ann. Intern. Med.* **51:**861–878.

73. **Rathinam, S. R., S. Rathnam, S. Selvaraj, D. Dean, R. A. Nozik, and P. Namperumalsamy.** 1997. Uveitis associated with an epidemic outbreak of leptospirosis. *Am. J. Ophthalmol.* **124:**71–79.

74. **Ribeiro, M. A., C. C. Souza, and S. H. Almeida.** 1995. Dot-ELISA for human leptospirosis employing immunodominant antigen. *J. Trop. Med. Hyg.* **98:**452–456.

75. **Ryu, E.** 1997. Rapid microscopic agglutination test for Leptospira without nonspecific reaction. *Bull. Off. Int. Epizoot.* **73:**49–58.

76. **Sanders, E. J., J. G. Rigau-Prez, H. Smits, C. Deseda, T. Aye, S. Bragg, R. Spiegel, and R. Weyant.** 1997. Hurricane-related leptospirosis in Dengue-negative patients, abstract 303, p.126. *In Program and Abstracts of the 35th Annual Meeting of the Infectious Diseases Society of America,* San Francisco.

77. **Sapiro-Hirsch, R., and W. Hirsch.** 1970. First isolation of Leptospira Icterohaemorrhagiae from man in Israel, with remarks on the paradoxical reaction in the serodiagnosis of leptospirosis. *Isr. J. Med. Sci.* **6:**399–402.

78. **Savio, M. L., C. Rossi, P. Fusi, S. Tagliabue, and M. L. Pacciarini.** 1994. Detection and identification of *Leptospira interrogans* serovars by PCR coupled with restriction endonuclease analysis of amplified DNA. *J. Clin. Microbiol.* **32:**935–941.

79. **Shenberg, E., and M. Torten.** 1973. A new leptospiral vaccine for use in man. I. Development of a vaccine from Leptospira grown on a chemically defined medium. *J. Infect. Dis.* **128:**642–646.

80. **Sinniah, R., V. Boonpucknovig, and B. Sinniah.** 1995. Spirochaetal and leptospiral diseases, p. 223–251. *In* D. Doerr and G. Seifert (ed.), *Tropical Pathology.* Springer-Verlag, Berlin.

81. **Solorzano, R. F.** 1964. A comparison of the rapid macroscopic slide agglutination test with the microscopic slide agglutination test for leptospirosis. *Proc. Annu. Meet. U.S. Animal Health Assoc.* **68:**440–444.

82. **Sperber, S. J., and C. J. Schleupner.** 1989. Leptospirosis: a forgotten cause of aseptic meningitis and multisystem febrile illness. *Southern Med. J.* **82:**1285–1288.

83. **Sulzer, C. R., J. W. Glosser, F. Rogers, W. L. Jones, and M. Frix.** 1975. Evaluation of an indirect hemagglutination test for the diagnosis of human leptospirosis. *J. Clin. Microbiol.* **2:**218–221.

84. **Terpstra, W. J., J. Jabboury-Postema, and H. Korver.** 1983. Immunoperoxidase staining of leptospires in blood and urine. *Zentralbl. Bakteriol. Mikrobiol. Hyg. Abt. 1 Orig. Reihe A* **254:**534–539.

85. **Terpstra, W. J., G. J. Schoone, G. S. Ligthart, and J. ter Schegget.** 1987. Detection of Leptospira interrogans in clinical specimens by in situ hybridization using biotin-labelled DNA probes. *J. Gen. Microbiol.* **133**(part 4):911–914.

86. **Torten, M., and R. B. Marshall.** 1994. Leptospirosis, p. 245–264. *In* G. W. Beran and J. H. Steele (ed.), *Handbook of Zoonoses.* CRC Press, Boca Raton, Fla.

87. **Torten, M., E. Shenberg, C. B. Gerichter, P. Neuman, and M. A. Klingberg.** 1973. A new leptospiral vaccine for use in man. II. Clinical and serologic evaluation of a field trial with volunteers. *J. Infect. Dis.* **128**:647–651.

88. **Torten, M., E. Shenberg, and J. Van der Hoeden.** 1966. The use of immunofluorescence in the diagnosis of human leptospirosis by a genus-specific antigen. *J. Infect. Dis.* **116**:537–543.

89. **van Crevel, R., P. Speelman, C. Gravekamp, and W. J. Terpstra.** 1994. Leptospirosis in travelers. *Clin. Infect. Dis.* **19**:132–134.

90. **Wang, C. P., C. W. Chu, and F. L. Lu.** 1965. Studies on anicteric leptospirosis. III. Roentgenologic observations of pulmonary changes. *Chin. Med. J.* **84**:298–306.

91. **Watt, G., L. M. Alquiza, L. P. Padre, M. L. Tuazon, and L.W. Laughlin.** 1988. The rapid diagnosis of leptospirosis: a prospective comparison of the dot enzyme-linked immunosorbent assay and the genus-specific microscopic agglutination test at different stages of illness. *J. Infect. Dis.* **157**:840–842.

92. **Watt, G., L. P. Padre, M. L. Tuazon, C. Calubaquib, E. Santiago, C. P. Ranoa, and L. W. Laughlin.** 1988. Placebo-controlled trial of intravenous penicillin for severe or late leptospirosis. *Lancet* **i**:433–435.

93. **Yasuda, P. H., A. G. Steigerwalt, K. R. Sulzer, A. F. Kaufman, F. Rogers, and D. J. Brenner.** 1987. Deoxyribonucleic acid relatedness between serogroups and serovars in the family *Leptospiraceae* with proposals for seven new *Leptospira* species. *Int. J. Syst. Bacteriol.* **37**:407–415.

94. **Zaki, S. R., and W. J. Shieh.** 1996. Leptospirosis associated with outbreak of acute febrile illness and pulmonary haemorrhage, Nicaragua, 1995. The Epidemic Working Group at Ministry of Health in Nicaragua. *Lancet* **347**:535–536. (Letter.)

95. **Zaki, S. R., and W. J. Shieh.** 1997. Outbreak of leptospirosis associated with pulmonary hemorrhage. *Lab. Invest.* **76**:142A.

chapter 5

Human Immunodeficiency Virus

Jeffrey Lennox and Mary Klassen

The current worldwide epidemic of retroviral infections in humans includes two related viruses: human immunodeficiency virus type 1 (HIV-1) and HIV-2. Infection with HIV-2 is generally limited to Western Africa and to areas where immigration from Western Africa has occurred. Clinical illness due to HIV-2 develops less rapidly, but is otherwise similar to that caused by HIV-1. The remainder of this discussion will therefore focus on HIV-1 infection.

HIV is a member of the lentivirus taxonomic group, from the Latin for slow. Lentiviruses accumulate in the cells of the host's immune system over many years. Destruction of the infected cells results in immunodeficiency. HIV is also a retrovirus, having an RNA genome that is converted into a DNA provirus. The virus consists of surface envelope and core proteins (Fig. 5.1). The genome is only 10 kb long and consists of two single strands of RNA that are positive strands like mRNA. The genome consists of three coding regions: *gag*, *env*, and *pol*. The *gag* region codes for capsid proteins. The *pol* region encodes the enzymes used for replication, including reverse transcriptase, which converts RNA into double-stranded DNA; integrase,

Jeffrey Lennox, Department of Medicine, Emory University School of Medicine, Atlanta, GA 30303. **Mary Klassen,** Department of Infectious and Parasitic Disease Pathology, Armed Forces Institute of Pathology, Washington, DC 20306-6000

Pathology of Emerging Infections 2
Edited by Ann Marie Nelson and C. Robert Horsburgh, Jr.
© 1998 American Society for Microbiology, Washington, D.C.

Infection of humans by HIV-1 was documented as early as the late 1950s

which incorporates viral DNA into host genome; and proteases, which cut viral proteins into pieces for incorporation into new viruses. Finally, *env* encodes the external glycoprotein. The genome has one promoter and one polyadenylation site with long terminal repeats.

Infection of humans by HIV-1 was documented as early as the late 1950s. The infection was probably limited to isolated populations until extensive urbanization occurred in the 1960s. The illness caused by HIV-1 was not described until the early 1980s, when an outbreak of opportunistic infections and unusual tumors occurred on both coasts of the United States. The same clinical syndrome, the acquired immunodeficiency syndrome (AIDS), was quickly recognized on the European and African continents. In the mid-1980s, HIV-1 was also documented to be present in South America and Australia. The Asian continent remained relatively unaffected until the late 1980s, when infections in Thailand and India were recognized.

It is now apparent that the strains of the HIV-1 virus present in different areas of the world differ substantially in their envelope sequences (41, 43). On the basis of these sequences, 11 subtypes of HIV-1 (subtypes A through J, and O) have been proposed. Subtype B is responsible for the majority of infections in North America, Australia, and Europe, with other subtypes becoming increasingly more common. In Africa all subtypes have been found. In South and Central America, subtypes B, C, D, and F have been isolated. In Asia, subtype B is predominant in drug abusers and their sexual contacts and subtypes E and C in patients who acquired their infection through heterosexual contact. Subtype E has recently been demonstrated to be a recombinant virus that contains portions of the envelope sequences of subtype A (43). In addition to Asia, subtype E has also been found in Africa and, less extensively, in Europe, the United States, and South America. Subtype G is also a recombinant with subtype A. Based on the available data it appears that multiple subtypes of HIV-1 may be circulating in a given population simultaneously, that dual infection and recombination events occur, and that some subtypes may be transmitted through the heterosexual route more easily than others (62).

The predominant mode of spread of the virus is by heterosexual sex. In some populations transmission by homosexual sex or by intravenous drug abuse is more common. Nosocomial acquisition of HIV-1 has occurred from contaminated clotting-factor concentrates, other blood components, and other fluids and tissues. Nosocomial transmission is now uncommon in the developed world due to donor screening. Occupational transmission to health care workers is an uncommon and potentially preventable event. The rate of occupational transmission of HIV-1 following a percutaneous injury is approximately 0.5%. The risk for percutaneous transmission is increased if the source patient has late stages of infection, if the injury was with a hollow-bore needle, if the needle was in the source's vein or had visible blood, and if the recipient received a deep injury or a blood injection.

Several factors have been reported to increase the likelihood of sexual transmission of HIV-1, the most important of which is the presence of ulcerative sexually transmitted diseases (46). Other factors include the stage of disease of the source patient, the type of sexual activity, nonulcerative sexually transmitted diseases, and certain genetic characteristics of the exposed person (23). The majority of children acquire the infection either in utero, during birth, or from exposure to the virus in breast milk. There are rare case reports of transmission between children (and adults) that probably occurred by exchange of saliva. However, in these cases the source patients had conditions that would cause larger than normal amounts of blood to be present in the saliva.

Epidemiology

The highest estimated prevalence of HIV is in sub-Saharan Africa (~5%), but all continents with permanent resident populations are affected. Of particular concern is the recent increase in HIV transmission in Asia, where most of the world's population resides. By 1996 the United Nations Program on HIV/AIDS (UNAIDS) estimated that approximately 30 million people had become infected with HIV worldwide (2). During 1996 the UNAIDS predicted that an additional 8,000 to 9,000 persons per day would acquire the infection, that the male:female ratio of these newly infected people would be approximately 1:1, and that children would account for approximately one in eight infections. These figures are estimates since testing for the virus is not considered a component of routine health care in most countries, including the United States.

Of particular concern is the recent increase in HIV transmission in Asia

In the United States, syndromic (AIDS) reporting began before the cause of the syndrome was recognized. Reporting of AIDS cases has continued as the main data collection method on the scope of the epidemic to date. The first 50,000 cases of AIDS were reported between 1981 and 1987 (13). In 1996, the most recent year for which data are available, an approximately equal number of cases (68,000) were reported (15). A comparison between these two groups of cases is illustrative of the changing epidemiology of HIV-1 infection in the United States over the last decade. In the cohort of the first 50,000 cases there was a male:female ratio of approximately 12:1. In 1996 the male:female ratio was 4:1. Whites made up 60% of the first 50,000 cases but <40% of the most recent cohort. In the first cohort, heterosexual transmission accounted for only 2.5% of cases, while in the most recent cohort it accounted for 19%. The proportion of cases that was reported to be due solely to homosexual contact fell from 64% to 44%. Those cases that were attributed solely to intravenous drug abuse increased from 17% to 26%. In both cohorts the majority of cases were reported in adults between the ages of 20 and 40 years.

Reporting of AIDS cases underestimates the true prevalence of HIV-1 infection in the U.S. population due to under-reporting and because it takes an average of 10 years from infection with the virus to the diagnosis of AIDS. In addition, treatments that became available in 1996 have profoundly altered the natural history of HIV infection. Reporting of HIV infection itself would therefore provide more accurate information about the scope of HIV-1 infection in the United States. Only 26 states presently

One method to estimate HIV-1 prevalence is by back-calculation from the number of reported AIDS cases

require such reporting. Direct information about the true scope of the epidemic in the United States is therefore limited.

One method to estimate HIV-1 prevalence is by back-calculation from the number of reported AIDS cases. Using this method, it was estimated that through 1992 there had been 630,000 to 897,000 cases of HIV-1 infection in the United States (59). To obtain a more accurate estimate of HIV-1 prevalence, a household survey was conducted between 1988 and 1994 (45). This 6-year survey sampled 31,311 adults between the ages of 18 and 59. The survey did not include those who were incarcerated or homeless people not living in shelters. Since these populations are known to have a high HIV-1 infection rate, the results were adjusted to account for this under-sampling. In the 6-year survey period it was estimated that 651,000 (409,000–1,000,000) adults were living with HIV-1 infection. The adjusted prevalence for the adult population was 0.04 cases per 100,000 population. The unadjusted prevalence was highest for black males (0.18 cases per 100,000). The rates were approximately equal for black females (0.06/100,000), Hispanic males (0.05/100,000), and white males (0.04/100,000). Prevalence rates were lower for Hispanic females (0.02/100,000) and were lowest for white females (0.006/100,000). The male:female ratio was approximately 3:1 for blacks and Hispanics and approximately 6:1 for whites.

One explanation for the changing epidemiology of HIV-1 infection as outlined above is the implementation of successful prevention strategies in populations of men who have sex with men. However, another contributing factor for the increase in the prevalence of HIV-1 in minority populations in the United States is the appearance of smokable "crack" cocaine in the mid-1980s. One study done in inner-city neighborhoods of New York, Miami, and San Francisco illustrates this (25). This study sampled 1,967 adults between the ages of 18 and 29 years who lived in the inner city and who had never used intravenous drugs. Crack smokers (1,137 participants) were compared with nonsmokers (830 participants). Crack smokers were 11 times more likely to have had greater than 50 sexual partners, 29 times more likely to have exchanged sex for drugs or money, and 3 times more likely to have a history of a genital ulcer disease than crack nonsmokers. The prevalence of HIV-1 infection was 15.7% for crack smokers and 5.2% for nonsmokers. The prevalence was highest for women who smoked crack and who had exchanged sex for money or drugs. In this subset, approximately 41% were HIV-1 infected. In the 6-year survey of U.S. households mentioned previously, the prevalence of cocaine in a serum or urine specimen was 8.8% for blacks, 1.7% for Hispanics, and 0.8% for whites. The prevalence of HIV-1 infection among cocaine-positive persons was highest for black females at 6.5%.

Data on the prevalence of HIV-1 infection in children and adolescents are derived primarily from AIDS reports and from anonymous testing of newborns. In the first 50,000 AIDS reports, children and adolescents accounted for 1.9% of cases. For cases reported from 1993 through October of 1995 this percentage remained relatively stable at 1.5% (15). Based on testing of newborns it is estimated that about 14,920 infants were born with

HIV-1 infection in the 15-year period between 1978 and 1993 (20). The rate of vertical transmission is declining due to recent treatment advances.

Data on the prevalence of HIV-1 infection in teenagers were recently published (65). Testing was done on 79,802 samples of blood from a nonrandomly selected group of 130 clinics catering to teenagers in 24 cities. The results are therefore illustrative of the problem in teens, but cannot be generalized to the entire teen population. The prevalence ranged from 0% to 4.8%, depending on the clinic location and type. Rates were highest in the Northeast and lowest in the Midwest, mirroring data from AIDS reporting. The combined median prevalence in adolescent medicine clinics, correctional facilities, and sexually transmitted disease clinics was 1.9% for females and 0.7% for males. Prevalence rates of 16% and 17% were found among homeless, homosexual male teens.

Clinical Features

Acute Infection

Primary infection with HIV-1 was first described in 1984 as a result of a percutaneous injury to a health care worker (1). The initial reports emphasized the similarities to mononucleosis. However, more recent case series have elucidated important differences between the primary manifestations of Epstein-Barr virus and HIV (39). The incubation period between exposure and symptoms is usually 2 to 6 weeks. However, one well-documented case has been reported in which the incubation period was 2 days (6). In rhesus monkeys inoculated with simian immunodeficiency virus (SIV), productively infected cells have been detected in lymph nodes at 4 days, which was the earliest time point sampled (16). In humans sampled during acute infection, the levels of HIV RNA measurable in blood frequently exceed several hundred thousand viral particles per milliliter of blood (47). The mean duration of the primary illness is 2 weeks, but it may last for up to several weeks.

Recent case series have elucidated important differences between the primary manifestations of Epstein-Barr virus and HIV

Fever is the most common initial symptom and sign and occurs in almost all symptomatic patients. Other common symptoms are sore throat (~50%), malaise and fatigue (~50%), myalgia (~40%), headache (~40%), diarrhea (~30%), nausea or vomiting (25%), and cough (~20%). Diffuse lymphadenopathy occurs in about 75% of patients and is usually accompanied by a nonexudative pharyngitis. Exudative pharyngitis, as is commonly observed in mononucleosis, is not characteristic of primary HIV-1 infection. A maculopapular rash is present in approximately 75% of patients. The rash is nonconfluent and distributed mainly over the upper thorax, face, scalp, and palate. Occasionally the rash may be vesicular or urticarial and may involve the palms and soles. The rash appears in the first few days of the illness and persists for 5 to 10 days, usually resolving without sequelae. Approximately 40% of patients will also have oral or genital ulcers. The ulcers are 5 to 10 mm in diameter, shallow, and either painless or painful. In the oropharynx the ulcers may involve the mucous membranes, gingiva, or palate. Ulcers of the rectum and esophagus have also been described. The triad of nonexudative pharyngitis, a nonconfluent, maculopapular rash of the upper trunk and scalp, and orogenital ulcers should suggest a diagnosis of acute HIV-1 infection. Other manifestations of primary HIV-1 infection include pneumonitis, meningoencephalitis, neuritis, Guillain-Barré syndrome, vasculitis, myositis, myopericarditis, hepatitis, and others. Coincident with the acute retroviral syndrome is an acute suppression of the number of CD4$^+$ T cells, otherwise known as T-helper cells. T-helper cell counts generally fall from normal limits to as low as ~150 cells/μl. Opportunistic infections may complicate this acute immune suppression. In one series of 31 patients oral candidiasis was present in 6 patients and esophageal candidiasis was present in 3 (39). Thrombocytopenia complicates the acute illness in about three-quarters of patients, leukopenia in about half, and anemia in about one-quarter of patients. As the symptomatic illness resolves, the T-helper counts and other laboratory abnormalities return toward baseline. The level of HIV-1 RNA in the blood also declines and frequently becomes undetectable. Those patients who do not have a decline in viral RNA to undetectable levels are more likely to progress rapidly to symptomatic HIV infection (47).

Chronic Infection

The hallmark of chronic infection with HIV-1 is the progressive depletion of CD4$^+$ T cells

The hallmark of chronic infection with HIV-1 is the progressive depletion of CD4$^+$ T cells. The rate of decline of the T-helper cell count averages about 50 cells/μl per year. Initially this depletion has no overt effect on the status of the patient's health. As the T-helper cell count continues to decline, however, patients develop recurrent viral, bacterial, and eventually opportunistic infections. In general, such complications are rare if the T-helper cell count is >500 cells/μl. At between 200 and 500 CD4$^+$ cells/μl, patients have an increased risk of developing common bacterial, viral, and fungal infections (63). These patients frequently show evidence of anergy and of an impaired ability to generate de novo antibody responses. At levels below 200 CD4$^+$ cells/μl patients are prone to develop the opportunistic infections and malignancies that define the AIDS case definition. For this reason the recent redefinition of the Centers for Disease Control and Prevention (CDC) criteria for AIDS includes any adult patient with <200 CD4$^+$ cells/μl (10). In infants the normal T-helper cell count range is higher than in adults, and AIDS manifestations develop at much higher T-helper cell counts.

The remainder of this brief discussion will focus on those manifestations that appear to be caused by HIV-1 replication (and the associated immune response) and are not simply a reflection of T-helper cell depletion. One of these manifestations is persistent generalized lymphadenopathy (PGL). PGL is characterized by enlargement of two or more extra-inguinal lymph nodes for greater than 3 months. PGL is usually bilateral and involves the cervical, axillary, epitrochlear, and femoral nodes. The presence or absence of PGL does not appear to have clinical significance.

Another manifestation related to viral replication is HIV-related immune thrombocytopenia (ITP). ITP may present at any stage of HIV-1 infection.

It is usually asymptomatic, rarely causing petechiae or significant bleeding. Platelet kinetic studies indicate that the ITP is due to peripheral destruction of platelets, rather than to hypoproduction. The destruction is due to autoantibodies and to anti-HIV antibodies on the surface of platelets.

Several neuromuscular complications are also described at all stages of HIV-1 infection. These include polymyositis, acute and chronic inflammatory demyelinating polyneuropathy, mononeuritis multiplex, and AIDS dementia complex. Polymyositis, which is one of the common manifestations of primary HIV infection, has also frequently been reported to complicate chronic infection. Such patients present with muscle weakness, fatigue, and tenderness. The inflammatory neuropathies and mononeuritis are rare compared to AIDS dementia complex (61). Inflammatory demyelinating polyneuropathy can be identified when patients in the early stages of HIV infection develop symmetric weakness and areflexia. The cerebrospinal fluid contains an increased amount of leukocytes and protein. In contrast, mononeuritis presents as an isolated peripheral or cranial neuropathy that resolves spontaneously. As its name suggests, the AIDS dementia complex is primarily a dementing process associated with late-stage HIV infection. When it does occur early in the course of the disease, it may present as mild cognitive impairment or memory dysfunction. In its early stages the dementia may be subtle, and diagnosis may be facilitated by neuropsychiatric testing. Magnetic resonance imaging of the brain characteristically shows gray matter atrophy and nonspecific abnormalities of the white matter. Lumbar puncture is useful clinically to exclude other infections, and recent evidence indicates that the levels of HIV-1 RNA are higher in the cerebrospinal fluid of those with dementia than those without (44).

Several neuromuscular complications are also described at all stages of HIV-1 infection

Pathogenesis

Virus-Host Interaction

The establishment and progression of HIV disease involve a complex array of multiphasic and multifactorial immunopathogenic mechanisms (29). HIV infects lymphocytes and macrophages. During the course of the disease the viral phenotype shifts from macrophage tropic to T-cell tropic. This phenomenon may have clinical implications and may account for variation in mode of transmission. The rate of virus production varies (Fig. 5.2). After primary infection there is a rapid increase in the number of circulating virions. During this early viremic phase, the virus is disseminated and trapped within the processes of follicular dendritic cells in the germinal centers of lymphoid tissue (29). Also, during this phase, some patients show major expansions of certain subsets of CD8$^+$ T lymphocytes that may be important in controlling the progression of HIV infection (29). The viral load decreases after the initial viremic period and remains at a plateau level for a period of time. This plateau may last for months to years. Suddenly and for unclear reasons, viral load rapidly increases and the CD4$^+$ cell count declines, correlating with progression to AIDS. The basis for these changes may be stimulation of the immune system by infection or vaccination. Long-term nonprogressors (persons who have stable T-helper cell counts and no progression despite years of HIV infection) have low viral burden (29).

Although persons infected with HIV show changes in all components of immunity, cellular immunity is affected most markedly. T-cell defects are the basis for much of the immune dysfunction. The number and function of T-helper cells are diminished, with loss of the ability to respond to antigens (37). Cytotoxic $CD8^+$ cells are also decreased. T-helper-1 (TH1) $CD4^+$ cells activate macrophages and promote T-cell proliferation. TH2 cells promote proliferation of B cells and induce immunoglobulin isotype switching. A switch from TH1 to TH2 correlates with clinical progression to AIDS.

While viral replication in $CD4^+$ T lymphocytes accounts for much of the immunosuppression, the virus-infected macrophage is also intimately involved in clinical manifestations of HIV infection (31). HIV infection results in numerous functional defects of macrophages (37). The monocyte/macrophage system functions of chemotaxis, phagocytosis, intracellular killing, and antigen presentation are defective. Even when intrinsic function is intact, lymphokine-dependent function can be abnormal because of loss of T-helper function. Infection of progenitor cells in bone marrow and the thymus contributes to the lack of regeneration of immunocompetent cells (29).

The initiation and propagation of HIV infection in $CD4^+$ cells involve dendritic cells (29). The interaction of dendritic cells and T cells in mucosa may support HIV-1 replication, even in subclinical stages of infection. The surface of the nasopharyngeal tonsil and adenoid tissue from persons with HIV infection contains many cells expressing Gag protein. The infected mucosal surface contains multinucleated syncytia of T cells and dendritic cells. These two cell types together support HIV-1 replication in culture (30). Histologic findings in the central nervous system and lymphatic tissue, as described below, typify pathology resulting from replication of HIV in macrophages (31).

One of the receptors for HIV is the CD4 protein. CD4 binds to the viral envelope protein gp120 and causes a conformational change that allows gp120 to bind to the chemokine receptor 5 protein (CCR5). CCR5 serves as a secondary receptor on $CD4^+$ lymphocytes and macrophages for certain strains of HIV-1 (23). Another secondary receptor is CXCR4 or fusin on the surface of T lymphocytes.

A 32-base-pair deletion is present at a frequency of approximately 0.10 in United States Caucasians. Patients homozygous for the deletion are frequently found among exposed HIV-1 antibody-negative individuals and rarely found among HIV-1-infected individuals. The frequency of deletion heterozygotes is significantly greater among individuals with HIV-1 infection of more than 10 years duration. It is less frequent among rapid progressors to AIDS. Survival analysis clearly shows that disease progression is slower in deletion-heterozygotic patients than in individuals homozygous for the normal gene. The deletion may act as a recessive restriction gene against HIV-1 infection and may exert a dominant phenotype of delaying progres-

Cellular immunity is affected most markedly

sion to AIDS among infected individuals. Mutation of other receptors in the CCR family may show similar decreased rates of progression.

The effects of HIV and of the agents of opportunistic infections can interact in a complex fashion on the immune system. In Africa the risk of seroconversion after exposure is greater and the rate of disease progression is faster. This phenomenon may be due in part to the increased state of immune activation associated with higher rate of parasite infestation and other infections (67). In cultures of dendritic cells and CD4$^+$ cells, 100 times less HIV is necessary to initiate productive infection if the cells had been activated by tetanus toxoid. Inappropriate immune activation and elevated secretion of certain proinflammatory cytokines occur during HIV infection; these cytokines play a role in the regulation of HIV expression in the tissues (29).

US28, a protein encoded by human cytomegalovirus (CMV), has homology to chemokine receptors (57). Its function in CMV pathogenesis is unknown. US28 can function as a receptor for RANTES, MIP-1 alpha, and MIP-1 beta, the ligands for the HIV-1 coreceptor CCR5. A human glioma cell that expresses CD4 and is ordinarily resistant to HIV infection can be infected by HIV in the presence of the coreceptors CCR5 or CXCR4. US28 can function similarly as a coreceptor for both HIV-1 and HIV-2 entry in this cell line. US28 facilitates entry of both macrophage- and T-cell-tropic HIV-1 isolates. These findings provide evidence for a role for CMV in HIV pathogenesis. Other studies have indicated that T-cell coinfection with HIV and CMV is uncommon. However, US28 might serve its coreceptor function without CMV cell entry. US28 may also expand the spectrum of cells able to be infected with HIV, such as in the central nervous system.

HIV has genes that most retroviruses lack. One of these genes codes for a protein called Vpr, which prevents infected cells from undergoing mitosis and proliferating (26). Vpr induces arrest of cells in the G2 phase of the cell cycle. Following the arrest of cells in G2, Vpr induces apoptosis in human fibroblasts, T cells, and primary peripheral blood lymphocytes (64). Both the initial arrest of cells and subsequent apoptosis may contribute to CD4$^+$ cell depletion. Vpr also plays a role in another unusual property of HIV-1, that is, its ability to enter the nucleus of a nondividing cell (26).

Apoptosis may be one of the major mechanisms of depletion of CD4$^+$ T cells. HIV-1-infected cells appear to be protected from apoptosis, whereas uninfected bystander cells show increased apoptosis (42). Addition of exogenous Tat protein induces apoptosis in uninfected T cells, but T cells stably expressing Tat are protected from activation-induced apoptosis. In vivo cell death in HIV-infected lymph nodes occurs predominantly through a novel pathway, related to but distinct from classical apoptosis and characterized by early and severe mitochondrial damage (7). Most dead cells from HIV-infected lymph nodes display combined features of apoptosis and necrosis, that is, chromatin condensation and mitochondrial swelling. Comparable levels of cell death are observed in other inflammatory lymphadenopathies not related to HIV. The incessant nature of HIV lymphadenopathy accounts for the progressive disruption and depletion of lymphoid tissues seen in HIV infection. Uninfected human macrophages

The effects of HIV and of the agents of opportunistic infections can interact in a complex fashion on the immune system

and, to a larger degree, HIV-infected macrophages mediate apoptosis of T cells from HIV-infected, but not from uninfected control individuals (14). Macrophage-dependent killing targets CD4$^+$ cells, but not CD8$^+$ cells, and it requires direct contact between macrophages and lymphocytes. Apoptosis-inducing ligands, FasL and tumor necrosis factor, mediate macrophage-induced apoptosis of CD4$^+$ cells. Mitogen-induced apoptosis is detectable in both infected and noninfected T cells before mitogenic responsiveness is reduced (60).

Polyclonal B-cell activation and impaired antibody responses to soluble antigens in vivo and in vitro are manifestations of impaired humoral immunity (37). Chronic nonspecific B-cell stimulation results in generalized lymphadenopathy and hypergammaglobulinemia. Hyperstimulated B cells are unable to respond to new antigens or to mount adequate immune responses, resulting in increased susceptibility to infections by encapsulated organisms such as *Streptococcus pneumoniae*, *Haemophilus influenzae*, and *Klebsiella* spp.

The innate defense system controls acute inflammation and can function in patients with humoral, cellular, or combined immune deficiencies. It may be the only response in patients with severe immunodeficiency in late-stage AIDS. However, granulocytopenia also occurs in a significant number of HIV-infected persons and can increase the risk and severity of bacterial and fungal infections.

Pathology

Histologically, there is a sequence of changes in the inflammatory response during the progression of HIV infection. Early in the disease, the inflammatory response is normal. With progression to AIDS, the response becomes hyporeactive and eventually anergic. An inappropriate suppurative response can occur. In infections that normally elicit a granulomatous response, giant cells are decreased or absent, numbers of organisms increase in both the intra- and extracellular environments, and there is regression to a suppurative response. Other atypical reactions include *Mycobacterium avium*-complex associated spindle cell- or granular cell-like lesions and CMV-associated pseudotumors.

While opportunistic infections are important causes of morbidity and mortality, noninfectious conditions frequently make substantial contributions to the disease course. Patients with HIV infection may be at increased risk for neoplastic disease. They do not, however, have an increased incidence of the most common tumors affecting the general population, such as breast, colon, and prostate carcinoma. Immunodeficiency results in increased susceptibility to malignant neoplasms by both decreased immunologic response to abnormal cells and increased susceptibility to infection by viruses. AIDS-indicator malignant neoplasms have associations with viruses: Kaposi's sarcoma with human herpesvirus 8, malignant lymphoma with Epstein-Barr virus, and cervical carcinoma with human papillomavirus. Patients with HIV infection also can develop reactive processes that are attributable to direct effects of HIV or immune system alterations. Such

Noninfectious conditions frequently make substantial contributions to the disease course

conditions include salivary gland cystic lymphoepithelial lesion, lymphadenopathy, lymphocytic interstitial pneumonitis, encephalopathy, enteropathy, nephropathy, hepatic conditions, dermatologic conditions, and anemia.

Mucosal Ulcers

Patients with HIV infection are prone to developing nonhealing ulcers of the oropharynx and the rest of the alimentary canal. HIV and other viruses have been investigated as etiologic agents, but in most lesions a cause is never identified. These lesions may result from immune dysfunction itself (e.g., ineffective cytokine modulation of healing).

Lymphadenopathy

Lymphadenopathy is one of the earliest manifestations of HIV infection. The histologic features fall into three stages (follicular hyperplasia, follicular involution, and lymphocyte depletion) that correlate to a certain extent with the patient's clinical and immunologic status (28, 54). Long-term nonprogressors do not show changes in lymph node architecture (29). None of the histologic findings is specific for HIV infection (53). In all stages, immunohistochemical staining shows HIV (p24) antigens in germinal centers, in follicular dendritic reticulum cells, in endothelial cells of paracortical venules, and in sinus macrophages (5) (Fig. 5.3).

In follicular hyperplasia there are large geographic follicles, follicle lysis, paracortical hyperplasia, focal hemorrhage, and preservation of tingible body macrophages (Fig. 5.4). The mantle zone lymphocytes invade follicles or are moderately to markedly decreased. Monocytoid B-lymphocyte hyperplasia and Warthin-Finkeldey-like multinucleated giant cells may be present. B lymphocytes and a small number of mature T lymphocytes comprise the germinal centers. Proliferation and activation of B lymphocytes correlate clinically with hypergammaglobulinemia (5).

During follicular involution there is diffuse lymphoid hyperplasia and loss of germinal centers. The mantle zone becomes thin and intrafollicular plasmacytosis and erythrophagocytosis occur (Fig. 5.5). Often there is vascular proliferation suggesting Castleman's disease or Kaposi's sarcoma. Fibrosis of capsule or subcapsular sinus begins.

Lymph nodes in the lymphocyte depletion or atrophic stage are small and not often biopsied. Follicles are absent and lymphocytes are depleted. Fibrosis becomes more marked. At this stage, patients are generally more immunodeficient; therefore, it is important to examine these lymph nodes for the presence of opportunistic infections and Kaposi's sarcoma.

Leukoencephalopathy and Encephalitis

There are two histologic patterns of AIDS dementia complex: leukoencephalopathy and encephalitis (33). HIV leukoencephalopathy is diffuse, noninflammatory, and degenerative. HIV encephalitis is multifocal and inflammatory. Histologically, both show multinucleated giant cells and involve the cortex and white matter (Fig. 5.6). HIV encephalitis is characterized by

There are two histologic patterns of AIDS dementia complex: leukoencephalopathy and encephalitis

microglial nodules composed of tight aggregates of microglia, astrocytes, and macrophages. Characteristic multinucleated giant cells and demyelination are present in only 50% of brain biopsies from patients with AIDS-related dementia (32, 68). Measurement of central nervous system viral burden is a more sensitive and earlier indicator of dementia.

Loss of neurons in AIDS-related dementia is not due to infection of these cells by HIV. Although other nervous system cell types can harbor HIV in vitro, only macrophages/microglia have been found to be significantly infected by immunohistochemical and in situ hybridization (66). Theories regarding the pathogenesis of HIV-associated neurologic disorders have thus focused on apoptosis due to toxins including HIV proteins, cellular metabolites, and cytokines. One putative toxic factor is the regulatory protein Tat, released from HIV-1-infected cells. Tat induces apoptosis in cultured human fetal neurons (51). The macrophages/microglia in the nervous systems of patients with HIV leukoencephalopathy and encephalitis produce tumor necrosis factor alpha (66). An increase in macrophage activity in HIV infection may be due to decreased production of cytokines such as interleukins 4 and 10 that inhibit macrophage activity.

Peripheral Neuropathy

Peripheral neuropathies are multifactorial in etiology and include acute or chronic demyelinating neuropathies (Guillain-Barré syndrome or chronic inflammatory demyelinating polyneuropathy), mononeuritis multiplex, ganglioneuronitis, autonomic neuropathy, and distal painful sensory neuropathy. HIV is not found within ganglionic neurons or Schwann cells but only rarely within the endoneurial macrophages (18, 66).

Some patients develop peripheral neuropathy as a manifestation of the diffuse infiltrative lymphocytosis syndrome, which is due to multivisceral CD8 cell infiltration (49). Nerve biopsy shows marked angiocentric CD8 infiltrates without mural necrosis and abundant expression of HIV p24 protein in macrophages.

Diagnosis and Monitoring

Initial screening for HIV infection is commonly done by detection of antibodies by enzyme-linked immunosorbent assay (ELISA) or agglutination (34). Current tests for anti-HIV antibodies are very sensitive. False-negative results may occur early in infection or with highly divergent strains such as HIV-1 subtype O (38, 48).

Reactive results are confirmed by Western blot (immunoblot) or further specific tests such as competitive ELISA which, when evaluated quantitatively, allow the differentiation of HIV types and, partially, subtypes (34).

Antibody tests performed on body fluids other than blood may prove to be as reliable and less invasive. A device designed to concentrate oral mucosal transudate from whole saliva produces samples that are as sensitive and as specific as serum for detection of HIV antibodies by ELISA (27).

Current tests for anti-HIV antibodies are very sensitive; false-negative results may occur

Laboratory monitoring of the progression of HIV infection involves enumeration of circulating $CD4^+$ cells by flow cytometry (37) and determination of viral load in plasma or serum. Absolute $CD4^+$ cell counts of less than 200/µl are diagnostic of AIDS.

Nucleic-acid-based assays are most useful for detection of infection of newborns, characterization of individual strains for subtyping and forensic identification, and therapeutic monitoring. Nucleic-acid-based assays narrow the serological diagnostic window period in early HIV infection and, when quantified, give some indication of clinical status (3, 47, 58). Nucleic acid amplification methodologies are able to detect very low levels of specific nucleic acids. Amplification techniques can be automated when combined with product detection systems designed for high throughput. PCR is used for diagnosis of HIV infection, and quantitative reverse transcriptase-PCR for viral RNA is useful for monitoring and determining prognosis. Self-sustained sequence replication amplification for detection of viral RNA is comparable to plasma culture for diagnosis of pediatric infections (3). Quantitative competitive PCR methods quantify HIV-1 RNA in plasma (56). Plasma virus levels determined by quantitative competitive PCR correlate with virus titers measured by endpoint dilution culture. Plasma virus level is significantly associated with disease stage and $CD4^+$ count and decreases with resolution of primary infection or institution of antiretroviral therapy.

Plasma virus level is significantly associated with disease stage and CD4 count

Treatment

The treatment of HIV-1 infection was revolutionized by three developments that occurred between 1993 and 1995. The first of these was the development and application of quantitative measures of blood and tissue viral RNA. Studies that applied these techniques demonstrated that the baseline level of plasma HIV-1 RNA correlates with disease progression, that HIV-1 replication is extraordinarily prolific, and that reduction of RNA levels due to therapy correlates with a slowing of disease progression (recently reviewed in reference 52). The second development was the publication of two studies that indicated that patients who were treated with two nucleoside analogs had a better clinical and virologic outcome than those who were treated with zidovudine alone (24, 35). The third major advance was the development of antiretroviral therapies with enhanced potency against HIV-1. These enhanced-potency antiretrovirals included nucleoside analog reverse transcriptase inhibitors (lamivudine [3TC]), non-nucleoside analog agents (nevirapine and delavirdine), and protease inhibitors (saquinavir, ritonavir, indinavir, and nelfinavir). The potency of these agents was initially demonstrated in monotherapy studies. In such studies it was shown that zidovudine reduced plasma HIV-1 RNA by approximately 0.7 $\log_{10}$. In contrast, both 3TC and nevirapine reduced viral replication by 1–1.5 $\log_{10}$. The results with protease inhibitors were even more dramatic, reducing HIV-1 RNA by 1.5–2 $\log_{10}$. However, monotherapy with nevirapine or a protease inhibitor rapidly

Patients who had previously been treated with a combination therapy that included a protease inhibitor had improved survival

resulted in the generation of mutations which were resistant to the antiretroviral agents. It was subsequently demonstrated that the emergence of this resistance could be delayed when combinations of two nucleoside analogs plus a protease inhibitor were used. In addition, many patients had a decline in viral RNA of greater than 2 $\log_{10}$ to below the limit of detection of the currently available assays. Simultaneously, the CD4$^+$ cell count rose on average by approximately 100 cells/µl.

Three large studies have since shown that patients who had previously been treated with a combination therapy that included a protease inhibitor had improved survival compared to similar patients who were not given such therapy (52). Epidemiological evidence indicates that a similar survival impact is being observed on a national scale in the United States (15). These impressive advances led to the 1997 revision of the National Institutes of Health Guidelines for the Use of Antiretroviral Agents. An update of these guidelines was released in June 1998 (52). The National Institutes of Health panel recommended that all HIV-infected patients with AIDS, thrush, or unexplained fever should receive combination antiretroviral therapy. The preferred combination includes two nucleoside analog reverse transcriptase inhibitors plus a protease inhibitor. The preferred protease inhibitors include indinavir, ritonavir, and nelfinavir, but not saquinavir due to its poor bioavailability. The panel further recommended that the same combination be given to those patients with a CD4$^+$ cell count of <500 cells/µl or an HIV RNA level greater than 10,000–20,000 RNA copies per ml of plasma (depending on which assay was used to measure RNA). A panel convened by the International AIDS Society-USA released similar recommendations (8). For those patients who do not meet the above criteria, the panel members were divided on whether therapy would be beneficial.

The NIH panel recommended that patients with acute or recent HIV infection (<6 months since seroconversion) receive therapy. It also recommended that pregnant women who fulfilled any of the treatment criteria listed above should consider combination therapy. Since the safety of triple combination therapy in pregnancy is unknown, the panel recommended extensive discussion with the patient and the delay of therapy until after 10 to 12 weeks of gestation.

The goal of antiretroviral therapy is to achieve sustained suppression of HIV RNA to below the limit of detection. A serious limitation of the currently available regimens is that they require strict adherence to a dosing schedule that is difficult to comply with. When patients are noncompliant, the virus becomes resistant to the medications, frequently within 4 to 6 months of starting therapy. For patients who fail to achieve sustained suppression on the initial combination regimen, the panel recommended that the therapy be changed to include two new reverse transcriptase inhibitors and a new protease inhibitor or combination of protease inhibitors. Cross-resistance between antiretroviral agents is common, however. For those unfamiliar with the use of these agents it is generally advisable that they refer patients to a specialist.

Prevention

There is currently no vaccine available to prevent HIV-1 infection. Several approaches to vaccine development are being tested, including inactivated, recombinant, and subunit vaccines. One approach that has been successful in the SIV model is an attenuated viral vaccine. Transmission of SIV to apes has been prevented by vaccination with an attenuated SIV strain that lacks an essential regulatory gene (19). These results have been bolstered by findings in a cohort of human patients who received blood products that contained an HIV-1 strain deficient in a similar gene (22). These patients and the source patient have remained free of disease. Whether they are protected from subsequent challenge is unknown, and dual infection of humans with different strains has been reported.

Sexual transmission of HIV-1 can be prevented through the use of condoms, which have been shown to be highly effective (21). Despite this evidence, condom usage rates in the United States remain low. Only 1.6% of sexually active adults who had more than one sexual partner in the last year reported "always" using condoms (40). Condom usage rates were lowest in married respondents who had greater than one partner in the previous year. Of those who reported "never" using condoms, 52% felt that they had "no chance" of developing HIV infection despite risky sexual behavior. On a community level there is evidence that an aggressive treatment program for other sexually transmitted diseases will lead to further reductions in HIV-1 transmission (36). There is also evidence that antiretroviral therapy reduces heterosexual transmission of HIV-1 (50).

Occupational acquisition of HIV-1 from percutaneous injury is reduced 79% by zidovudine therapy (12). Currently the U.S. Public Health Service recommends that individuals with high-risk injuries receive triple drug therapy as soon as possible after the injury (14). This therapy should continue for at least 4 weeks. Ideally the triple drug regimen should include zidovudine, a protease inhibitor, and another antiretroviral that has never been used to treat the source patient.

Perinatal transmission of HIV-1 is reduced by two-thirds when the mother and infant both receive zidovudine treatment (17). Trials are ongoing to determine whether treatment with combination regimens is even more effective. Breast-feeding also increases the risk of transmission and is therefore to be avoided in areas where a safe water supply is available for mixing artificial substitutes. There is debate over whether delivery of children by cesarean section further reduces HIV-1 transmission.

There is currently no vaccine available to prevent HIV-1 infection

Figure 5.1   Simplified life cycle of HIV.

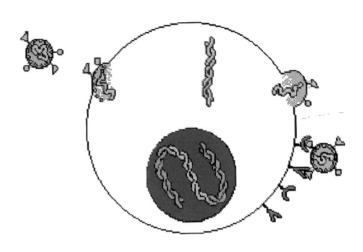

Figure 5.2   Graph of viremia versus CD4 count.

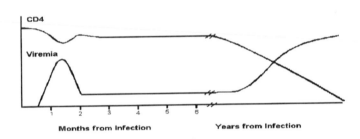

Figure 5.3   Hyperplastic stage of HIV-related lymphadenopathy showing follicular hyperplasia with geographic follicles, follicle lysis, preservation of mantle zone, and paracortical hyperplasia. Hematoxylin and eosin (H&E) stain; ×25.

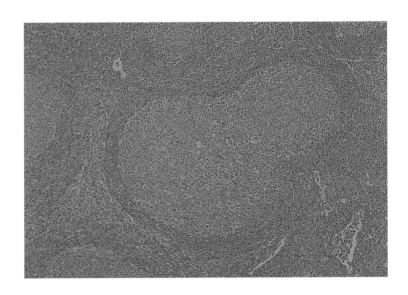

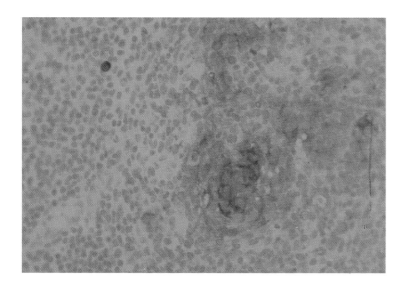

Figure 5.4   Hyperplastic stage of HIV-related lymphadenopathy, HIV p24 (*gag*) antigen staining. Note the follicular "network" staining and the cytoplasmic staining of individual cells in the paracortical areas. ×100.

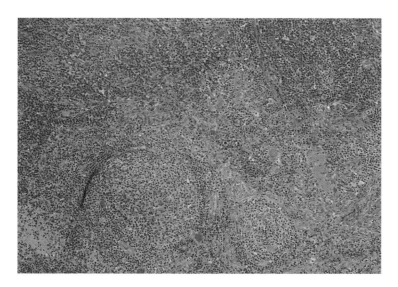

Figure 5.5   Involution stage of HIV-related lymph showing loss of germinal centers and mantle zones, diffuse lymphoid and monocytoid B-cell hyperplasia, plasmacytosis, and vascular proliferation. H&E stain; ×25.

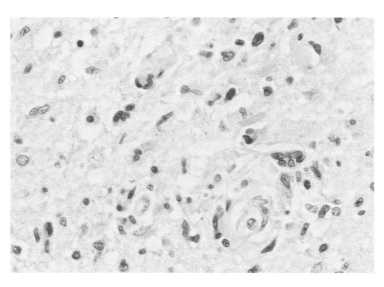

Figure 5.6   HIV-associated encephalitis showing microglial nodules with multinucleated giant cells. H&E stain; ×100.

References

1. **Anonymous.** 1984. Needlestick transmission of HTLV-III from a patient infected in Africa. *Lancet* **2:**1376–1377.

2. **Anonymous.** 1996. Fact sheet. United Nations Program on HIV/AIDS, New York.

3. **Arens, M.** 1993. Use of probes and amplification techniques for the diagnosis and prognosis of human immunodeficiency virus (HIV-1) infections. *Diagn. Microbiol. Infect. Dis.* **16:**165–172.

4. **Badley, A. D., D. Dockrell, M. Simpson, R. Schut, D. H. Lynch, P. Leibson, and C. V. Paya.** 1997. Macrophage-dependent apoptosis of CD4+ T lymphocytes from HIV-infected individuals is mediated by FasL and tumor necrosis factor. *J. Exp. Med.* **185:**55–64.

5. **Baroni, C. D., and S. Uccini.** 1993. The lymphadenopathy of HIV infection. *Am. J. Clin. Pathol.* **99:**397–401.

6. **Ben-Galim, P., Y. Shaked, A. Vonsover, and M. Garty.** 1996. Immediate immunosuppression caused by acute HIV-1 infection: a fulminant multisystemic disease 2 days post infection. *Infection* **24:**332–335.

7. **Carbonari, M., A. M. Pesce, M. Cibati, A. Modica, L. Dell'Anna, G. D'Offizi, A. Angelici, S. Uccini, A. Modesti, and M. Fiorilli.** 1997. Death of bystander cells by a novel pathway involving early mitochondrial damage in human immunodeficiency virus-related lymphadenopathy. *Blood* **90:**209–216.

8. **Carpenter, C. C. J., M. A. Fischl, S. M. Hammer, M. S. Hirsch, D. M. Jacobsen, D. A. Katzenstein, J. S. G. Montaner, D. R. Richman, M. S. Saag, R. T. Schooley, M. A. Thompson, S. Vella, P. G. Yeni, and P. A. Volberding.** 1997. Antiretroviral therapy for HIV infection in 1997: updated recommendations of the International AIDS Society-USA panel. *JAMA* **277:**1962–1969.

9. **Celentano, D., K. E. Nelson, S. Suprasert, S. Eiumtrakul, S. Tulvatana, S. Kuntolbutra, P. Akarasewi, A. Matanasarawoot, N. H. Wright, N. Sirisopana, and C. Theetranont.** 1996. Risk factors for HIV-1 seroconversion among men in northern Thailand. *JAMA* **275:**122–127.

10. **Centers for Disease Control and Prevention.** 1992. 1993 revised classification system for HIV infection and expanded surveillance case definition for AIDS among adults and adolescents. *Morbid. Mortal. Weekly Rep.* **41**(RR-17):1–19.

11. **Centers for Disease Control and Prevention.** 1993. HIV transmission between two adolescent brothers with hemophilia. *Morbid. Mortal. Weekly Rep.* **42:**948–951.

12. **Centers for Disease Control and Prevention.** 1995. Case-control study of HIV seroconversion in health-care workers after percutaneous exposure to HIV-infected blood: France, United Kingdom, and United States, January 1988–August 1994. *Morbid. Mortal. Weekly Rep.* **44:**929–933.

13. **Centers for Disease Control and Prevention.** 1995. First 50,000 AIDS cases—United States, 1995. *Morbid. Mortal. Weekly Rep.* **44:**849–853.

14. **Centers for Disease Control and Prevention.** 1996. Update: provisional recommendations for chemoprophylaxis after occupational exposure to human immunodeficiency virus. *Morbid. Mortal. Weekly Rep.* **45:**468–472.

15. **Centers for Disease Control and Prevention.** 1997. Update: trends in AIDS incidence, deaths, and prevalence—United States, 1996. *Morbid. Mortal. Weekly Rep.* **46:**165–173.

16. Chakrabarti, L., M.-C. Cumont, L. Montagnier, and B. Hurtrel. 1994. Kinetics of primary SIV infection in lymph nodes. *J. Med. Primatol.* **23:**117–124.

17. Connor, E. M., R. S. Sperling, R. Gelber, P. Kiselev, G. Scott, M. J. O'Sullivan, R. VanDyke, M. Bey, W. Shearer, R. L. Jacobson, E. Jimenez, E. O'Neill, B. Bazin, J.-F. Delfraissy, M. Culnane, R. Coombs, M. Elkins, J. Moye, P. Stratton, and J. Balsley for The Pediatric AIDS Clinical Trials Group Protocol 076 Study Group. 1994. Reduction of maternal-infant transmission of human immunodeficiency virus type 1 with zidovudine treatment. *N. Engl. J. Med.* **331:**1173–1180.

18. Dalakas, M. C., and E. J. Cupler. 1996. Neuropathies in HIV infection. *Baillieres Clin. Neurol.* **5:**199–218.

19. Daniel, M. D., F. Kirchoff, S. C. Czajak, P. K. Sehgal, and R. C. Desrosiers. 1992. Protective effects of a live attenuated SIV vaccine with a deletion in the nef gene. *Science* **258:**1880–1881.

20. Davis, S. F., R. H. Byers, M. L. Lindegren, B. Caldwell, J. M. Karon, and M. Gwinn. 1995. Prevalence and incidence of vertically acquired HIV infection in the United States. *JAMA* **247:**952–955.

21. de Vincenzi, I., for The European Study Group on Heterosexual Transmission of HIV-1. 1994. A longitudinal study of human immunodeficiency virus transmission by heterosexual partners. *N. Engl. J. Med.* **331:**341–346.

22. Deacon, N. J., A. Tsykin, A. Solomon, K. Smith, M. Ludford-Menting, D. J. Hooker, D. A. McPhee, A. L. Greenway, A. Ellett, C. Chatfield, V. A. Lawson, S. Crowe, A. Maerz, S. Sonza, J. Learmont, J. S. Sullivan, A. Cunningham, D. Dwyer, D. Dowton, and J. Mills. 1995. Genomic structure of an attenuated quasi species of HIV-1 from a blood transfusion donor and recipients. *Science* **270:**988–991.

23. Dean, M., M. Carrington, C. Winkler, G. A. Huttley, M. W. Smith, R. Allikmets, J. J. Goedert, S. P. Buchbinder, E. Vittinghoff, E. Gomperts, S. Donfield, D. Vlahov, R. Klaslow, A. Saah, C. Rinaldo, R. Detels, Hemophilia Growth and Development Study, Multicenter AIDS Cohort Study, Multicenter Hemophilia Cohort Study, San Francisco City Cohort, Alive Study, and S. J. O'Brien. 1996. Genetic restriction of HIV-1 infection and progression to AIDS by a deletion allele of the CKR5 structural gene. *Science* **273:**1856–1862.

24. Delta Coordinating Committee. 1996. Delta: a randomized double-blind controlled trial comparing combinations of zidovudine plus didanosine or zalcitabine with zidovudine alone in HIV-infected individuals. *Lancet* **348:**283–291.

25. Edlin, B. R., K. I. Irwin, S. Faruque, C. B. McCoy, C. Word, Y. Serrano, J. A. Inciardi, B. P. Bowser, R. F. Schilling, S. D. Holmberg, and The Multicenter Crack Cocaine and HIV Infection Study Team. 1994. Intersecting epidemics—crack cocaine use and HIV infection among inner-city young adults. *N. Engl. J. Med.* **331:**1422–1427.

26. Emerman, M. 1996. HIV-1, Vpr and the cell cycle. *Curr. Biol.* **6:**1096–1103.

27. Emmons, W. W., S. F. Paparello, C. F. Decker, J. M. Sheffield, and F. H. Lowe-Bey. 1995. A modified ELISA and western blot accurately determine anti-human immunodeficiency virus type 1 antibodies in oral fluids obtained with a special collecting device. *J. Infect. Dis.* **171:**1406–1410.

28. Ewing, E. P., Jr., F. W. Chandler, T. J. Spira, R. K. Brynes, and W. C. Chan. 1985. Primary lymph node pathology in AIDS and AIDS-related lymphadenopathy. *Arch. Pathol. Lab. Med.* **109:**977–981.

29. **Fauci, A. S., G. Pantaleo, S. Stanley, and D. Weissman.** 1996. Immunopathogenic mechanisms of HIV infection. *Ann. Intern. Med.* **124:**654–663.

30. **Frankel, S. S., B. M. Wenig, A. P. Burke, P. Mannan, L. D. Thompson, S. L. Abbondanzo, A. M. Nelson, M. Pope, and R. M. Steinman.** 1996. Replication of HIV-1 in dendritic cell-derived syncytia at the mucosal surface of the adenoid. *Science* **272:**115–117.

31. **Gendelman, H. E., J. M. Orenstein, D. C. Kalter, and C. Roberts.** 1992. Pathogenesis of HIV-1 infection, p. 57–75. *In* G. P. Wormser (ed.), *AIDS and Other Manifestations of HIV Infection*, 2nd ed. Raven Press, New York.

32. **Glass, J. D., S. L. Wesselingh, O. A. Selnes, and J. C. McArthur.** 1993. Clinical-neuropathologic correlation in HIV-associated dementia. *Neurology* **43:**2230–2237.

33. **Grassi, M. P., F. Clerici, R. Boldorini, C. Perin, L. Vago, A. D'Arminio Monforte, M. Borella, M. Nebuloni, and A. Mangoni.** 1997. HIV encephalitis and HIV leukoencephalopathy are associated with distinct clinical and radiological subtypes of the AIDS dementia complex. *AIDS* **11:**690–691.

34. **Gurtler, L.** 1996. Difficulties and strategies of HIV diagnosis. *Lancet* **348:** 176–179.

35. **Hammer, S. M., D. A. Katzenstein, M. D. Hughes, H. Gundacker, R. T. Schooley, R. H. Haubrich, K. Henry, M. M. Lederman, J. P. Phair, M. Niu, M. S. Hirsch, and T. C. Merigan for The AIDS Clinical Trials Group 175 Study Team.** 1996. A trial comparing nucleoside monotherapy with combination 1 therapy in HIV-infected adults with CD4 cell counts from 200–500 per cubic millimeter. *N. Engl. J. Med.* **335:**1081–1090.

36. **Hayes, R., F. Mosha, H. Grosskurth, J. Todd, A. Gavyole, A. Klokke, R. Gabone, and P. Mayaud.** 1996. Treatment of symptomatic STDs to prevent HIV: results of a randomized control trial, abstr. S46, p. 49. *In 3rd Conference on Retroviruses and Opportunistic Infections*, January 28-February 1, Washington, D.C.

37. **Horsburgh, C. R., Jr.** 1989. Immunologic evaluation of persons infected with human immunodeficiency virus. *Clin. Lab. Med.* **9:**393–403.

38. **Hu, D. J., T. J. Dondero, M. A. Rayfield, J. R. George, G. Schochetman, H. W. Jaffe, C. C. Luo, M. L. Kalish, B. G. Weniger, C. P. Pau, C. A. Schable, and J. W. Curran.** 1996. The emerging genetic diversity of HIV. The importance of global surveillance for diagnostics, research, and prevention. *JAMA* **275:**210–216.

39. **Kinloch-de Loes, S., P. de Saussure, J.-H. Saurat, H. Stalder, B. Hirschel, and L. H. Perrin.** 1993. Symptomatic primary infection due to human immunodeficiency virus type 1: review of 31 cases. *Clin. Infect. Dis.* **17:**59–65.

40. **Leigh, B. C., M. T. Temple, and K. F. Trocki.** 1993. The sexual behavior of US adults: results from a national survey. *Am. J. Public Health* **83:**1400–1408.

41. **Louwagie, J., F. E. McCutchan, M. Peeters, T. P. Brennan, E. Sanders-Buell, G. A. Eddy, G. van der Groen, K. Fransen, G. M. Gershy-Damet, and R. Deleys.** 1993. Phylogenetic analysis of gag genes from 70 international HIV-1 isolates provides evidence for multiple genotypes. *AIDS* **7:**769–780.

42. **McCloskey, T. W., M. Ött, E. Tribble, S. A. Khan, S. Teichberg, M. O. Paul, S. Pahwa, E. Verdin, and N. Chirmule.** 1997. Dual role of HIV Tat in regulation of apoptosis in T cells. *J. Immunol.* **158:**1014–1019.

43. **McCutchan, F. E., M. O. Salminen, J. K. Carr, and D. Burke.** 1996. HIV-1 genetic diversity. *AIDS* **10:**S13–S20.

44. **McCutchan, J. A., R. Ellis, K. Hsia, R. Heaton, M. Wallace, J. Nelson, T. Wolfson, I. Grant, and S. A. Spector.** 1997. Relationship of cerebrospinal fluid HIV-1 RNA levels (CSF RNA) to plasma RNA, CSF pleocytosis, stage of HIV infection and cognitive functioning, abstr. 7, p. 66. *In 4th Conference on Retroviruses and Opportunistic Infections*, January 22–26, Washington, D.C.

45. **McQuillan, M. C., M. Kahare, J. M. Karon, C. A. Schable, and D. Vlahov.** 1997. Update on the seroepidemiology of human immunodeficiency virus in the United States household population: NHANES III, 1988–1994. *J. AIDS* **14:**355–360.

46. **Mehendale, S. M., J. J. Rodrigues, R. S. Brookmeyer, R. R. Gangakhedkar, A. D. Divekar, M. R. Gokhale, A. R. Risbud, R. S. Paranjape, M. E. Shepherd, A. E. Rompalo, R. R. Sule, S. N. Tolat, V. D. Jadhav, T. C. Quinn, and R. C. Bollinger.** 1995. Incidence and predictors of human immunodeficiency virus type 1 seroconversion in patients attending sexually transmitted disease clinics in India. *J. Infect. Dis.* **72:**1486–1491.

47. **Mellors, J. W., L. A. Kingsley, C. R. Rinaldo, J. A. Todd, B. S. Hoo, R. P. Kokka, and P. Gupta.** 1995. Quantitation of HIV-1 RNA in plasma predicts outcome after seroconversion. *Ann. Intern. Med.* **122:**573–579.

48. **Mortimer, P. P.** 1996. Ten years of laboratory diagnosis of HIV: how accurate is it now? *J. Antimicrob. Chemother.* **37**(Suppl. B)**:**27–32.

49. **Moulignier, A., F. J. Authier, M. Baudrimont, G. Pialoux, L. Belec, M. Polivka, B. Clair, F. Gray, J. Mikol, and R. K. Gherardi.** 1997. Peripheral neuropathy in human immunodeficiency virus-infected patients with the diffuse infiltrative lymphocytosis syndrome. *Ann. Neurol.* **41:**438–445.

50. **Musicco, M., A. Lazzarin, A. Nicolosi, M. Gasparini, P. Costigliola, C. Arici, and A. Saracco for The Italian Study Group on HIV Heterosexual Transmission.** 1994. Antiretroviral treatment of men infected with human immunodeficiency virus type 1 reduces the incidence of heterosexual transmission. *Arch. Intern. Med.* **154:**1971–1976.

51. **New, D. R., M. Ma, L. G. Epstein, A. Nath, and H. A. Gelbard.** 1997. Human immunodeficiency virus type 1 Tat protein induces death by apoptosis in primary human neuron cultures. *J. Neurovirol.* **3:**168–173.

52. **NIH Panel To Define Principles of Therapy of HIV Infection.** 1998. Report of the NIH panel to define principles of therapy of HIV infection. *Ann. Intern. Med.* **128:**1057–1078.

53. **O'Murchadha, M. T., B. C. Wolf, and R. S. Neiman.** 1987. The histologic features of hyperplastic lymphadenopathy in AIDS-related complex are nonspecific. *Am. J. Surg. Pathol.* **11:**94–99.

54. **Öst, Å., C. D. Baroni, P. Biberfeld, J. Diebold, A. Moragas, H. Noël, G. Pallesen, P. Rácz, M. Schipper, and K. Tenner-Rácz.** 1989. Lymphadenopathy in HIV infection: histological classification and staging. *APMIS* **8**(Suppl.)**:**7–15.

55. **Panel on Clinical Practices for the Treatment of HIV Infection.** 1998. Guidelines for the use of antiretroviral agents in HIV-infected adults and adolescents. *Ann. Intern. Med.* **128:**1079–1100.

56. **Piatak, M., Jr., M. S. Saag, L. C. Yang, S. J. Clark, J. C. Kappes, K. C. Luk, B. H. Hahn, G. M. Shaw, and J. D. Lifson.** 1993. High levels of HIV-1 in plasma during all stages of infection determined by competitive PCR. *Science* **259:**1749–1754.

57. **Pleskokk, O., C. Treboute, A. Brelot, N. Heveker, M. Seman, and M. Alizon.** 1997. Identification of a chemokine receptor encoded by human cytomegalovirus as a cofactor for HIV-1 entry. *Science* **276:**1874–1878.

58. **Roberts, C. R.** 1991. Laboratory diagnosis of retroviral infections. *Dermatol. Clin.* **9:**453–464.

59. **Rosenberg, P. S.** 1995. Scope of the AIDS epidemic in the United States. *Science* **270:**1372–1375.

60. **Rothern, M., S. Gratzl, H. H. Hirsch, and C. Moroni.** 1997. Apoptosis in HIV-infected individuals is an early marker occurring independently of high viremia. *AIDS Res. Hum. Retroviruses* **13:**771–779.

61. **Simpson, D. A., and M. Tagliati.** 1994. Neurologic manifestations of HIV infection. *Ann. Intern. Med.* **121:**769–785.

62. **Soto-Ramirez, L. E., B. Renjifo, M. F. McLane, R. Marlink, C. O'Hara, R. Sutthent, C. Wasi, P. Vithayasai, C. Apichartpiyakul, P. Auerwarakul, V. Pena Cruz, D. S. Chui, R. Osathanondh, K. Mayer, T. H. Lee, and M. Essex.** 1996. HIV-1 Langerhans' cell tropism associated with heterosexual transmission of HIV. *Science* **271:**1291–1293.

63. **Stein, D. S., J. A. Korvick, and S. H. Vermund.** 1992. CD4$^+$ lymphocyte cell enumeration for prediction of clinical course of human immunodeficiency virus disease: a review. *J. Infect. Dis.* **165:**352–363.

64. **Stewart, S. A., B. Poon, J. B. Jowett, and I. S. Chen.** 1997. Human immunodeficiency virus type 1 Vpr induces apoptosis following cell cycle arrest. *J. Virol.* **71:**5579–5592.

65. **Sweeney, P., M. L. Lindegren, J. W. Buehler, I. M. Onorato, and R. S. Janssen.** 1995. Teenagers at risk of human immunodeficiency virus type 1 infection. *Arch. Pediatr. Adolesc. Med.* **149:**521–528.

66. **Tyor, W. R., S. L. Wesselingh, J. W. Griffin, J. C. McArthur, and D. E. Griffen.** 1995. Unifying hypothesis for the pathogenesis of HIV-associated dementia complex, vacuolar myelopathy, and sensory neuropathy. *J. Acquired Immune Defic. Syndr. Hum. Retrovir.* **9:**379–388.

67. **Weissman, D., T. D. Barker, and A. S. Fauci.** 1996. The efficiency of acute infection of CD4$^+$ T cells is markedly enhanced in the setting of antigen-specific immune activation. *J. Exp. Med.* **183:**687–692.

68. **Wiley, C. A., and C. Achim.** 1994. Human immunodeficiency virus encephalitis is the pathological correlate of dementia in acquired immunodeficiency syndrome. *Ann. Neurol.* **36:**673–676.

chapter 6

Emerging Fungal Infections: Histoplasmosis, Phaeohyphomycosis, and Sporotrichosis

Francis W. Chandler, Michael M. McNeil, and Leo Kaufman

Histoplasmosis, phaeohyphomycosis, and sporotrichosis are cosmopolitan fungal infections acquired from the environment. Although there is no national surveillance for these or other invasive mycotic infections, there have been increasing reports of severe and opportunistic diseases caused by them. The population of severely immunocompromised patients who are at highest risk for these infections continues to increase due to medical advances that have effectively prolonged the survival of critically ill patients and because of the ongoing AIDS epidemic. The clinical presentation of these infections may be variable and nonspecific, and is dependent upon the route of inoculation, dose of inoculum, immunologic status of the patient, and organ distribution of lesions. Clinical laboratories and physicians must be alert to consider these infections

Francis W. Chandler, Department of Pathology - BF230, Medical College of Georgia, Augusta, GA 30912-3605. **Michael M. McNeil,** Division of Bacterial and Mycotic Diseases, Centers for Disease Control and Prevention, Mailstop C-23, 1600 Clifton Road, Atlanta, GA 30333. **Leo Kaufman,** Division of Bacterial and Mycotic Diseases, Centers for Disease Control and Prevention, Mailstop G-11, 1600 Clifton Road, Atlanta, GA 30333.

Pathology of Emerging Infections 2
Edited by Ann Marie Nelson and C. Robert Horsburgh, Jr.
© 1998 American Society for Microbiology, Washington, D.C.

in susceptible patients. Despite the development of newer rapid, noninvasive, diagnostic laboratory tests for some of these infections, a clinical diagnosis may still be difficult; either cultural identification of the fungus or determination of its characteristic appearance on histologic examination of biopsy specimens may be essential. Therapy for histoplasmosis and sporotrichosis has recently changed with the advent of newer, more effective, oral azole medications; however, prolonged (lifelong) antifungal therapy or prophylaxis may be indicated, particularly for HIV-infected patients. The prognosis for patients with invasive phaeohyphomycosis may still be guarded despite combination antifungal therapy and surgical excision of lesions. Recurrences and drug-resistant infections may occur in these patients.

Epidemiology

Histoplasmosis

Histoplasmosis is caused by the dimorphic fungus *Histoplasma capsulatum*. The fungus exists in nature as a mold and in tissue as small, oval to round, budding cells. Histoplasmosis is caused by two varieties of *H. capsulatum*, the small-celled (2- to 5-μm) form (var. *capsulatum*), which occurs globally, and the large-celled (8- to 15-μm) form (var. *duboisii*), which is confined to the African continent and Madagascar. The areas in the United States in which *H. capsulatum* var. *capsulatum* is most highly endemic are in the Mississippi and Ohio River valley states, in particular Kentucky, Missouri, Ohio, and Tennessee. The natural habitat of *H. capsulatum* is soil, particularly soil enriched with bird or bat droppings. If contaminated soil or bird roosts are disturbed during building, renovation, construction, or demolition, large numbers of conidia may be aerosolized, possibly exposing many individuals to the risk of infection. Bat-roosting sites, such as caves, also are important sources of *H. capsulatum*, particularly in the tropics. It is estimated that 50,000 to 200,000 persons are infected per year in the United States; 550 of these may experience severe, disseminated infections, making histoplasmosis capsulati the most common endemic mycosis (78). In areas of the United States with endemic disease, more than 80% of the population have had subclinical infection (24). Several outbreaks of histoplasmosis also have been reported (57, 64, 66, 73, 78, 80). Although infections due to *H. capsulatum* var. *duboisii* have been confined to the central region of Africa (and termed African histoplasmosis), infections with var. *capsulatum* also have been reported from parts of that continent.

*T*he major route of acquisition of histoplasmosis is inhalation

The major route of acquisition of histoplasmosis is inhalation. Otherwise healthy individuals generally experience a mild, transient influenza-like infection. However, in predisposed patients, illness can proceed to chronic, progressive infection of the lungs or more widespread infection.

Phaeohyphomycosis

The term phaeohyphomycosis was coined by Ajello et al. in 1974 (2) to refer to subcutaneous and deep-seated infections caused by a number of brown-pigmented (dematiaceous) molds that are found as yeasts, septate hyphae, or a mixture of these forms in tissue (1, 54). Thus, the term reflects a similarity in histopathologic features seen with numerous fungal etiologic agents that vary greatly in their specific morphology and taxonomic classification. Fungi representing 60 genera and over 110 species have been confirmed as agents of phaeohyphomycosis (Table 6.1)

Table 6.1   Currently known agents of phaeohyphomycosis

Genera and species	Genera and species	Genera and species	Genera and species
Acrophialophora	*Cladosporium*	*Myceliophthora*	*Phyllosticta*
A. fusispora	C. cladosporioides	M. thermophila	P. citricarpa
Alternaria	C. elatum	*Mycocentrospora*	*Phyllostictina*
A. alternata	C. oxysporum	M. acerina	P. species
A. chartarum	C. sphaerospermum	*Mycoleptodiscus*	*Pleurophoma*
A. chlamydospora	*Colletotrichum*	M. indicus	P. pleurospora
A. dianthicola	C. coccodes	*Nattrassia*	*Pleurophomopsis*
A. infectoria	C. dematium	N. mangiferae	P. lignicola
A. longipes	*Coniothyrium*	*Nigrospora*	*Pseudomicrodochium*
A. stemphylioides	C. fuckelii	N. sphaerica	P. suttonii
A. tenuissima	*Curvularia*	*Ochroconis*	*Pyrenochaeta*
Anthopsis	C. brachyspora	O. constricta	P. unguis-hominis
A. deltoidea	C. clavata	O. gallopava	*Ramichloridium*
Arnium	C. geniculata	O. tshawytschae	R. obovoideum
A. leporinum	C. lunata	*Oidiodendron*	*Rhinocladiella*
Arthrinium	C. pallescens	O. cerealis	R. atrovirens
A. phaeospermum	C. senegalensis	*Onychocola*	R. schulzeri
Ascotrichosporon	C. verruculosa	O. canadensis	*Sarcinomyces*
A. chartarum	*Dichotomophthora*	*Phaeoacremonium*	S. phaeomuriformis
Aureobasidium	D. portulacae	P. inflatipes	*Scytalidium*
A. pullulans	*Dichotomophthoropsis*	P. parasitica	S. infestans
Bipolaris	D. nymphearum	*Phaeoannellomyces*	S. japonicum
B. australiensis	*Dissitimurus*	P. elegans	*Sphaeropsis*
B. hawaiiensis	D. exedrus	P. werneckii	S. subglobosa
B. spicifera	*Drechslera*	*Phaeosclera*	*Staphylotrichum*
Botryomyces	D. biseptata	P. dematioides	S. coccosporum
B. caespitosus	*Exophiala*	*Phaeotrichonis*	*Taeniolella*
Cephaliophora	E. dermatitidis	P. crotalariae	T. stilbospora
C. irregularis	E. jeanselmei	*Phialemonium*	*Tetraploa*
Chaetomium	E. pisciphila	P. obovatum	T. aristata
C. arthrobrunneum	E. salmonis	*Phialophora*	*Thermomyces*
C. funicolum	E. spinifera	P. americana	T. lanuginosus
C. globosum	*Exserohilum*	P. bubakii	*Trichomaris*
C. perpulchrum	E. longirostratum	P. repens	T. invadens
C. strumarium	E. mcginnisii	P. richardsiae	*Ulocladium*
Cladophialophora	E. rostratum	P. verrucosa	U. chartarum
C. arxii	*Fonsecaea*	*Phoma*	*Veronaea*
C. bantianum	F. pedrosoi	P. cava	V. botryosa
C. boppii	*Hormonema*	P. cruris-hominis	
C. carrionii	H. dematioides	P. eupyrena	
C. devriesii	*Lasiodiplodia*	P. glomerata	
Cladorrhinum	L. theobromae	P. herbarum	
C. bulbillosum	*Moniliella*	P. hibernica	
	M. suaveolens	P. minutella	
		P. oculo-hominis	

(L. Ajello, personal communication). This number of organisms has markedly increased in the last 10 years, and it most likely will continue to enlarge (1, 62).

Phaeohyphomycosis has a worldwide distribution. Opportunistic infections in severely immunocompromised patients have been reported with increasing frequency (53). In these infections, specific identification can only be accomplished through isolation and identification of the etiologic agents. The most prevalent agents of phaeohyphomycosis include *Alternaria* spp., *Bipolaris* spp., *Cladophialophora bantiana* (*Xylohypha bantiana*, *Cladosporium bantianum*), *Curvularia* spp., *Exophiala* spp., *Exserohilum* spp., *Ochroconis* spp., *Phialophora* spp., and *Exophiala* (*Wangiella*) *dermatitidis*. These fungi are saprophytes of soil and have also been isolated from decaying vegetable debris; others are plant pathogens (43, 54, 55). Human infection typically follows traumatic percutaneous implantation of the fungus from the soil, but inhalation may be an alternative route for acquiring infection. An unusual property of these fungi is melanin formation in the cell wall in culture (and, in most cases, in human tissue), which may have importance as a virulence factor.

Sporotrichosis

Sporotrichosis is a subacute or chronic fungal infection of worldwide distribution in which lesions are usually confined to the skin and subcutaneous tissues. Sporotrichosis is caused by the dimorphic fungus *Sporothrix schenckii*, which grows in nature as a mold, but in tissue forms small, budding, yeastlike cells. A variety of the species, *S. schenckii* var. *luriei*, has recently been identified in India, Italy, and South Africa (3, 4, 59). *S. schenckii* is usually found in the soil and as a saprophyte on plants, decomposing wood, and sphagnum moss (44). Human lymphocutaneous infection, the classic clinical form of sporotrichosis, usually results from minor trauma and soil contamination, such as abrasions or wounds due to thorns or wood splinters, and is characterized by skin ulcers and painless lymphangitis. Rarely, primary pulmonary sporotrichosis resulting from inhalation may occur (25, 26, 74). In occasional cases, disseminated infection may occur. Invasive and widely disseminated disease has been associated with AIDS (19).

Sporotrichosis is worldwide in distribution but occurs most frequently in temperate, humid climatic regions. Currently, the majority of reported cases are from North America (44). Other regions where the infection is endemic include South America, South Africa, and Southeast Asia. It is difficult to estimate the actual public health burden of disease, since there is no national surveillance; however, several outbreaks have been reported to date, and the disease can result in significant morbidity, especially in occupational groups who routinely handle soil or plant materials such as gardeners, florists, and carpenters (17, 18, 20, 31). For this reason, sporotrichosis has been regarded as an occupational disease. There are no clear associations with age, race, or sex; however, children are less often affected than adults. Sporotrichosis is not a transmissible disease.

Human lymphocutaneous infection, the classic clinical form of sporotrichosis, usually results from minor trauma and soil contamination

Clinical Features

Histoplasmosis

Acute Pulmonary Histoplasmosis

Most normal individuals remain asymptomatic following inhalation of low levels of *H. capsulatum* conidia. Inhalation of higher levels of conidia results, after an incubation period of 1 to 3 weeks, in an acute, symptomatic infection. The most common symptoms are fever, chills, headache, myalgia, anorexia, cough, and retrosternal or pleuritic chest pain. Approximately 10% of patients present with arthritis or severe arthralgia associated with erythema nodosum. Chest radiographs reveal small, scattered, reticulonodular infiltrates; hilar lymphadenopathy is often evident, and a pleural effusion may be present. The lung infiltrates tend to resolve over several months, leaving scattered calcifications throughout both lung fields. Most patients will recover without treatment, usually within 1 to 3 weeks. However, less commonly, their convalescence may be prolonged for several months. Healing of a localized, necrotic infiltrate may form a rounded, residual nodule, termed a histoplasmoma, which may itself enlarge with the deposition of surrounding scar tissue. The presence of intralesional calcification on chest radiographs may aid in distinguishing this benign entity from a pulmonary neoplasm.

Individuals reinfected with *H. capsulatum* develop a similar but milder illness, and the incubation period may be significantly shortened (less than 1 week). These patients present with abrupt onset of malaise, headache, chills, fever, and cough. On chest radiograph, multiple, small, interstitial, miliary nodules may be observed; however, mediastinal lymphadenopathy is absent, pleural effusions are not seen, and late calcification does not occur.

Individuals reinfected with H. capsulatum develop a similar but milder illness

Complications that may occur include hilar or mediastinal lymphadenitis that persists after clearing of the radiographic infiltrates, development of mediastinal fibrosis, and pericarditis secondary to erosion of the pericardium by enlarged mediastinal lymph nodes.

Chronic Pulmonary Histoplasmosis

Chronic pulmonary histoplasmosis is a slowly progressive illness that usually occurs in middle-aged men with underlying chronic obstructive lung disease. The initial symptoms often include a cough productive of sputum, fever, weight loss, malaise, and pleuritic chest pain. Frequently the patient's course extends over several weeks or months. The patient's clinical findings can mimic those of tuberculosis. The commonest findings on chest radiograph are interstitial pulmonary infiltrates in the apical segments of the upper lobes. Interstitial infiltrates often disappear, but chronic fibrosis and cavitation may develop. Lesions are more common in the right upper lobe, but bilateral upper lobe lesions develop in approximately 25% of patients, and in time, the infection will spread to the lower lobes (80). Pleural effusion is uncommon, but pleural thickening adjacent to lesions is found in more than 45% of patients (80). Without specific antifungal therapy, the patient's course is one of insidious pulmonary infection resulting in hemoptysis, recurrent bacterial infection with abscess formation, and death resulting from progressive lung failure.

Disseminated Histoplasmosis

Disseminated histoplasmosis is a progressive, often lethal illness that tends to develop in immunocompromised patients or other predisposed groups of individuals, particularly infants and persons over 55 years of age (28, 64). The clinical manifestations of disseminated histoplasmosis range from a fulminant illness that is fatal within a few weeks if untreated (often seen in infants and immunocompromised patients) to an indolent, chronic illness that can involve multiple different sites and persist for months or years. Symptomatic illness lasting more than 3 weeks suggests disseminated infection because most cases of acute histoplasmosis resolve in less than 2 weeks.

Infants and immunocompromised patients often present with fever, chills, prostration, malaise, anorexia, and weight loss. Common clinical findings include hepatosplenomegaly, abnormal liver function tests, and anemia. Chest radiographs are often normal or demonstrate diffuse interstitial infiltrates, rather than focal infiltrates (64). Pleural effusions are uncommon.

In contrast, in immunocompetent individuals, disseminated histoplasmosis follows an indolent, chronic course. Often chest radiographs are normal. Hepatic infection is common, but hepatosplenomegaly is less evident than in patients with the fulminant infection. Adrenal gland destruction is a frequent complication. Mucosal ulcers are found in over 60% of patients with indolent infection (7). Usually patients have a single lesion, painless at first, in the mouth or throat, with a characteristic, distinct heaped-up margin. Similar lesions in the gastrointestinal tract may cause bleeding, perforation, or, less often, obstruction. Meningitis or focal cerebral lesions occur in 10 to 25% of patients with indolent disseminated histoplasmosis (76). The main symptoms are headache and altered mental status, and often the diagnosis may be delayed in these patients. Most patients have abnormal cerebrospinal fluid (CSF) findings, including elevated protein concentration, lowered glucose concentration, and mild pleocytosis (76). Computed tomogram scans will reveal cerebral lesions. Chronic disseminated histoplasmosis may also cause endocarditis with typical large vegetations.

African Histoplasmosis

The clinical illness of *H. capsulatum* var. *duboisii* infection is usually indolent in onset and the predominant sites affected are the skin and bones (16, 47). Patients with more widespread infection involving the liver, spleen, and other organs have a febrile, wasting illness that is fatal within weeks or months if untreated. Bone lesions that are often painless usually involve the spine, ribs, cranial bones, sternum, and long bones. Multiple lesions are often found. The infection can spread into contiguous joints, causing arthritis, or into adjacent soft tissue, causing a purulent subcutaneous abscess. Other cutaneous manifestations of African histoplasmosis are subcutaneous

In immunocompetent individuals, disseminated histoplasmosis follows an indolent, chronic course

granulomata and nodular or papular lesions. Papules are common on the face and trunk. Both nodules and papules often enlarge and ulcerate.

Histoplasmosis in Special Hosts

Disseminated histoplasmosis is a particularly serious infection in AIDS patients who have resided in or traveled through regions with endemic disease (56). Fever and weight loss are the most common presenting symptoms. Up to 25% of infected patients demonstrate hepatosplenomegaly, and a similar proportion have anemia, leukopenia, and thrombocytopenia (34). Mucosal lesions are uncommon. Chest radiographs reveal diffuse interstitial or reticulonodular infiltrates in about 50% of AIDS patients with histoplasmosis (34, 77). However, approximately 30% of infected AIDS patients may present with a normal chest radiograph. Meningitis may be an uncommon complication in AIDS patients with histoplasmosis. Although the illness is usually gradual in onset, up to 10% of patients have presented with disseminated intravascular coagulation, often with multiple organ failure leading to rapid death (77, 79).

Disseminated histoplasmosis is a particularly serious infection in AIDS patients

Differential Diagnosis

The clinical presentation of patients with acute pulmonary histoplasmosis is quite nonspecific. Thus, for a patient with a febrile illness and a history of residence in or travel to an area of endemicity, it is essential that the clinician maintain a high index of suspicion; history taking may reveal a possible environmental exposure to *H. capsulatum* conidia. There may also be remarkable similarity in the clinical and radiologic findings of patients with chronic pulmonary histoplasmosis and those with tuberculosis, blastomycosis, and coccidioidomycosis, and these diagnoses may have to be excluded.

Phaeohyphomycosis

The major clinical forms of phaeohyphomycosis include subcutaneous infections, paranasal sinusitis, and systemic (cerebral) infections; however, cutaneous infections, endocarditis following cardiac valve surgery, peritonitis complicating chronic ambulatory peritoneal dialysis, and posttraumatic osteomyelitis and arthritis have rarely been reported (53, 55). The majority of reports concern patients with subcutaneous phaeohyphomycosis. This form of the disease most often occurs as a single lesion on an extremity and usually follows the traumatic implantation of the fungus into the subcutaneous tissues. Infection may result from relatively minor trauma, such as wounds due to thorns or wood splinters; however, patients may also not recall a specific injury because the lesion is very slow to progress, which may significantly delay them from seeking medical attention (i.e., months or years). The principal etiologic agents include *Exophiala jeanselmei*, *Exophiala spinifera*, *Exophiala* (*Wangiella*) *dermatitidis*, *Phialophora richardsiae*, and *Phialophora parasitica*. The initial lesion is a firm, sometimes tender, subcutaneous nodule, which may enlarge slowly to form a painless cystic abscess (5). Lesions are attached to the skin, but not to underlying structures. The overlying skin may often remain unaffected unless the cyst ruptures. In immunocompromised patients with subcutaneous phaeohyphomycosis, sinus formation and disseminated disease may occur.

Paranasal sinus infection is usually chronic and may remain confined to the sinuses or spread to involve contiguous structures. Patients may give a history of prolonged symptoms of allergic rhinitis, nasal polyps, or intermittent sinus pain (45). The principal etiologic agents include *Alternaria* spp., *Bipolaris spicifera*, *Bipolaris hawaiiensis*, *Curvularia lunata*, and *Exserohilum rostratum*. Clinical features may include nasal obstruction and facial pain, with or without proptosis. The sinuses often are filled with a dark, tenacious, inspissated mucus. In addition, *Alternaria* and *Curvularia* species have caused necrotic lesions of the nasal septum in occasional patients with leukemia or AIDS.

The cerebral form of phaeohyphomycosis may result from hematogenous dissemination from a primary pulmonary focus, or it may complicate a preexisting paranasal sinusitis. Most cases are due to *Cladophialophora bantiana* (*Xylohypha bantiana*, *Cladosporium bantianum*) (22). Other etiologic agents include *Bipolaris* spp. and *Exophiala dermatitidis*. Often patients with cerebral *C. bantiana* infection have no apparent predisposing factors. Initially, these patients may present with a gradual onset of persistent headache, but fever may be minimal or absent. Clinical findings may include focal neurologic signs, hemiparesis, and seizures. A computed tomographic scan of the head may reveal a unilateral, well-circumscribed lesion, usually in the frontal lobes of the brain. CSF findings may include an elevated opening pressure, increased protein concentration, reduced glucose concentration, and a pleocytosis. Rarely, the fungus may be isolated from CSF (22). However, usually a definitive diagnosis is established only at the time of neurosurgical resection of the lesion.

Cutaneous *Alternaria* sp. infections may be associated with crusted, ulcerated, or scaling skin lesions (51). These infections may follow traumatic implantation and have often occurred in patients with leukemia or transplant recipients. The extremities are the commonest sites of infection.

Differential Diagnosis

The lesions of subcutaneous phaeohyphomycosis may be confused with the early lesions of blastomycosis, chromoblastomycosis, coccidioidomycosis, sporotrichosis and paracoccidioidomycosis, and cutaneous leishmaniasis (62). Lack of lymphangitic involvement, as occurs in sporotrichosis, and infrequent development of verrucous lesions, as occurs in these other conditions, suggest phaeohyphomycosis. In nonimmunocompromised individuals, the clinical presentation of paranasal phaeohyphomycotic sinusitis may closely resemble that of an *Aspergillus* infection. In immunocompromised patients, unlike phaeohyphomycotic sinusitis, aspergillus sinusitis is usually a fulminant, often lethal condition; however, both groups of fungi can cause black necrotic lesions of the nasal septum. The clinical presentation of a patient with cerebral phaeohyphomycosis may most closely resemble that of a patient with a bacterial brain abscess. Rarely, the diagnosis of crypto-

The lesions of subcutaneous phaeohyphomycosis may be confused with the early lesions of several fungal and parasitic infections

coccosis, coccidioidomycosis, histoplasmosis, or sporotrichosis must be excluded in these patients.

Sporotrichosis

Sporotrichosis may be associated with various clinical presentations. Lymphocutaneous infection is the most common clinical form of the disease. Rarely, the fungus may cause infection of the lungs, joints, bones, eyes, and meninges. Invasive, disseminated infection has been reported to occur particularly in diabetics, alcoholics, intravenous drug abusers, and AIDS patients.

Cutaneous sporotrichosis typically affects the extremities, especially the hands and fingers. Initially, a painless nodule develops at the site of implantation of the fungus. The skin overlying the nodule becomes progressively erythematous, ulcerates, and discharges a serous or purulent fluid (44). Within a few days to several weeks, additional lesions may develop around the primary lesion and also along the course of the draining lymphatics. These soon become palpable and may ulcerate through the skin. Usually, however, the lymphangitis heals or remains unchanged for a long time without ulcers forming. Commonly, the regional lymph nodes are uninvolved; however, involvement of these lymph nodes may also result from a superimposed bacterial infection. Lesions may be described as papulopustular, nodulopustular, papillomatous or verrucous, infiltrative, or ulcerative, and several ulcers may be interconnected by subcutaneous fistulae (44). Confluent lesions may form a purulent and warty plaque with an expanding margin and central cutaneous atrophy. Although the lesions of sporotrichosis are generally painless, they may often be pruritic. Primary cutaneous lesions may heal spontaneously but may leave residual scars that are disfiguring and cause a functional impairment. Secondary lesions may be more chronic and persist for several years.

Pulmonary sporotrichosis is a rare but well-recognized condition. It may be primary, following the inhalation of conidia, and be accompanied by enlargement of the hilar or tracheobronchial lymph nodes, but it also may be secondary to hematogenous dissemination. The symptoms are nonspecific and include cough, sputum production, fever, and weight loss. Hemoptysis may occur and can be massive and fatal. The course may be chronic. The typical radiologic finding is a single, nodular, upper lobe lesion which may or may not cavitate. The natural course of the lung lesion is gradual progression to death.

Pulmonary sporotrichosis is a rare but well-recognized condition

Most patients with osteoarticular sporotrichosis also have preceding cutaneous lesions. This condition presents as stiffness and pain in a large joint which is indolent in onset. In almost all cases of arthritis, the knee, elbow, ankle, or wrist is involved. Osteomyelitis seldom occurs without arthritis; the lesions are usually confined to the long bones near affected joints (60). Endophthalmitis, although rare, may result in blindness; chorioretinitis has also been reported, as well as have cases of meningitis.

Differential Diagnosis

The development of a cutaneous lesion on the limbs following trauma is suggestive of sporotrichosis if the patient resides in an endemic disease region.

The development of multiple ulcers along the course of lymphatics is also suspicious. During the latter stages of development, lesions of sporotrichosis must be distinguished from those of mycoses such as blastomycosis, chromoblastomycosis, or paracoccidioidomycosis, and from leishmaniasis, verrucous tuberculosis, and tertiary syphilis. The diagnosis ultimately depends on mycologic and histologic examination.

Diagnosis

Histoplasmosis

Direct Examination
The detection of single, budding, yeastlike cells, 2 to 5 μm in diameter, which are primarily intracellular, by direct examination or histologic study of biopsy specimens should raise strong suspicion that the fungus is *H. capsulatum* var. *capsulatum*. This finding, however, is not diagnostic per se, since several other fungal pathogens mimic the intracellular forms of *H. capsulatum* var. *capsulatum*. Giemsa- or Wright-stained preparations may be useful with bronchoalveolar lavage fluid, bone marrow aspirates, or blood smears (42), while the periodic acid-Schiff (PAS) and Gomori's methenamine silver (GMS) stains are useful with tissues. The use of immunofluorescent reagents allows the specific identification of the yeast form of *H. capsulatum* var. *capsulatum* and its differentiation from mycotic and nonmycotic look-alikes (39). If clinical specimens contain large, thick-walled yeast cells and come from patients with a history of visiting or residing in Africa or Madagascar, then *H. capsulatum* var. *duboisii* should be considered as the pathogen. In vivo, the *duboisii* variety of *H. capsulatum* morphologically resembles *Blastomyces dermatitidis*, which also causes disease in parts of Africa. *H. capsulatum* var. *duboisii* may be identified by its narrow-based buds, by its uninucleate character, or by immunofluorescent staining (38, 39).

Isolation and Identification

Isolation and identification of H. capsulatum from clinical materials may take 2 to 4 weeks and require special media

Isolation and identification of *H. capsulatum* from clinical materials may take 2 to 4 weeks and require special media to reduce contamination by bacteria and a variety of saprophytic fungi. CSF, blood, and bone marrow are excellent sources of the fungus in immunocompromised patients. The lysis-centrifugation technique is very useful for concentrating blood for the isolation of *H. capsulatum* (42). The isolation of downy white to brownish colonies, characterized by production of tuberculate macroconidia, is only suggestive of *H. capsulatum*, since saprophytic species in the genera *Arthroderma*, *Chrysosporium*, *Renispora*, and *Sepedonium* also produce tuberculate conidia. To further complicate identification, atypical nonsporulating and red- and yellow-pigmented isolates of *H. capsulatum* var. *capsulatum* have been encountered, and these may be confused with other saprophytic and pathogenic fungi (38, 70).

Unequivocal identification of a mycelial isolate as an *H. capsulatum* variety requires conversion to the yeast form, which can take 3 to 6 weeks, or identification by commercially available exoantigen immunoidentification tests or the more rapid DNA probe (Gen-Probe, San Diego, Calif.). Conversion may occur on brain heart infusion agar or other suitable medium at 37°C after approximately 1 to 4 weeks of incubation. With the exoantigen test, definitive results are achievable within 48 to 72 h of receipt of a mature culture. Only isolates of *H. capsulatum* produce the diagnostic H and M antigens. The DNA probe is 100% sensitive and specific for *H. capsulatum*. It allows an unequivocal identification of the pathogen 2 h after testing 1 to 2 µl of a yeast or mycelial colony. None of the methods, however, allows differentiation of the two varieties of *H. capsulatum* (38).

Immunodiagnosis

Immunologic evidence often provides the first clues in establishing a definitive diagnosis of histoplasmosis. Such evidence may be obtained through commercially available complement fixation (CF), immunodiffusion (ID), and latex agglutination (LA) antibody kits or by the double-antibody sandwich radioimmunoassay or enzyme immunoassay (EIA) tests (23, 40) for *H. capsulatum* polysaccharide antigen. The CF tests, although sensitive, are not entirely specific. The CF and ID tests with histoplasmin as antigen have a sensitivity of about 80%, whereas the CF test with the yeast-form antigens has a greater sensitivity. The CF test, when run in conjunction with the ID test, yields reliable results. Because H and M antigens of histoplasmin are specific for *H. capsulatum*, the ID test provides a more accurate diagnosis with sera that have low titers or cross-react in CF tests. In the absence of a recent histoplasmin skin test, the detection of the M precipitin may serve as an indicator of early histoplasmosis. The demonstration of both H and M precipitins is highly suggestive of active disease, regardless of other serologic test results. The detection of such precipitins in CSF specimens may be considered evidence of meningeal histoplasmosis. CF titers of 1:8 or greater with either antigen are generally considered presumptive evidence of histoplasmosis. Titers of 1:32 or greater and increasing titers offer stronger presumptive evidence (38). The histoplasmin LA test may help detect early acute primary histoplasmosis, but it is frequently negative with sera from patients with chronic histoplasmosis.

One must be aware that levels of histoplasmin antibodies detected by CF, ID, or LA tests may be induced or significantly increased in histoplasmin-sensitized persons after a single histoplasmin skin test. Detection of *H. capsulatum* polysaccharide antigen provides a rapid means of diagnosing disseminated histoplasmosis in AIDS patients and in those otherwise immunocompromised. The antigen is found in the urine of 90% and in the blood of 50% of patients with disseminated disease. Antigenuria detection offers an opportunity for early diagnosis of histoplasmosis since it is usually present at the time of clinical illness, whereas cultures may not become positive until 2 to 4 weeks later. Unfortunately, cross-reactivity with antigens of other endemic mycotic agents must be considered in interpreting a positive reaction, since specimens from patients with blastomycosis, coccidioidomycosis, paracoccidioidomycosis, and penicilliosis marneffei may also be positive (40).

Levels of histoplasmin antibodies detected by CF, ID, or LA tests may be induced or significantly increased in histoplasmin-sensitized persons

Phaeohyphomycosis

Isolation and Identification

Because the agents of phaeohyphomycosis cannot be identified on the basis of their morphologic appearance in clinical materials, isolation is necessary for their identification. Care must be taken to avoid isolation of contaminants from clinical material. The isolate should be morphologically consistent with the fungus recognized in the clinical specimen. Clinical specimens such as those submitted for direct examination should be cultured on Sabouraud dextrose agar (SDA) containing chloramphenicol, on SDA containing both chloramphenicol and cycloheximide, and on corn meal agar. Cultures should be incubated at 30°C and 37°C. Growth is usually apparent after 7 to 10 days. Negative cultures should be incubated for 6 weeks. After 7 days of incubation, the cultures should be characterized on the basis of their colonial and microscopic features. Colonies should manifest a yeastlike, velvety, or woolly appearance and be deeply pigmented, grey, olive, or black in color. On SDA they should consist of septate, branched, yellow-brown hyphae with or without conidia. If conidia are absent, they can be induced on corn meal agar. Identification of a phaeoid fungus can be difficult. Important characteristics to be considered include type of conidiation, proteolysis, decomposition of casein and tyrosine, thermotolerance, and resistance to cycloheximide. Because of the extensive diversity demonstrated by the agents of phaeohyphomycosis, specific identification of the etiologic agents is beyond the scope of this presentation, and the reader is referred to reference 65.

Immunodiagnosis

Standardized serologic tests are not available for the diseases caused by the phaeohyphomycotic agents

Standardized serologic tests are not available for the diseases caused by the phaeohyphomycotic agents. Preliminary studies, however, suggest that such tests may be useful. Studies with sera from a patient with a brain abscess due to *Cladophialophora bantiana* and from a patient with pulmonary disease due to *Ochroconis gallopava* indicated that precipitins to these agents could be detected. Reliable exoantigen tests for the immunoidentification of cultures have been developed (41, 67). These tests have been used for the rapid and accurate identification of *Cladophialophora bantiana*, *Exophiala jeanselmei*, *Exophiala spinifera*, *Ochroconis gallopava*, and *Exophiala dermatitidis*. Exoantigen tests have also proved valuable for studying antigenic and taxonomic relationships among fungi. Such studies have revealed that *E. jeanselmei* has three serotypes. Isolates that cause mycetomas have been identified as serotype 1, whereas those that cause phaeohyphomycosis belong to serotypes 1, 2, or 3. In addition, exoantigen analyses revealed that *C. bantiana* and *C. trichoides* are antigenically identical and support their synonymy.

Sporotrichosis

Direct Examination

In most human lesions due to *S. schenckii* it is difficult to find the organisms. Gram-stained smears are of little value as the few organisms present are difficult to differentiate from other tissue elements. With biopsy specimens, PAS or GMS stains and specific fluorescent-antibody tests (40, 59) are more helpful because even a few fungal cells stand out clearly. With the fluorescent-antibody procedure, lesional exudates and histologic materials may be specifically stained. The morphology of the yeast cells of *S. schenckii* varies from globose budding cells to cigar-shaped cells; these range in size from 2 to 6 μm or 3 to 10 μm, respectively. *S. schenckii*, although hyaline in tissue, is considered by some to be phaeoid since in tissue, melanin can be demonstrated in the yeast cells with the Fontana-Masson stain, and in culture the fungus is phaeoid (65). *S. schenckii* var. *luriei* in tissue demonstrates large, thick-walled cells measuring 10 to 30 μm in diameter which divide by fission; many show the classical eyeglass-shaped form produced by incomplete separation of a septate cell. Yeastlike cells similar to those of *S. schenckii* var. *schenckii* are also produced in tissue.

Isolation and Identification

The fungus may be isolated from pus obtained from skin lesions, from ground-up biopsy tissues, or from other clinical specimens. Culture is important since several fungal pathogens are morphologically similar in clinical specimens. *S. schenckii* develops rapidly on SDA at 25°C. Since it is not inhibited by either chloramphenicol or cycloheximide, media containing these antibiotics are useful in selectively isolating the fungus from clinical materials. Within 3 to 7 days, moist white colonies appear that soon develop wrinkled surfaces. After 1 to 2 weeks of growth, the colony becomes brownish and finally black. Microscopic examination reveals narrow (2-μm-diameter), branching, septate hyphae. Single-celled conidia are produced from slender, tapering conidiophores rising at right angles from the hyphae. The conidia (2 to 3 by 3 to 6 μm) are pyriform or oval and are borne on delicate sterigmata as "flower-like petals." Conidia may be hyaline or pigmented. Except for being longer, the conidial structures of *S. schenckii* var. *luriei* are essentially similar to those of *S. schenckii* var. *schenckii*. These are best demonstrated in slide culture preparations. It is essential to demonstrate the tissue form to identify the pathogen. This can be accomplished by conversion of the mycelial form to the yeast form on BHI agar incubated at 37°C. Creamy, white yeastlike growth composed of budding cells (2 to 6 μm) will be apparent. The yeast form of *S. schenckii* var. *luriei* is indistinguishable from that of the typical variety.

Immunodiagnosis

Serologic tests may be useful in the diagnosis of sporotrichosis, especially in extracutaneous or disseminated disease, when distinct clinical features are lacking. Serologic tests may be applied to sera from patients with skin lesions, subcutaneous nodules, lymphadenopathy, or pulmonary disease, and to CSF from patients with undiagnosed chronic meningitis. Three tests have proved satisfactory: EIA, tube agglutination, and LA. The antigen that is the basis for these tests is most likely the peptido-L-rhamno-D-mannan found in the cell wall of the fungus. The LA and EIA tests are

Serologic tests may be useful in the diagnosis of sporotrichosis, especially in extracutaneous or disseminated disease

highly recommended because of their excellent sensitivity, high specificity, and ability to provide rapid results. The tube agglutination test has good sensitivity, but sera from patients with leishmaniasis may show false-positive reactions at low titers. An EIA titer of 1:16 in serum or 1:8 in CSF is considered positive. CSF titers of 1:8 or greater are considered specific. A positive titer in CSF is strong evidence for meningeal sporotrichosis. LA titers of 1:4 or greater are considered presumptive evidence of sporotrichosis. Sera from patients with localized cutaneous, subcutaneous, disseminated subcutaneous, or systemic sporotrichosis may show titers ranging from 1:4 to 1:512. LA titers of 1:4 or greater with CSF are helpful in diagnosing chronic meningitis due to *S. schenckii*. The LA test has limited prognostic value, whereas EIA antibody titers frequently decline with successful treatment (40).

Pathology

Histoplasmosis

In tissue sections, the yeastlike cells of *H. capsulatum* var. *capsulatum* are hyaline, spherical to oval, and 2 to 4 μm in diameter and produce single buds attached to parent cells by relatively narrow bases. The fungal cells are remarkably uniform in appearance, and they are often clustered within large mononuclear phagocytes (6, 12). Rarely, short hyphae and huge, thick-walled, bizarre yeast forms of *H. capsulatum* var. *capsulatum* can be found along with typical-sized forms on or near the surface of valvular vegetations in histoplasma endocarditis (71). This morphologic diversity of histoplasma cells appears to be an intravascular phenomenon (32).

In acute pulmonary histoplasmosis capsulati, alveolar spaces are filled with large macrophages that are packed with spherical to oval, single and budding yeast forms of *H. capsulatum* var. *capsulatum* (11, 63) (Fig. 6.1). Alveolar spaces also may contain cellular debris, fibrin, and fewer extracellular yeasts. Mild interstitial inflammation is usually noted. In hematoxylin and eosin (H&E)-stained tissue sections, the hematoxylinophilic cytoplasm of individual fungal cells is retracted from the thin, poorly stained but rigid cell wall, giving the false impression of an unstained capsule or optically clear "halo." With the special stains for fungi (GMS, PAS, or Gridley), the pseudocapsular effect is not evident because fungal cell walls are uniformly colored by these procedures (11, 63) (Fig. 6.2).

Organs most commonly involved in disseminated histoplasmosis capsulati are the lungs, lymph nodes, spleen, liver, bone marrow, gastrointestinal tract, and adrenal glands

Organs most commonly involved in disseminated histoplasmosis capsulati are the lungs, lymph nodes, spleen, liver, bone marrow, gastrointestinal tract, and adrenal glands, all of which contain abundant mononuclear phagocytes (12, 30). Microscopically, single and budding yeast forms of *H. capsulatum* var. *capsulatum* are almost always seen within the cytoplasm of these cells, hence the designation "histiocytomycotic" or "reticuloendothelial cytomycotic" disease in the older literature. Marked infiltration and proliferation of histiocytes in many organs often obliterates normal histologic architecture, and bland necrosis also may be seen. Necrosis of the adrenal glands due to histiocytic proliferation may cause symptoms of Addison's disease (30). Fewer lymphocytes and plasma cells may be present, but polymorphonuclear leukocytes are rare. In general, numerous cells of *H. capsulatum* var. *capsulatum* proliferate extracellularly and within bland, loosely arranged histiocytes in the profoundly immunodeficient host (35, 52, 79) (Fig. 6.2), whereas in the immunocompetent host fungal elements are less numerous and elicit an epithelioid and giant cell granulomatous reaction with or without caseation (11, 63) (Fig. 6.3). In immunodeficient patients, especially those with AIDS, the yeast-form cells are often more variable in size and shape; germ tubes and pseudohyphae may be produced by the rapidly proliferating fungal cells.

Many patients with active histoplasmosis capsulati have latent, asymptomatic disease that is not recognized until old, "healed," necrotic and sometimes calcified lesions are noted as an incidental finding at autopsy or at biopsy to rule out malignancy (29). These residual lesions have been variously termed "tuberculomas," histoplasmomas, fibrocaseous nodules, and burned-out granulomas (11, 72). They are usually located in the lungs, just beneath the pleura, and are less frequently found in the spleen, liver, lymph nodes, and other organs. Microscopically, the nodules consist of large, caseous, often irregularly calcified centers surrounded by thick fibrotic capsules that may contain scattered epithelioid histiocytes, multinucleated giant cells, and peripheral lymphoid aggregates (11, 12) (Fig. 6.3). When present, fungal cells are usually sparse and located within the central caseous residuum as extracellular forms; they appear singly or in small clusters, the latter due to their intracellular confinement before death of their host cells. Fungal elements are almost impossible to demonstrate with the H&E stain. However, a careful search with the GMS stain usually reveals varying numbers of yeast forms that are generally distorted, fragmented, and poorly stained ("ghost" forms); budding is infrequent, and attempts to culture the fungus from residual lesions are often unsuccessful (Fig. 6.4). Granular calcifications (calcific bodies) within the central caseous material are hematoxylinophilic and PAS positive and can resemble small yeasts. However, the former are generally more pleomorphic, and they do not stain with GMS (11, 12).

Intracellular, capsule-deficient cryptococci mimic the intracellular forms of *H. capsulatum* var. *capsulatum* and present a diagnostic challenge. Cryptococci, however, are more pleomorphic and range in size from 2 to 20 μm. Also, most capsule-deficient cryptococci are at least weakly carminophilic when tissue sections containing these fungi are stained with Mayer's mucicarmine procedure. Small tissue forms ("microforms") of *Blastomyces dermatitidis* also may be confused with the yeast-form cells of *H. capsulatum* var. *capsulatum*, but the former are usually more pleomorphic, bud by a much broader base, have thick "double-contoured" walls, are multinucleated, and are often mixed with *B. dermatitidis* cells of typical size. In tissue, the yeast-like cells of *Torulopsis* (*Candida*) *glabrata* can be easily confused with those of *H. capsulatum* var. *capsulatum* because they are comparable in size and both may occur intracellularly. *T. glabrata* cells often are slightly larger than those

Intracellular, capsule-deficient cryptococci mimic the intracellular forms of H. capsulatum *var.* capsulatum

of *H. capsulatum* var. *capsulatum*, oval to elongated yeast forms of *T. glabrata* are more common, budding occurs with greater frequency, and individual yeast forms are amphophilic and stain entirely with H&E; there is no pseudocapsular or "halo" effect. In all of these instances, immunohistologic techniques are valuable adjuncts for confirming a presumptive histologic diagnosis (11).

Intracellular forms of the protozoan *Leishmania donovani* appear similar to cells of *H. capsulatum* var. *capsulatum*, but under oil immersion, bar-shaped kinetoplasts (paranuclear bodies) can be seen within the *L. donovani* cells, especially with Wolbach's Giemsa and Wilder's reticulum stains. The fungal cells have no such structure. Clusters of *Toxoplasma gondii* cells within mononuclear phagocytes also can mimic the yeast forms of *H. capsulatum* var. *capsulatum*, but under oil immersion the *T. gondii* cells are slightly smaller and lack an optically clear zone or "halo" around each organism. GMS and other special stains for fungi do not reliably stain individual cells of these two protozoans.

Phaeohyphomycosis

Subcutaneous lesions (phaeomycotic cysts) develop at the site of inoculation and are usually located on the extremities. They generally enlarge slowly, ranging from 0.4 to 7.0 cm or more in diameter, and can be mistaken clinically for a synovial cyst or giant cell tumor of the tendon sheath (58). Lymphangitis and regional lymphadenopathy are uncommon. Progressive disseminated phaeohyphomycosis following percutaneous infection is very rare (10).

In systemic (cerebral) phaeohyphomycosis, the route of infection is generally via the respiratory tract, and the most commonly encountered agent is *Cladophialophora bantiana* (formerly *Xylohypha bantiana*, *Cladosporium bantianum*). This fungus is particularly neurotropic, and most infections are confined to the brain and meninges, with only rare involvement of other organs. The primary pulmonary infection is usually inapparent (15, 21). Cerebral lesions are either solitary or multiple, up to 5 cm in diameter, and appear as encapsulated abscesses similar to those encountered in phaeomycotic cysts, or as generalized inflammatory infiltrates with necrosis (61).

The host reaction in phaeohyphomycosis is similar regardless of the causative agent or the tissues affected (10, 13). It is characterized by the formation of cystic or dispersed granulomas that are usually solitary and encapsulated and contain foci of suppurative necrosis (Fig. 6.5). A histopathologic diagnosis is made by demonstrating phaeoid (brown), moniliform hyphae within the walls and necrotic centers of the granulomas (Fig. 6.6 and 6.7). The hyphae range from 2 to 6 μm in width and may be branched; they are often closely septate and constricted at their prominent septations, and they sometimes contain bizarre, thick-walled, vesicular swellings that reach a diameter of 25 μm or more and resemble chlamydoconidia (10, 13). Budding yeastlike cells also may be present. Occasionally, the natural brown pigmentation of the fungi may not be readily apparent, but a detailed search will almost always reveal at least some phaeoid fungal

In systemic (cerebral) phaeohyphomycosis, the route of infection is generally via the respiratory tract

elements in H&E-stained or unstained (cleared and mounted) tissue sections. When pigmentation is not observed or is equivocal in H&E-stained sections, the Fontana-Masson stain for melanin can sometimes accentuate and confirm the presence of melanoid pigments in the fungal cell walls (10, 82). The agents of phaeohyphomycosis are easily demonstrated with the special stains for fungi, especially the GMS procedure. However, special stains are usually unnecessary because the brown pigmentation of the cell walls highlights the phaeoid fungal elements. Because special stains mask the natural brown color of the fungi (Fig. 6.8), a diagnosis of phaeohyphomycosis may be missed unless a replicate H&E-stained or unstained tissue section is carefully examined.

H&E-stained sections of an excised phaeomycotic cyst typically reveal a cystic granuloma surrounded by dense fibrous connective tissue in the deep dermis and subcutaneous tissue (13, 83) (Fig. 6.5). The wall of the granuloma consists of compact epithelioid histiocytes admixed with numerous multinucleated giant cells of both the foreign body and Langhans' types (Fig. 6.6). Centrally, there are one or more geographic and stellate areas of suppurative necrosis. Within epithelioid and giant cells in the wall of the granuloma, and extracellularly amid the central cellular debris, are polymorphous fungal elements that are naturally pigmented, appearing light to dark brown. The fungi are distinctly moniliform and easily highlighted by their natural pigmentation. Foreign materials, such as splinters or thorns, are sometimes located within the lesion and are presumed to be the vehicles of percutaneous inoculation (13, 33).

Because the multiple recognized agents of phaeohyphomycosis are morphologically and tinctorially similar in infected tissue, they cannot be differentiated from each other. Nevertheless, a disease diagnosis can be based on the natural brown color of morphologically typical, phaeoid fungi within suppurative and granulomatous lesions, or forming fungus balls within sinuses and cavities (Fig. 6.7). Immunohistochemical reagents for identifying these fungi are not currently available; culture is needed for their specific identification.

An important consideration in the histopathologic differential diagnosis of phaeohyphomycosis is chromoblastomycosis, a chronic cutaneous and subcutaneous mycosis of humans caused by any one of several dematiaceous fungi—*Fonsecaea pedrosoi*, *Phialophora verrucosa*, *Cladophialophora carrionii*, *Fonsecaea compacta*, and *Rhinocladiella aquaspersa* (27, 54). A diagnosis of chromoblastomycosis can be based on the presence of dark brown, spherical to polyhedral muriform cells or "sclerotic bodies" that characteristically have thick walls, divide by septation in two planes, and do not form chains of cells (10). Because the septate muriform cells of chromoblastomycosis are morphologically distinctive, they should not be mistaken for the phaeoid, polymorphous fungal elements of phaeohyphomycosis.

In tissue sections, phaeohyphomycosis also can be confused with black grain mycetomas caused by dematiaceous fungi (10, 13). However, the causative agents of mycetomas form distinct granules. The causative agents of phaeohyphomycosis do not form true granules but appear as individual

An important consideration in the histopathologic differential diagnosis of phaeohyphomycosis is chromoblastomycosis

fungal elements or small but loose aggregates of elements that may rarely be ensheathed by Splendore-Hoeppli material. These fungi are often intracellular, whereas granules of the mycetomas are nearly always extracellular.

Sporotrichosis

Microscopically, *S. schenckii* usually provokes a mixed suppurative and granulomatous inflammatory reaction that is often accompanied by fibrosis (9, 48). This mixed inflammatory response is typical of both cutaneous and disseminated forms of the disease (Fig. 6.9), but it is not specific (8). A similar pattern of inflammation may be seen in certain other mycoses, e.g., blastomycosis and coccidioidomycosis, and in certain bacterial diseases, e.g., tuberculosis, syphilis, cat scratch disease, and tularemia. In tissue sections, *S. schenckii* appears as spherical, oval, or elongated (cigar-shaped) single or budding yeastlike cells, 2 to 6 μm or more in diameter (Fig. 6.10). The fungal cells bud by a relatively narrow base, and in some instances multiple budding is seen. Although considered by some to be the classic form of the organism in tissue, cigar-shaped forms (cigar bodies) are, in our experience, not regularly found (9, 14). When present, they are mixed with a predominant population of spherical to oval forms and are most often observed in disseminated lesions. Large, spherical, yeastlike cells up to 10 μm in diameter, germinating forms, and hyphae of *S. schenckii* may occasionally be found, particularly in disseminated lesions or experimental lesions of animals (9, 50).

Lesions of cutaneous sporotrichosis are usually characterized by segmental hyperkeratosis, acanthosis, and pseudoepitheliomatous hyperplasia overlying an intense dermal inflammatory reaction composed of neutrophils, lymphocytes, plasma cells, macrophages, fibroblasts, and multinucleated giant cells of both the foreign body and Langhans' types (9, 50) (Fig. 6.9). Fungal cells are difficult to demonstrate with H&E, but the GMS stain reveals small numbers of spherical, oval, and elongated single or budding yeast forms 3 to 6 μm in diameter in the dermis and within intraepidermal microabscesses. Fungal elements are both intracellular and extracellular, and *S. schenckii* cells often bear elongated ("teardrop" or "pipestem") buds (9, 14). An interesting and rare finding in lesions of cutaneous sporotrichosis is the presence of slender hyphae bearing conidia within transepidermal elimination channels and in the hyperkeratotic layer of the epidermis (7). Generally, only a few *S. schenckii* cells are found in cutaneous lesions of humans, and special stains, preferably GMS, complemented by specific immunohistologic procedures (Fig. 6.11), are needed to identify the fungus in formalin-fixed, paraffin-embedded tissues (9, 14).

The asteroid body of sporotrichosis consists of one or more fungal cells intimately surrounded by a stellate, radial corona of Splendore-Hoeppli material that is refractile and brightly eosinophilic and measures up to 100 μm in diameter (9, 49) (Fig. 6.12). Asteroid bodies are almost always located within microabscesses in the dermis and epidermis or within suppurative centers of granulomas in other organs. Occasionally, the centrally located fungal cell(s) will not be visible, even in sections stained with the GMS procedure. The asteroid body is not pathognomonic for sporotrichosis. Splendore-

Generally, only a few S. schenckii cells are found in cutaneous lesions of humans

Hoeppli material may be seen surrounding microcolonies of bacteria in actinomycosis and botryomycosis, parasite ova, foreign objects such as suture material, and other species of fungi, particularly *Coccidioides immitis*, *Aspergillus* spp., *Candida* spp., agents of entomophthoromycosis, and some of the agents that cause mycetomas (9, 46). Therefore, a diagnosis of sporotrichosis cannot be based solely on the presence of asteroid bodies. Because asteroid formation does not occur in many cases of sporotrichosis, the absence of asteroid bodies does not rule out the possibility of this mycosis.

We and others have examined tissues from several patients with pulmonary sporotrichosis that was presumed to be primary (25, 26, 74). Histopathologically, the pulmonary lesions closely resembled those of histoplasmosis capsulati and tuberculosis and consisted of large and sometimes confluent necrotizing and nonnecrotizing granulomas (9, 25). Organisms, sometimes abundant and easily mistaken for other small yeast forms, were usually located in the necrotic or suppurative centers of the granulomas or within giant and epithelioid cells at the periphery. We also have seen solitary, peripheral, pulmonary nodules of sporotrichosis that, in H&E-stained sections, were indistinguishable from the fibrocaseous nodules (histoplasmomas) seen in residual pulmonary histoplasmosis capsulati (9, 74). However, unlike the latter, calcification was not observed within the central caseous material of the sporotrichomas. In all of these cases, immunohistologic procedures were required for a definitive histologic diagnosis of sporotrichosis (9, 74).

A new and unique variety of *S. schenckii*, named *S. schenckii* var. *luriei*, was first isolated from a cutaneous lesion of a South African in 1969. Since its first description by Ajello and Kaplan (3), several other cases caused by this variety have been reported. Most of these cases have originated in Europe, India, or South Africa (4). In tissue, *S. schenckii* var. *luriei* produces typical, small, yeastlike cells that divide by budding and large (up to 20 μm), spherical, thick-walled cells that divide by either budding or septation. In the latter process, daughter cells separate by dissolution of the parent cell wall (9).

Treatment

Histoplasmosis
Specific antifungal therapy is rarely indicated for patients with acute pulmonary histoplasmosis, and often spontaneous clinical improvement has begun before the diagnosis is made (75). Only those patients with severe acute pulmonary histoplasmosis, pneumonia that fails to resolve in several months, or chronic cavitary pulmonary histoplasmosis should receive antifungal therapy. Chronic, progressive, disseminated histoplasmosis requires therapy. Itraconazole (generally a dose of 200 mg/day) is the treatment of choice for most types of histoplasmosis except meningitis, endocarditis, and life-threatening pulmonary or disseminated histoplasmosis (20). If the patient fails to respond after several weeks, the dose may be increased to 200 mg twice daily. The total duration of therapy required is not known. Most

Specific antifungal therapy is rarely indicated for patients with acute pulmonary histoplasmosis

*F*or life-threatening forms of histoplasmosis, amphotericin B remains the treatment of choice

patients should receive therapy for at least 6 months. Chronic cavitary pulmonary histoplasmosis is the most difficult form of the disease to treat, which is probably related to underlying chronic obstructive pulmonary disease in these patients (29); often therapy is required for at least 1 year. For life-threatening forms of histoplasmosis, amphotericin B remains the treatment of choice (75). The management of HIV-infected patients with histoplasmosis may be especially difficult. Itraconazole (200 mg three times a day for 3 days and then 200 mg twice daily, and after an initial 12-week course, 200 mg daily for lifelong maintenance) can be used if patients are not acutely ill and do not have meningeal involvement (35, 36). Patients with moderately severe or life-threatening infection or meningeal disease, or patients unable to take oral drugs, should be treated initially with amphotericin B. Then, when cultures are negative for *H. capsulatum* in these patients and their clinical parameters have stabilized, this therapy can be changed to itraconazole (35, 36).

Phaeohyphomycosis

Subcutaneous phaeohyphomycosis requires complete surgical excision of the lesion. Incision and drainage of subcutaneous lesions is unlikely to be successful (i.e., the lesions may recur) (62). Systemic antifungal therapy with amphotericin B has cured or improved nonresectable lesions; however, relapsing infection has been common in these patients (45, 62). Paranasal sinus infection also responds best to the combination of complete surgical debridement and systemic antifungal therapy (amphotericin B) (45). Nevertheless, despite this combination of therapies, it is not uncommon for the condition to recur. Repeated surgical debridement may be essential for patients with disabling symptoms or erosion of the bone separating the paranasal sinus from the brain. Oral itraconazole (100 to 400 mg/day) appears to constitute promising therapy; however, the optimum dosage and duration of this treatment have not yet been defined (68). Necrotic lesions of the nasal septum due to *Alternaria* or *Curvularia* species have been cured following surgical excision (45). Complete surgical resection is essential in all patients with cerebral phaeohyphomycosis; lesions that have not been completely removed have usually proved fatal.

Sporotrichosis

Saturated potassium iodide solution (SSKI) remains an easily administered, low-cost, and effective drug for treating patients with lymphocutaneous or cutaneous sporotrichosis. However, the use of SSKI is associated with a relatively high incidence of side effects. The SSKI starting dose is 5 to 10 drops in water three times daily, and this is increased by 5 drops each week until a total of 40 to 50 drops is administered three times daily if tolerated by the patient (44). Treatment should be continued for at least a month after clinical cure is obtained, which may take 2 to 4 months. Local heat, alone or in combination with drug treatment, has been shown to improve cutaneous lesions. Although not approved by the Food and Drug Administration for the treatment of sporotrichosis, itraconazole is better tolerated than SSKI and has become the drug of choice for this infection (36, 69, 81). The usual dose is 200 mg/day for 3 to 6 months. A higher dose (200 mg twice daily) and longer course (1 year) are recommended for the therapy for osteoarticular sporotrichosis, and surgical debridement may also be indicated. Therapy for pulmonary sporotrichosis with either itraconazole (200 mg twice daily) or amphotericin B has been problematic; response rates may be <50%, and some patients may require lifelong therapy. Patients with meningeal sporotrichosis or those who are severely ill should be initially treated with amphotericin B. Fluconazole should be considered only as second-line therapy and could be used for patients who do not tolerate or cannot absorb itraconazole (37).

Prevention

Histoplasmosis
Prevention efforts should be directed at educating the public in regions of endemic histoplasmosis about measures to avoid either occupational or recreational exposures to microfoci of soil that may be contaminated with bird or bat excrement. Public education about the risks of disturbing such foci may prevent many exposures, especially those associated with building construction and renovation projects. Soil known to be heavily contaminated by *H. capsulatum* that must be disturbed can be decontaminated by treatment with a 3% formalin solution, with strict observation of state and local regulations pertaining to its use. Development of an effective vaccine against histoplasmosis should be made a priority. It is not known if chronic prophylactic administration of an azole can prevent the development of disseminated histoplasmosis in the HIV-infected population.

Prevention efforts should be directed at educating the public in regions of endemic histoplasmosis about measures to avoid exposures

Phaeohyphomycosis
Prevention efforts for phaeohyphomycosis should emphasize educating the public about measures to avoid either occupational or recreational exposures that may result in traumatic injury to the skin that may be contaminated with soil. Routine wound care measures should also be emphasized.

Sporotrichosis
Prevention efforts for sporotrichosis should emphasize educating the public about precautions to avoid occupational or recreational exposure to thorny plants or sphagnum moss, as these may serve as vehicles of inoculation of contaminated soil. In particular, individuals should be encouraged to wear long sleeves and, preferably, puncture-resistant gloves when working with plants or sphagnum moss. Routine wound care measures should also be emphasized.

Figure 6.1 Acute pulmonary histoplasmosis capsulati. Alveolar macrophages contain innumerable spherical to oval yeast forms, 2 to 4 μm in diameter. There is no pseudocapsular effect because fungal cell walls are uniformly colored with the GMS stain. GMS with H&E counterstain; ×250.

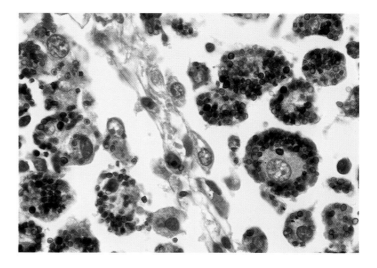

Figure 6.2 Severe, disseminated histoplasmosis capsulati in an AIDS patient. Large extracellular aggregates ("yeast lakes") of proliferating histoplasma cells partially efface the bone marrow. In profoundly immunodeficient hosts, there is greater variation in size and shape of the fungal cells. GMS with H&E counterstain; ×250.

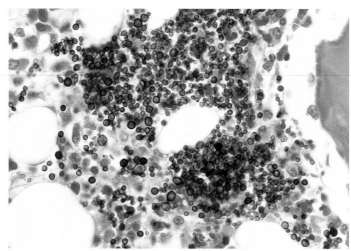

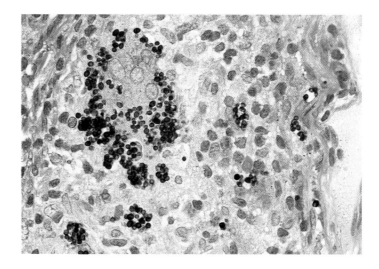

Figure 6.3 Disseminated histoplasmosis capsulati involving a cervical lymph node in an immunocompetent spelunker. Note clustering of uniform, spherical to oval fungal cells within epithelioid histiocytes and multinucleated giant cells. GMS with H&E counterstain; ×160.

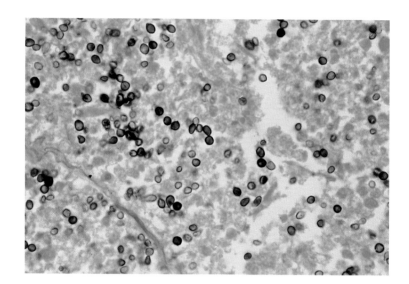

Figure 6.4   Residual pulmonary histoplasmosis capsulati. Histoplasma cells within the central caseous residuum of a histoplasmoma are distorted and unevenly stained. Budding is infrequent. GMS; ×250.

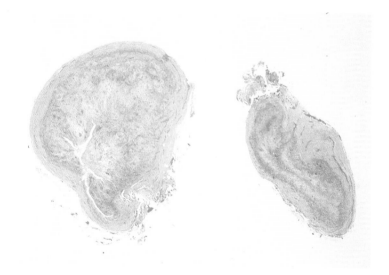

Figure 6.5   Phaeomycotic cyst. Two sharply circumscribed cystic granulomas are surrounded by prominent fibrous capsules. These excisional biopsy specimens were located in the subcutaneous tissue. H&E; ×3.

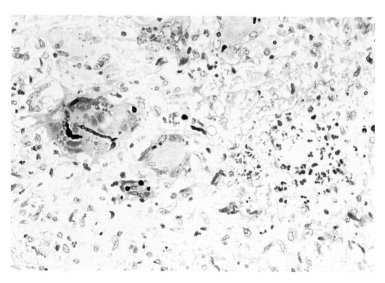

Figure 6.6   Polymorphous fungal elements of *Exophiala jeanselmei* in fibrogranulomatous wall of phaeomycotic cyst. Special stains for fungi mask the brown color of the phaeoid fungi. GMS with H&E counterstain; ×50.

Figure 6.7 Systemic (cerebral) phaeohyphomycosis caused by *Cladophialophora bantiana*. Numerous phaeoid (brown) hyphae in wall of cerebral granuloma are constricted at their prominent septations. Yeastlike cells and larger, thick-walled chlamydoconidia are also present. H&E; ×160.

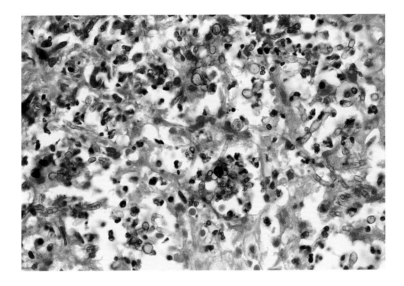

Figure 6.8 Systemic (cerebral) phaeohyphomycosis. The natural brown color of polymorphous fungal elements is masked when special stains for fungi are used, as illustrated here. Note the numerous, spherical, thick-walled chlamydoconidia. GMS; ×160.

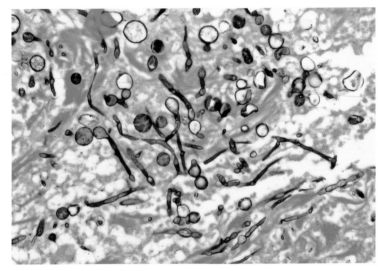

Figure 6.9 Cutaneous sporotrichosis. There is pseudoepitheliomatous hyperplasia of the epidermis and a mixed suppurative and granulomatous inflammatory infiltrate in the dermis. Clinically, this lesion had been mistaken for a squamous cell carcinoma. H&E; ×3.

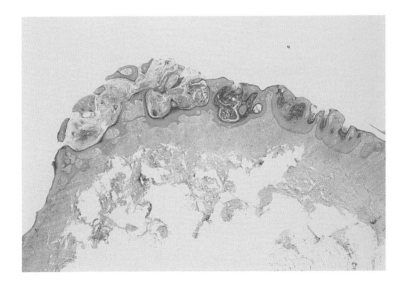

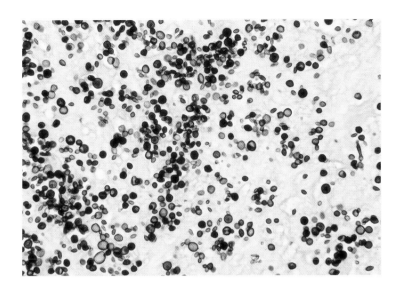

Figure 6.10 Pleomorphic spherical, oval, and elongated yeastlike cells of S. *schenckii* in a dermal granuloma. Budding forms are numerous. In this case, an unusually large number of fungal cells are present. GMS; ×160.

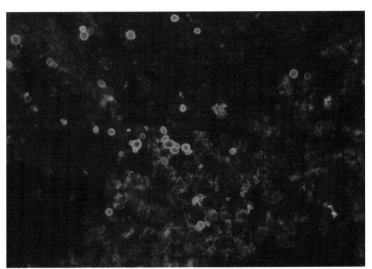

Figure 6.11 Immunofluorescence staining of S. *schenckii* in deparaffinized section of formalin-fixed skin lesion. Fungal cell walls are brightly decorated using a species-specific conjugate. A yeast-like cell with multiple buds is seen at center. Direct immunofluorescence; ×160.

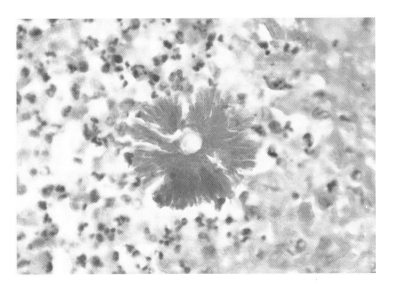

Figure 6.12 Asteroid body of sporotrichosis within the suppurative center of a pulmonary granuloma. A single, weakly stained fungal cell is ensheathed by radiating, brightly eosinophilic spicules of Splendore-Hoeppli material. H&E; ×400.

References

1. **Ajello, L.** 1986. Hyalohyphomycosis and phaeohyphomycosis: two global disease entities of public health importance. *Eur. J. Epidemiol.* **2:**243–251.

2. **Ajello, L., L. K. Georg, R. T. Steigbigel, and J. K. Wang.** 1974. A case of phaeohyphomycosis caused by a new species of *Phialophora. Mycopathologia* **66:**490–498.

3. **Ajello, L., and W. Kaplan.** 1969. A new variant of *Sporothrix schenckii. Mykosen* **12:**633–644.

4. **Alberici, F., C. T. Paties, G. Lombardi, L. Ajello, L. Kaufman, and F. Chandler.** 1989. *Sporothrix schenckii* var. *luriei* as the cause of sporotrichosis in Italy. *Eur. J. Epidemiol.* **5:**173–177.

5. **Bambirra, E. A., D. Miranda, A. M. F. Nogueira, and C. S. P. Barbosa.** 1983. Phaeohyphomycotic cyst: a clinicopathologic study of the first four cases described from Brazil. *Am. J. Trop. Med. Hyg.* **32:**794–798.

6. **Binford, C. H.** 1955. Histoplasmosis: tissue reactions and morphologic variations of the fungus. *Am. J. Clin. Pathol.* **25:**25–36.

7. **Bullock, W. E.** 1995. Histoplasma capsulatum, p. 2340–2353. *In* G. L. Mandell, J. E. Bennett, and R. Dolin (ed.), *Principles and Practice of Infectious Diseases,* 4th ed. Churchill Livingstone, New York.

8. **Bullpitt, P., and D. Weedon.** 1978. Sporotrichosis: a review of 39 cases. *Pathology* **10:**249–256.

9. **Chandler, F. W., and J. C. Watts.** 1987. *Pathologic Diagnosis of Fungal Infections,* p. 193–202. ASCP Press, Chicago.

10. **Chandler, F. W., and J. C. Watts.** 1987. *Pathologic Diagnosis of Fungal Infections,* p. 233–263. ASCP Press, Chicago.

11. **Chandler, F. W., and J. C. Watts.** 1993. Fungal infections, p. 355–362. *In* D. H. Dail and S. P. Hammar (ed.), *Pulmonary Pathology,* 2nd ed. Springer-Verlag, New York.

12. **Chandler, F. W., and J. C. Watts.** 1997. Histoplasmosis capsulati, p. 1007–1016. *In* D. Connor and F. W. Chandler (ed.), *Pathology of Infectious Diseases.* Appleton and Lange, Norwalk, Conn.

13. **Chandler, F. W., and J. C. Watts.** 1997. Phaeohyphomycosis, p. 1059–1066. *In* D. Connor and F. W. Chandler (ed.), *Pathology of Infectious Diseases.* Appleton and Lange, Norwalk, Conn.

14. **Chandler, F. W., and J. C. Watts.** 1997. Sporotrichosis, p. 1089–1096. *In* D. Connor and F. W. Chandler (ed.), *Pathology of Infectious Diseases.* Appleton and Lange, Norwalk, Conn.

15. **Chandramukhi, A., M. G. Ramadevi, and S. K. Shankar.** 1983. Cerebral cladosporiosis: a neuropathological and microbiological study. *Clin. Neurol. Neurosurg.* **85:**245–253.

16. **Cockshott, W. P., and A. O. Lucas.** 1964. Histoplasmosis duboisii. *Q. J. Med.* **133:**223–238.

17. **Coles, F. B., A. Schuchat, J. R. Hibbs, S. F. Kondraki, I. F. Salkin, D. M. Dixon, H. G. Chang, R. A. Duncan, N. J. Hurd, and D. L. Morse.** 1992. A multistate outbreak of sporotrichosis associated with sphagnum moss. *Am. J. Epidemiol.* **136:**475–487.

18. **Cooper, C. R., Jr., B. J. Breslin, D. M. Dixon, and I. F. Salkin.** 1992. DNA typing of isolates associated with the 1988 sporotrichosis epidemic. *J. Clin. Microbiol.* **30:**1631–1635.

19. **Davis, B. A.** 1996. Sporotrichosis. *Dermatol. Clin.* **14:**69–76.

20. **Dismukes, W. E., R. W. Bradsher, Jr., G. C. Cloud, C. A. Kauffman, S. W. Chapman, R. B. George, D. A. Stevens, W. M. Girard, M. S. Saag, and C. Bowles-Patton.** 1992. Itraconazole therapy for blastomycosis and histoplasmosis. *Am. J. Med.* **93:**489–497.

21. **Dixon, D. M., I. F. Salkin, R. A. Duncan, N. J. Hurd, J. H. Haines, M. E. Kemna, and F. B. Coles.** 1991. Isolation and characterization of *Sporothrix schenckii* from clinical and environmental sources associated with the largest U.S. epidemic of sporotrichosis. *J. Clin. Microbiol.* **29:**1106–1113.

22. **Dixon, D. M., T. J. Walsh, W. G. Merz, and M. R. McGinnis.** 1989. Infections due to *Xylohypha bantiana* (*Cladosporium trichoides*). *Rev. Infect. Dis.* **11:**515–525.

23. **Durkin, M. M., P. A. Connolly, and L. J. Wheat.** 1997. Comparison of radioimmunoassay and enzyme-linked immunoassay methods for detection of *Histoplasma capsulatum* var. *capsulatum* antigens. *J. Clin. Microbiol.* **35:** 2252–2255.

24. **Edwards, L. B., F. A. Acquaviva, V. T. Livesay, F. W. Cross, and C. E. Palmer.** 1969. An atlas of sensitivity to tuberculin, PPD-B, and histoplasmin in the United States. *Am. Rev. Respir. Dis.* **99**(Suppl.)**:**1–132.

25. **England, D. M., and L. Hochholzer.** 1985. Primary pulmonary sporotrichosis: report of eight cases with clinicopathologic review. *Am. J. Surg. Pathol.* **9:**193–204.

26. **England, D. M., and L. Hochholzer.** 1987. Sporothrix infection of the lung without cutaneous disease: primary pulmonary sporotrichosis. *Arch. Pathol. Lab. Med.* **111:**298–300.

27. **Fader, R. C., and M. R. McGinnis.** 1988. Infections caused by dematiaceous fungi: chromoblastomycosis and phaeohyphomycosis. *Infect. Dis. Clin. North Am.* **2:**925–938.

28. **Goodwin, R. A., Jr., and R. M. Des Prez.** 1973. Pathogenesis and clinical spectrum of histoplasmosis. *South. Med. J.* **66:**13–25.

29. **Goodwin, R. A., Jr., F. T. Owens, J. D. Snell, W. W. Hubbard, R. D. Buchanan, R. T. Perry, and R. M. Des Prez.** 1976. Chronic pulmonary histoplasmosis. *Medicine* (Baltimore) **55:**413–452.

30. **Goodwin, R. A., Jr., J. L. Shapiro, G. H. Thurman, S. S. Thurman, and R. M. Des Prez.** 1980. Disseminated histoplasmosis: clinical and pathologic correlations. *Medicine* (Baltimore) **59:**1–33.

31. **Hajjeh, R., S. McDonnell, S. Reef, C. Licitra, M. Hankins, B. Toth, A. Padhye, L. Kaufman, L. Pasarell, C. Cooper, L. Hutwanger, R. Hopkins, and M. McNeil.** 1997. Outbreak of sporotrichosis among tree nursery workers. *J. Infect. Dis.* **176:**499–504.

32. **Hutton, J. P., J. B. Durham, D. P. Miller, and E. D. Everett.** 1985. Hyphal forms of *Histoplasma capsulatum*: a common manifestation of intravascular infections. *Arch. Pathol. Lab. Med.* **109:**330–332.

33. **Iwatsu, T., and M. Miyaji.** 1984. Phaeomycotic cyst: a case with a lesion containing a wooden splinter. *Arch. Dermatol.* **120:**1209–1211.

34. **Johnson, P. C., N. Khardori, A. F. Najjar, P. W. A. Mansell, and G. A. Sarosi.** 1988. Progressive disseminated histoplasmosis in patients with acquired immunodeficiency syndrome. *Am. J. Med.* **85:**152–158.

35. **Kauffman, C. A.** 1994. Newer developments in therapy for endemic mycoses. *Clin. Infect. Dis.* **19**(Suppl.)**:**S28–S32.

36. **Kauffman, C. A.** 1996. Role of azoles in antifungal therapy. *Clin. Infect. Dis.* **22**(Suppl.)**:**S148–S153.

37. **Kauffman, C. A., P. G. Pappas, D. S. McKinsey, R. A. Greenfield, J. R. Perfect, G. A. Cloud, C. J. Thomas, and W. E. Dismukes.** 1996. Treatment of lymphocutaneous and visceral sporotrichosis with fluconazole. *Clin. Infect. Dis.* **22:**46–50.

38. **Kaufman, L.** 1992. Laboratory methods for the diagnosis and confirmation of systemic mycoses. *Clin. Infect. Dis.* **14**(Suppl. 1)**:**S23–S29.

39. **Kaufman, L.** 1992. Immunohistologic diagnosis of systemic mycoses: an update. *Eur. J. Epidemiol.* **8:**377–382.

40. **Kaufman, L., J. A. Kovacs, and E. Reiss.** 1997. Clinical immunomycology, p.585–604. *In* N. R. Rose, E. Conway de Macario, J. D. Folds, H. C. Lane, and R. M. Nakamura (ed.), *Manual of Clinical Laboratory Immunology*, 5th ed. American Society for Microbiology, Washington, D.C.

41. **Kaufman, L., and P. G. Standard.** 1987. Specific and rapid identification of medically important fungi by exoantigen detection. *Ann. Rev. Microbiol.* **41:**209–225.

42. **Kwon-Chung, K. J., and J. E. Bennett.** 1992. Histoplasmosis (Darling's disease, reticuloendothelial cytomycosis, Ohio Valley disease), p. 464–513. *In Medical Mycology.* Lea & Febiger, Philadelphia.

43. **Kwon-Chung, K. J., and J. E. Bennett.** 1992. Phaeohyphomycosis (chromomycosis, phaeosporotrichosis, cerebral chromomycosis), p. 620–677. *In Medical Mycology.* Lea & Febiger, Philadelphia.

44. **Kwon-Chung, K. J., and J. E. Bennett.** 1992. Sporotrichosis, p. 716–718. *In Medical Mycology.* Lea & Febiger, Philadelphia.

45. **Lawson, W., and A. Blitzer.** 1993. Fungal infections of the nose and paranasal sinuses. Part II. *Otolaryng. Clin. North Am.* **26:**1037–1068.

46. **Liber, A. F., and H. H. Choi.** 1973. Splendore-Hoeppli phenomenon about silk sutures in tissue. *Arch. Pathol.* **95:**217–220.

47. **Lucas, A. O.** 1970. Cutaneous manifestations of African histoplasmosis. *Br. J. Dermatol.* **82:**435–447.

48. **Lurie, H. I.** 1963. Histopathology of sporotrichosis. *Arch. Pathol.* **75:**92–109.

49. **Lurie, H. I., and W. J. S. Still.** 1969. The "capsule" of *Sporotrichum schenckii* and the evolution of the asteroid body: a light and electron microscopic study. *Sabouraudia* **7:**64–70.

50. **Maberry, J. D., J. F. Mullins, and O. J. Stone.** 1966. Sporotrichosis with demonstration of hyphae in human tissue. *Arch. Dermatol.* **93:**65–67.

51. **Male, O., and H. Pehamberger.** 1985. The cutaneous alternariosis. Case reports and synopsis of literature tissue. *Mykosen* **28:**278–305.

52. **Mandell, W., D. M. Goldberg, and H. C. Neu.** 1986. Histoplasmosis in patients with the acquired immune deficiency syndrome. *Am. J. Med.* **81:**974–978.

53. **Matsumoto, T., L. Ajello, T. Matsuda, P. J. Szanszlo, and T. J. Walsh.** 1994. Developments in hyalohyphomycosis and phaeohyphomycosis. *J. Med. Vet. Mycol.* **32:**329–349.

54. **McGinnis, M. R.** 1983. Chromoblastomycosis and phaeohyphomycosis: new concepts, diagnosis, and mycology. *J. Am. Acad. Dermatol.* **8:**1–16.

55. **McGinnis, M. R., M. G. Rinaldi, and R. E. Winn.** 1986. Emerging agents of phaeohyphomycosis: pathogenic species of *Bipolaris* and *Exserohilum*. *J. Clin. Microbiol.* **24:**250–259.

56. **McKinsey, D. S., R. A. Spiegel, L. Hutwanger, J. Stanford, M. R. Driks, J. Brewer, M. R. Gupta, D. L. Smith, M. C. O'Connor, and L. Dall.** 1997. Prospective study of histoplasmosis in patients infected with human immunodeficiency virus: incidence, risk factors, and pathophysiology. *Clin. Infect. Dis.* **24:**1195–1203.

57. **Morse, D. L., M. A. Gordon, T. Matte, and G. Eadie.** 1985. An outbreak of histoplasmosis in a prison. *Am. J. Epidemiol.* **122:**253–261.

58. **Moskowitz, L. B., T. J. Cleary, M. R. McGinnis, and C. B. Thomson.** 1983. *Phialophora richardsiae* in a lesion appearing as a giant cell tumor of the tendon sheath. *Arch. Pathol. Lab. Med.* **107:**374–376.

59. **Padhye, A. A., L. Kaufman, E. Durry, C. K. Banerjee, S. K. Jindal, P. Talwar, and A. Chakrabarti.** 1992. Fatal pulmonary sporotrichosis caused by *Sporothrix schenckii* var. *luriei* in India. *J. Clin. Microbiol.* **30:**2492–2494.

60. **Purvis, R. S., D. G. Diven, R. D. Dreschel, J. H. Calhoun, and S. K. Tyring.** 1993. Sporotrichosis presenting as arthritis and subcutaneous nodules. *J. Am. Acad. Dermatol.* **28:**879–884.

61. **Riley, O., Jr., and S. H. Mann.** 1960. Brain abscess caused by *Cladosporium trichoides*: review of 3 cases and report of a fourth case. *Am. J. Clin. Pathol.* **33:**525–531.

62. **Rinaldi, M. G.** 1996. Phaeohyphomycosis. *Dermatol. Clin.* **14:**147–153.

63. **Sarosi, G. A., and S. F. Davies.** 1983. *Histoplasma capsulatum* pneumonia, p. 375–379. *In* J. E. Pennington (ed.), *Respiratory Infections: Diagnosis and Management.* Raven Press, New York.

64. **Sathapatayavongs, B., B. E. Batteiger, J. Wheat, T. G. Slama, and J. L. Wass.** 1983. Clinical and laboratory features of disseminated histoplasmosis during two large urban outbreaks. *Medicine* (Baltimore) **62:**263–270.

65. **Schell, W. A., L. Pasarell, I. F. Salkin, and M. R. McGinnis.** 1995. *Bipolaris, Exophiala, Scedosporium, Sporothrix,* and other dematiaceous fungi, p. 825–846. *In* P. R. Murray, E. J. Baron, M. A. Pfaller, F. C. Tenover, and R. H. Yolken (ed.), *Manual of Clinical Microbiology,* 6th ed. American Society for Microbiology, Washington, D.C.

66. **Schlech, W. F., III, L. J. Wheat, J. L. Ho, M. L. V. French, R. J. Weeks, R. B. Kohler, C. E. Deane, H. E. Eitzen, and J. D. Band.** 1983. Recurrent urban histoplasmosis, Indianapolis, Indiana, 1980–1981. *Am. J. Epidemiol.* **118:**301–312.

67. **Sekhon, A. S., A. A. Padhye, P. G. Standard, L. Kaufman, L. Ajello, and A. K. Garg.** 1990. Antigenic relationship of *Dactylaria gallopava* to *Scolecobasidium constrictum*. *J. Med. Vet. Mycol.* **28:**59–66.

68. **Sharkey, P. K., J. R. Graybill, M. G. Rinaldi, D. A. Stevens, R. M. Tucker, J. D. Peterie, P. D. Hoeprich, D. L. Greer, L. Frenkel, G. W. Counts, J. Goodrich, S. Zellner, R. W. Bradsher, C. M. van der Horst, K. Israel, G. A. Pankey, and C. P. Barranco.** 1990. Itraconazole treatment of phaeohyphomycosis. *J. Am. Acad. Dermatol.* **23:**577–586.

69. Sharkey-Mathis, P. K., C. A. Kauffman, J. R. Graybill, D. A. Stevens, J. S. Hostetler, G. Cloud, and W. E. Dismukes. 1993. Treatment of sporotrichosis with itraconazole. NIAID Mycoses Study Group. *Am. J. Med.* **95**:279–285.

70. Sutton, D.A., A. A. Padhye, P. G. Standard, and M. G. Rinaldi. 1997. An aberrant variant of *Histoplasma capsulatum* var. *capsulatum*. *J. Clin. Microbiol.* **35**:734–735.

71. Svirbely, J. R., L. W. Ayers, and W. J. Buesching. 1985. Filamentous *Histoplasma capsulatum* endocarditis involving mitral and aortic valve porcine bioprostheses. *Arch. Pathol. Lab. Med.* **109**:273–276.

72. Ulbright, T. M., and A. L. A. Katzenstein. 1980. Solitary necrotizing granulomas of the lung. *Am. J. Surg. Pathol.* **4**:13–28.

73. Waldman, R. J., A. C. England, R. Tauxe, T. Line, R. J. Weeks, L. Ajello, L. Kaufman, B. Wentworth, and D. W. Fraser. 1983. A winter outbreak of acute histoplasmosis in northern Michigan. *Am. J. Epidemiol.* **117**:68–75.

74. Watts, J. C., and F. W. Chandler. 1987. Primary pulmonary sporotrichosis (editorial). *Arch. Pathol. Lab. Med.* **111**:215–217.

75. Wheat, L. J. 1992. Histoplasmosis—diagnosis and management. *Infect. Dis. Clin. Prac.* **1**:277–280.

76. Wheat, L. J., B. E. Batteiger, and B. Sathapatayavongs. 1990. *Histoplasma capsulatum* infections of the central nervous system. *Medicine* (Baltimore) **69**:244–260.

77. Wheat, L. J., P. A. Connolly-Stringfield, R. L. Baker, M. F. Curfman, M. E. Eads, K. S. Israel, S. A. Norris, D. H. Webb, and M. L. Zeckel. 1990. Disseminated histoplasmosis in the acquired immune deficiency syndrome: clinical findings, diagnosis and treatment, and review of the literature. *Medicine* (Baltimore) **69**:361–374.

78. Wheat, L. J., T. G. Slama, H. E. Eitzen, R. B. Kohler, M. L. V. French, and J. L. Biesecker. 1981. A large urban outbreak of histoplasmosis: clinical features. *Ann. Intern. Med.* **94**:331–337.

79. Wheat, L. J., T. G. Slama, and M. L. Zeckel. 1985. Histoplasmosis in the acquired immune deficiency syndrome. *Am. J. Med.* **78**:203–210.

80. Wheat, L. J., J. Wass, J. Norton, R. B. Kohler, and M. L. V. French. 1984. Cavitary histoplasmosis occurring during two large urban outbreaks. Analysis of clinical, epidemiologic, roentgenographic, and laboratory features. *Medicine* (Baltimore) **63**:201–209.

81. Winn, R. E. 1995. A contemporary view of sporotrichosis. *Curr. Top. Med. Mycol.* **6**:73–94.

82. Wood, C., and B. Russel-Bell. 1983. Characterization of pigmented fungi by melanin staining. *Am. J. Dermatopathol.* **5**:77–81.

83. Ziefer, A., and D. H. Connor. 1980. Phaeomycotic cyst: a clinicopathologic study of twenty-five patients. *Am. J. Trop. Med. Hyg.* **29**:901–911.

chapter 7

Diphtheria

David A. Schwartz and Melinda Wharton

> "...Sluggish resisting phlegm was found which covered the trachea like a membrane and the entry and exit of air to the exterior was not free"

The history of the identification of the bacterial agent of diphtheria, the unraveling of the epidemiology of this lethal disease, and the subsequent development of an effective vaccine is one of the most interesting in the annals of bacteriology. Descriptions of a syndrome of sore throat, membrane production, and suffocation appear as early as the Hippocratic writings (50). The autopsy findings of diphtheria recorded by the French physician Guillaume de Baillou during the Paris diphtheria epidemic of 1576 constitute one of the earliest descriptions of an epidemic disease from autopsy. Following the post-mortem examination of a 7-year-old boy whose pharynx was slightly swollen before death, de Baillou identified the false membrane characteristic of the disease. His autopsy description stated that "sluggish resisting phlegm was found which covered the trachea like a membrane and the entry and exit of air to the exterior was not free" (71). Diphtheria was

David A. Schwartz, Departments of Pathology and Medicine (Infectious Diseases), Emory University School of Medicine, 69 Butler Street, S.E., Atlanta, GA 30303. Melinda Wharton, National Immunization Program, Centers for Disease Control and Prevention, Mailstop E-61, 1600 Clifton Road, N.E., Atlanta, GA 30333.

Pathology of Emerging Infections 2
Edited by Ann Marie Nelson and C. Robert Horsburgh, Jr.
© 1998 American Society for Microbiology, Washington, D.C.

initially established as a specific clinical entity in 1826 after publication of a classic monograph by Pierre Bretonneau.

The first modern accounts date to the 16th and 17th centuries, when repeated outbreaks occurred in Spain (25). In the 18th century, an epidemic of "throat distemper" occurred in the New England colonies with high mortality among children; during a 12-month period in 1735–1736, 1 in 20 residents of New Hampshire died of diphtheria (14). Severe epidemics recurred in Europe and the United States in the 19th century, and at the beginning of the 20th century, diphtheria remained one of the major causes of death among children in the United States.

The bacterial etiology of the disease was not completely established until Klebs described seeing chaining cocci and bacilli in microscopic preparations of diphtheritic membranes in 1883 (2). While working in Robert Koch's laboratory a year later, Friedrich Loeffler isolated and morphologically characterized the diphtheria bacillus in a culture medium that bears his name (48). Loeffler then demonstrated that the organism could produce disease when inoculated into guinea pigs, and fulfilled Koch's postulates for proof that it was the etiological agent of diphtheria. Loeffler made other significant new observations as well. He demonstrated that healthy asymptomatic persons could harbor the organism in their throats and established the existence of a carrier state; observed that the bacillus remained localized to the pseudomembrane and did not invade the tissues; and predicted that the neurologic and cardiologic manifestations of disease were caused by a toxin elaborated by the diphtheria bacillus (48). This was confirmed at the Pasteur Institute in 1888, when Roux and Yersin separated the toxin from the bacillus by filtration (69). Two years later, von Behring demonstrated that antiserum against the toxin was capable of protecting infected animals from death after experimental infection. Following this, Roux reported in 1894 that antitoxin produced in horses reduced mortality from diphtheria among foundlings in Paris from 51% to 24%. An unfortunate complication of the administration of horse antiserum to diphtheria patients was development of acute serum sickness in approximately 10% of persons vaccinated. Horses were ideal animals in which to produce antitoxin because they were not only large and highly reactive to diphtheria toxin, but also relatively insensitive to the effects of the toxin. Unfortunately, the horses used for long-term antibody production eventually died of amyloidosis. In 1897, Ehrlich developed a bioassay for the toxin, using guinea pigs to determine the minimum lethal dose (24).

The earliest diphtheria vaccines were balanced mixtures of toxin and antitoxin

The earliest diphtheria vaccines were balanced mixtures of toxin and antitoxin. Formalin-treated toxoid vaccine was introduced in 1913, and the vaccine became available in the United States in the 1920s. With introduction of vaccination with diphtheria toxoid, diphtheria incidence decreased dramatically. However, outbreaks have occurred in recent years in both developed and developing countries, demonstrating the continued threat that diphtheria presents (19, 36, 78, 85). In 1990, a massive diphtheria epidemic began in Russia that subsequently spread throughout the countries of the former Soviet Union (35).

Microbiology

Corynebacteria are a heterogeneous genus of gram-positive, catalase-positive, aerobic or facultatively anaerobic, nonsporulating rods that are usually nonmotile. *Corynebacterium* species are widely distributed in nature, commonly found in soil and water, and reside on the skin and mucous membranes of humans and animals. In some species, the bacterial cell wall is weaker at one end, resulting in a bacillus that is club shaped. The genus name is derived from the Greek words *koryne*, meaning club, and *bacterion*, little rod. *C. diphtheriae* is the only major human pathogen in this genus, which includes a number of opportunistic species as well as nonpathogenic, poorly described saprophytes frequently found on the surfaces of mucous membranes. Other potentially pathogenic corynebacterial species and the diseases they produce include *C. ulcerans* (pharyngitis), *C. pseudotuberculosis* (lymphadenitis), *C. pseudodiphtheriticum* (pharyngitis, endocarditis, lower respiratory infections), *C. minutissimum* (erythrasma), *Corynebacterium* sp. group D2 (urinary tract infections), and *C. jeikeium* (wound infections and septicemia). The exact family affiliation of this genus is unclear, but the corynebacteria are taxonomically related to the mycobacteria and nocardia based on similarity in the composition of their cell walls.

C. ulcerans and C. pseudotuberculosis have been demonstrated to be closely related to *C. diphtheriae* based on 16S rRNA gene sequence analysis (63). Of note, strains of both *C. ulcerans* and *C. pseudotuberculosis* have been demonstrated to produce diphtheria toxin (84). Cases of exudative pharyngitis with pseudomembrane formation due to *C. ulcerans*, clinically indistinguishable from those due to *C. diphtheriae*, have been documented (16, 41). DNA hybridization studies demonstrate homology of the *tox* gene among these species and *C. diphtheriae*, and in toxigenic strains of *C. ulcerans*, DNA restriction fragments hybridize with ß corynebacteriophage (33). Nontoxigenic strains of both *C. ulcerans* and *C. pseudotuberculosis* can be converted to toxigenicity by ß-like phages (51).

C. imitans is the proposed name for an organism which was recently isolated from the nasopharynx of a 5-month-old Romanian boy who developed an upper respiratory disease which was clinically suspected of being diphtheria. Seven adults who had contact with either the infant or an adult contact person also developed symptoms of pharyngeal diphtheria. All were treated with antidiphtheria antitoxin and recovered. Biochemical and chemotaxonomic analysis revealed that a corynebacterial organism was present in throat swabs from the infant index case and three adults; these *Corynebacterium* isolates were clonal and were different from all other species in this genus. Comparative 16S rRNA gene sequence analysis revealed this agent to represent a new subline in the genus *Corynebacterium* (27).

C. diphtheriae is a slender, gram-positive, nonsporulating, nonencapsulated, and nonmotile pleomorphic bacillus. The species name is derived from the Greek word *diphtheria*, meaning leather hide, and refers to the characteristic leathery membrane which it forms in infected tissues. The bacillus is club shaped at both ends and measures approximately 1.5 to 5 μm long

C. ulcerans and C. pseudotuberculosis have been demonstrated to be closely related to C. diphtheriae based on 16S rRNA gene sequence analysis

Special diagnostic reagents are required for isolation of C. diphtheriae by culture and subsequent subculture for toxigenicity and biochemical testing

and 0.5 to 1 μm wide. In Gram-stained smears of organisms grown on Loeffler's medium, the bacilli may show metachromatic granules, and the bacteria are characteristically arranged in palisades or at sharp angles to one another in "V" and "L" configurations. These "Chinese character" arrangements result from a "snapping" movement involving two cells during cell division. Special diagnostic reagents are required for isolation of *C. diphtheriae* by culture and subsequent subculture for toxigenicity and biochemical testing. On selective media containing potassium tellurite, many of the normal throat commensals are inhibited and *C. diphtheriae* appears as gray-black colonies containing reduced tellurite. The species is divided into four types—*gravis*, *intermedius*, *mitis*, and *belfanti*—based on differences in colonial morphology on tellurite agar, fermentation reactions, and hemolytic patterns. Similar to other corynebacterial species as well as the nocardia and mycobacteria, the peptidoglycans of the cell wall of *C. diphtheriae* contain meso-α,ϵ-diaminopimelic acid and the major cell wall sugars are arabinose and galactose. The lipids associated with the outer envelope also contain significant amounts of mycolic acids, which are similar to the large saturated, α-branched, β-hydroxy fatty acids of the mycobacteria.

Current knowledge of the toxigenic characteristics of the diphtheria toxin is extensive (52, 61, 62). Exotoxin production by *C. diphtheriae* is dependent on the presence of a lysogenic bacteriophage which carries the gene coding for production of toxin (*tox*$^+$). During the lysogenic phase, the bacteriophage's circular DNA strand integrates with the genetic material of the host bacterium as a prophage, resulting in the ability of the bacillus to express the gene necessary for production of the toxin polypeptide. The exotoxin is a 62,000-kDa polypeptide composed of two parts: an enzymatically active part (fragment A) at its amino terminus and a carboxy-terminal fragment (fragment B) which attaches to specific receptors on susceptible host cell membranes. Diphtheria toxin binds to the precursor of a heparin-binding epidural growth factor on the surface of a susceptible eukaryotic host cell. After internalization and attachment to cell membranes by the B fragment, the A fragment is translocated into the cytosol of the cell. Fragment A inactivates the tRNA translocase elongation factor 2, which is present in eukaryotic but not bacterial cells. The loss of this enzyme prevents the interaction of mRNA and tRNA, halting further addition of amino acids to elongating polypeptide chains.

Significant toxin production not only depends upon the presence of the lysogenic *tox*$^+$ bacteriophage, but is dependent upon bacterial growth being slowed by exhaustion of iron in the environment. Although diphtheria toxin affects all cells in the body, it exerts its most prominent effects on the nerves, kidneys, and heart. Minuscule amounts of toxin halt protein synthesis in cultured HeLa cells within 3 h, and only 0.1 μg/kg is necessary to kill a susceptible animal. These properties make diphtheria toxin one of the most potent known.

Immunity against clinical diphtheria is dependent upon the presence of antitoxin in the blood, produced either following clinical or subclinical infection or by artificial active immunization with toxoid. Infants under the age of 6 months are passively protected from diphtheria by the transplacental passage of antitoxin from immune mothers. Although immunized individuals can still develop diphtheria, prior immunization reduces the frequency and severity of clinical disease.

Strains of C. *diphtheriae* which lack lysogenic phage do not produce toxin. However, these strains can be converted to toxin production in vitro by infection with the lysogenic *tox*⁺ phage, a process termed lysogenization. Significantly, there is evidence that this process can also occur in nature (62).

Although diphtheria toxin is the major virulence factor in C. *diphtheriae*, other virulence factors exist as well. Infection with nontoxigenic strains of C. *diphtheriae* can cause an illness clinically indistinguishable from that caused by toxigenic strains, with pharyngitis and pseudomembrane, but toxin-mediated complications such as myocarditis and neuropathy are not seen (3, 23). In addition, invasive disease due to nontoxigenic strains is well documented (1, 64, 86). Beta-hemolytic streptococci are often isolated from patients with respiratory or cutaneous diphtheria, but the role of these organisms in pathogenesis is unclear.

Epidemiology

Infections due to C. *diphtheriae* are worldwide in distribution. In most developed countries, diphtheria is only rarely recognized. In the United States, only 41 cases of respiratory diphtheria were reported during the period 1980–1995 (9). Small outbreaks have occurred in the United States and Western Europe among disadvantaged urban populations, and sporadic infections have been identified among travelers to developing countries (19, 36, 76). This pattern of disease incidence suggests that circulation of toxigenic strains of C. *diphtheriae* is not widespread in developed countries. However, communities with ongoing endemic transmission of toxigenic C. *diphtheriae* have been identified in both the United States and Canada, demonstrating the continued risk that diphtheria presents, even in countries with little recognized disease due to the organism (13, 17, 83).

Since the 1970s, infant vaccination with diphtheria toxoid has been implemented as part of the Expanded Program on Immunization (EPI) of the World Health Organization (WHO), with dramatic reductions in diphtheria incidence in developing countries. During the 1970s, 70,000 to 90,000 cases of diphtheria were reported annually worldwide to the WHO; by 1990–1992, this had decreased to 20,000 to 27,000 cases reported annually, reflecting reduced disease incidence in developing countries (29). With introduction of EPI, diphtheria shifted from being a disease concentrated among young children to older children, adolescents, and young adults (28, 49). Outbreaks among adolescents and young adults have occurred in several developing countries 5 to 10 years following implementation of childhood vaccination programs (28, 46, 78, 85).

In 1990, a major diphtheria epidemic began in the Russian Federation and subsequently spread to the other countries of the former Soviet Union. From 1990 through the first quarter of 1996, approximately 125,000 cases

Since the 1970s, infant vaccination with diphtheria toxoid has been implemented, with dramatic reductions in diphtheria incidence in developing countries

and 4,000 deaths were reported in the newly independent states (15, 66). In most of the countries of the former Soviet Union, a majority of cases were reported among adults, a group not previously targeted for diphtheria vaccination (35). In Russia, the predominant strains were of biotype *gravis*, and emergence of an epidemic clone was demonstrated (65). However, in some countries of the former Soviet Union *mitis* strains predominated, suggesting that microbial factors alone were unlikely to account for the epidemic. In two case-control studies, Russian-manufactured diphtheria toxoid was highly effective in prevention of diphtheria among children (35). The toxin gene and the gene encoding its regulatory element, *dtxR*, have been sequenced in strains from the Russian epidemic and compared with those of the Park-Williams no. 8 strain. Only silent mutations were found in the *tox* gene, but some differences in predicted amino acid sequence in *dtxR* were found in some strains; the functional significance of these differences is unknown (58). Although the causes of the epidemic are not fully understood, contributing factors were inadequate population immunity and social and economic conditions and population movements that facilitated spread (35). For control of the epidemic, the European Regional Office of WHO recommended rapidly increasing population immunity by increasing coverage among children through routine childhood vaccination programs and administering a single dose of diphtheria toxoid to the entire population for outbreak control. With implementation of these strategies, the epidemic has begun to come under control (21).

The primary reservoir of C. diphtheriae in endemic areas is thought to be cutaneous disease

The primary reservoir of C. *diphtheriae* in endemic areas is thought to be cutaneous disease. Because toxin is poorly absorbed from cutaneous sites of infection, serious complications due to diphtheria are uncommon in cases of cutaneous infections, but can occur in susceptible persons (30, 47). In developing countries prior to the widespread use of vaccine, C. *diphtheriae* was commonly isolated from skin lesions of children (8, 11, 54, 56, 74). The occurrence of frequent, repeated skin infections in children is thought to account for the absence of epidemic respiratory diphtheria in many countries in the absence of high vaccination coverage among children. Repeated cutaneous infections with C. *diphtheriae* confer immunity, and as long as the organism remains endemic in the population, reinfection throughout life probably occurs, with maintenance of immunity. Cutaneous infection probably has also played an important role in the transmission of infection in developed countries. In the southeastern United States, cutaneous cases of diphtheria were important in maintaining circulation of the organism during the 1960s and 1970s (4–6). In Seattle, Washington, an outbreak of diphtheria among alcoholic urban adults occurred during the period 1972 to 1982, with a predominance of cutaneous infection (36). Cutaneous infection with nontoxigenic strains of C. *diphtheriae* has been documented among intravenous drug users in Zurich and is thought to be important in recent cases of invasive disease due to nontoxigenic strains in France (34, 64).

Diphtheria is transmitted from person to person by respiratory droplets. Both asymptomatically infected persons and persons with clinical disease can transmit C. *diphtheriae* to others. The organism remains viable in the environment for some time, and transmission by fomites can occur (4, 20). This may account for the high transmissibility of cutaneous diphtheria, especially in environments of crowding and poor hygiene (5, 6).

Diphtheria toxoid is highly effective in preventing clinical diphtheria, but does not prevent infection with C. diphtheriae. The impact of vaccination on circulation of the organism is complex and not fully understood. In the United States during the 1920s and early 1930s, vaccine coverage of >50% among school-age children and of 30% among pre-school-age children resulted in dramatic decreases in diphtheria incidence in many communities (32). Pappenheimer proposed that in a vaccinated population, the presence of the *tox* gene would confer no selective advantage to the organism and over time would be lost, converting toxigenic to nontoxigenic strains (60).

Because selective media are required for isolation of C. diphtheriae, the organism is unlikely to be found unless specifically sought from cultures of nonsterile sites, and recent data on the prevalence of nontoxigenic strains are limited. In 1970, nontoxigenic C. diphtheriae strains were found in throat or nasal specimens from 28 of 818 schoolchildren in Athens (77). A similar survey was repeated in 1980, and only 7 of 895 children were found to be carriers of the organism (44). Typical C. diphtheriae was not found in nasal and pharyngeal specimens from 515 adults in central Italy (53). Following identification of a cluster of cases of invasive disease due to nontoxigenic C. diphtheriae biotype *mitis* among intravenous drug users, Gruner et al. found the organism in 5 of 117 pharyngeal specimens and 5 of 28 specimens from superficial wounds from intravenous drug users. In contrast, the organism was not found among 200 patients with pharyngitis who were not intravenous drug users (34). Six of 578 homosexual men attending a sexually transmitted disease clinic in the U.K. were found to have pharyngeal infection with nontoxigenic C. diphtheriae strains, while 1 of 653 heterosexual men and none of 1,043 women were found to harbor the organism (82). The role of immunity to bacterial components other than toxin in prevention of infection is not well understood.

Recent data on the prevalence of nontoxigenic strains are limited

Clinical Features

The classic clinical feature of respiratory diphtheria is the pseudomembrane, typically white or gray in color (Fig. 7.1). The membrane is firmly adherent, and bleeding will result if it is forcibly removed. Following an incubation period of 2 to 5 days, the membrane most commonly begins on the tonsils, soft palate, or uvula and may extend to the posterior oropharynx, upward to the nasopharynx, or downward into the larynx (see Fig. 7.2); laryngeal diphtheria may also occur in the absence of involvement of the upper respiratory tract. If extensive, the membrane may result in obstruction of the airway. In nasal diphtheria, no pharyngeal membrane may be visible. In severe cases of respiratory diphtheria, cervical lymphadenopathy and extensive soft tissue swelling lead to the "bull neck" appearance (see Fig. 7.3), and in the most severe cases, edema may extend below the clavicles.

Symptoms of respiratory diphtheria vary by the site of local infection

Symptoms of respiratory diphtheria vary by the site of local infection. Nasal infection results in mucoid or serosanguineous nasal discharge accompanied by few constitutional symptoms (see Fig. 7.6). Pharyngeal infection results in sore throat, dysphagia, and low-grade fever. In laryngeal diphtheria, patients present with hoarseness, stridor, and dyspnea. Other signs and symptoms are due to systemically absorbed toxin. In susceptible persons, diphtheria toxin results in weakness, rapid pulse, and circulatory collapse. Death may occur early in the course (within the first week) or due to delayed manifestations of myocarditis or neuropathy, which may occur weeks after initial onset of disease.

Diphtheria myocarditis is a common complication of respiratory diphtheria. Evidence of myocardial involvement has been reported in 32 to 66% of patients studied; the proportion of patients with myocarditis is even higher in patients with severe diphtheria, with virtually all patients having electrocardiographic evidence of myocarditis (7, 10, 37, 55). Onset may be early, within the first few days of illness, or late, 3 to 4 weeks after onset of disease. Electrocardiographic abnormalities include T-wave abnormalities, ST segment shifts, and conduction abnormalities, including complete heart block (55). Conduction abnormalities, especially third-degree atrioventricular block, are associated with a poor prognosis, even with use of ventricular pacing (73). Permanent myocardial damage following diphtheria myocarditis is thought to be rare (70).

Neurological complications of diphtheria include cranial nerve palsies and paralysis of the extremities. Mechanical ventilation may be required in patients with involvement of the phrenic nerve. Neurological symptoms may occur early in the course of illness or late, with paralysis of the soft palate occurring relatively early in the course (during the first 1 to 4 weeks), other cranial nerve palsies later (during weeks 3 to 6), and weakness of the limbs during week 4 or later (68, 75). Autonomic dysfunction has been demonstrated in patients with diphtheria and may contribute to cardiovascular instability (42). Electrophysiologic studies demonstrate slowing of conduction, prolongation of distal motor latency, and, in severe cases, conduction block (31).

In severe cases of diphtheria, hemorrhagic complications and disseminated intravascular coagulation may occur (80). Renal involvement is common in severe cases; in the prevaccine era, proteinuria was considered a grave prognostic sign due to its frequent association with myocarditis and death (40).

Although primary infection of the skin with C. *diphtheriae* does occur, the organism most commonly results in secondary infection of a cutaneous site of preexisting injury or another infection. Primary cutaneous diphtheria begins as a pustule which progresses to form a deep punched-out ulcer with a pseudomembranous base. The ulcer is initially painful but later becomes anesthetic (38). Group A streptococci are often isolated concurrently. In cutaneous diphtheria, complications related to absorption of diphtheria toxin are uncommon but can occur in susceptible persons (30, 47). Rarely, C. *diphtheriae* may result in infections in other sites, including the genital tract, conjunctiva, and ear (39, 45).

Pathology

The clinicopathological presentations of diphtheria can be divided into two major types, respiratory tract and extrarespiratory infections (72). Faucial diphtheria is the most common clinical presentation and can involve infection of the posterior structures of the mouth, tonsils, and proximal pharynx. Following exposure of the mucosal surface to *C. diphtheriae*, the organism multiplies rapidly on epithelial cells at the infected site. Production of exotoxin results in necrosis of the cells in the area of infection. An inflammatory reaction occurs, accompanied by development of a fibrin-rich exudate. This process results in the abrupt onset of sore throat, mild pharyngeal injection, malaise, and low-grade fever. Development of the characteristic pseudomembrane of diphtheria usually begins on one or both tonsils and extends to involve one or more of the following structures: uvula, tonsillar pillars, oropharynx, soft palate, and nasopharynx. The pseudomembrane initially is white and glossy, but later becomes gray with focal areas of green or black necrosis. The extent of pseudomembrane formation correlates with the severity of symptoms. Thus, localized tonsillar disease is often mild, but extension of the pseudomembrane into the posterior pharynx, soft palate, and periglottal mucosa is associated with severe malaise, prostration, and weakness. The initial exudate is initially white, shiny, and patchy, but later the local exudative lesions coalesce to form a resilient pseudomembrane which tightly adheres to the underlying ulcerated tissue. It is composed of lymphocytes, neutrophils, erythrocytes, and necrotic epithelial cells in a matrix of fibrin. Tissue Gram staining can reveal large numbers of gram-positive, club-shaped bacilli within the exudate, especially in early stages of infection.

The extent of pseudomembrane formation correlates with the severity of symptoms

With progression of disease, neutrophilic infiltration of the underlying tissues becomes more intense and is accompanied by edema, vascular congestion, fibrin exudation, and perivascular cuffing. Infection of the larynx can develop as a primary site of infection or as a result of distal spread from the pharynx. Laryngeal involvement produces hoarseness, dyspnea, respiratory stridor, and cough, resulting from involvement of the epiglottis, false cords, and true cords by a pseudomembrane which can extend distally into the trachea. In laryngeal involvement, the submucosal seromucinous glands underlying the pseudomembrane often are necrotic. Because the larynx contains columnar respiratory epithelium, the membrane peels or is coughed easily off the basement membrane. However, in the squamous epithelium-lined vocal cords the pseudomembrane separates with difficulty, and airway obstruction can occur. In some cases, inflammation and necrosis of subjacent tissues result in spontaneous separation of the pseudomembrane, resulting in aspiration and respiratory embarrassment. Following resolution of the infection with treatment, the pseudomembrane is either expelled or enzymatically digested, the inflammatory reaction subsides, and the ulcerated mucosa heals by regeneration (72).

Extrarespiratory diphtheria occurs most commonly in the tropical regions of the world. Cutaneous infection is the most common extrarespiratory manifestation of diphtheria. The classic diphtheritic cutaneous ulcer is nonhealing and covered with a dirty gray pseudomembrane. However, 85% of diphtheritic ulcers cannot reliably be clinically distinguished from other dermatologic conditions including eczema and psoriasis. The clinical presentation of cutaneous diphtheria is indolent and is rarely associated with systemic signs of toxicity. Most cases of cutaneous diphtheria are associated with *Staphylococcus aureus* and group A streptococci. The cornea and conjunctiva can occasionally be involved in diphtheria. The diphtheritic pseudomembrane on the mucosal surfaces of the eye appear similar to those in other parts of the body, and may be accompanied by hemorrhage ("bloody tears") when the pseudomembrane is torn or shed (see Fig. 7.4).

The systemic complications of diphtheria which result from elaboration of diphtheria toxin are most severe in the cardiac and nervous tissues. The first evidence of cardiac involvement usually begins after 1 to 2 weeks of illness, and evidence of myocarditis can occur in as many as two-thirds of patients. In a recent series of 212 adult patients with diphtheria from Russia, 90 (42%) had cardiac complications (67). Cardiac dysfunction associated with diphtheria can present clinically as congestive heart failure, circulatory collapse, progressive dyspnea, or weakness. A recent autopsy study of 102 adults dying of diphtheria on disease day 1 to 102 revealed interesting data on the natural history of cardiac pathology (43). Dystrophic and necrotic lesions in the cardiac conduction system and myocardium were found on disease days 1 to 8. The severity and extent of these lesions were related to ventilation respiratory failure. The authors found that progression of diphtheritic myocarditis had two stages. The early stage (exudative) began on disease day 3, and the late (productive) stage began on disease day 9, with the disease eventually resulting in myocardiosclerosis after disease day 28. In patients with diphtheritic myocarditis who were autopsied, hearts were pale and flabby and yellow streaking was present in the myocardium (22). Microscopically, myofibrils can show hyaline, granular, and fatty changes. Myocarditis can be present, consisting of necrosis of single or clusters of myofibers associated with mixed mononuclear and polymorphonuclear interstitial inflammation.

The severity of neurologic toxicity is proportional to the severity of primary infection

Similar to cardiac toxicity, the severity of neurologic toxicity is proportional to the severity of primary infection. Although mild cases of diphtheria will only infrequently develop neurological manifestations, as many as 75% of persons with severe disease develop neuropathy. Neurological involvement usually begins with local paralysis of the soft palate and posterior pharyngeal wall. Following this, cranial neuropathies can develop, and later, peripheral neuritis. Occasionally, motor nerves of the upper extremities, neck, and trunk are involved (50). The pathological findings of nerves in cases with diphtheritic neurotoxicity are nonspecific and include degeneration of myelin sheaths and axon cylinders.

Bacteremia with *C. diphtheriae* is a less well-known complication of infection with this agent. Cases include both children and adults of all ages. Most patients will have diphtheritic endocarditis, with the mitral valve most frequently affected, followed by the aortic and, less commonly, tricuspid valve (64).

Other unusual sites of diphtheria include the vagina, nose, and ear. Infection of these sites is almost always associated with pharyngeal or cutaneous infection. As a result of the systemic effects of exotoxin, patients with diphtheria can develop generalized reticuloendothelial hyperplasia of spleen and lymph nodes. The regional lymph nodes of the neck can enlarge dramatically in patients with respiratory tract infection, resulting in a "bull neck" appearance. In cases of severe infection, fatty change and focal necrosis of parenchymal cells in the liver, adrenal glands, and kidneys may occur. The kidneys may show interstitial inflammation, nephrocalcinosis, and degenerative and regenerative changes of renal tubules with epithelial casts (72).

Diagnosis

In all cases in which diphtheria is suspected, the laboratory should be told the specimen may contain toxigenic C. *diphtheriae*. Specimens should be inoculated onto blood agar and tellurite media (Downie's medium) immediately. Tellurite medium is whole sheep blood in an agar base and supports the characteristic morphology of C. *diphtheriae* while suppressing other bacteria. After incubating overnight in tellurite media, *gravis* colonies are large, flat, and gray to black with a dull surface; *mitis* organisms produce medium-sized colonies that are blacker, glossy, and more convex; and *intermedius* colonies are very small and either smooth or rough. Each colony type is subcultured on Columbia blood agar plates for toxigenicity and biochemical testing. To determine microscopic morphology, the colonies are further subcultured on Dorset's egg medium and then smeared on slides. The slides are stained by Loeffler's methylene blue stain and Albert's stain, both of which allow identification of metachromatic granules. However, immediate microscopic diagnosis of C. *diphtheriae* from culture by morphological features may be difficult. In some microbiological media, the bacteria may stain variably or negatively, unlike classical textbook descriptions of organisms grown on Loeffler's serum medium or Dorset's egg medium. In fact, the organisms may have to be cultured on the more classical (Loeffler's) medium before they can be recognized by their morphologic features. C. *diphtheriae* initially outgrows other throat flora when inoculated onto Loeffler's medium, so that the plate should be examined within 24 h for evidence of growth.

Although biochemical testing is irrelevant to patient management, it is an essential tool for biotyping purposes, for contact tracing, and for epidemiological studies. Biotyping is best performed on cultures that have been incubated for 24 to 28 h.

Toxigenicity testing of isolated strains is important and should be performed immediately. Although the test can be performed in vivo using guinea pigs, the results obtained are relatively slow to develop. A more rapid method involves in vitro testing using the modified Elek's immunodiffusion method which can be run in a clinical laboratory. Results are available within 24 to 36 h.

PCR (polymerase chain reaction) has emerged as a rapid and highly reliable technique for the detection of the diphtheria toxin gene *tox*. Using this

> *In all cases in which diphtheria is suspected, the laboratory should be told the specimen may contain toxigenic C. diphtheriae*

method, differentiation between toxigenic and nontoxigenic bacterial strains can be quickly performed. In a recent study of clinical samples from patients with diphtheria and other respiratory tract infections and healthy controls, PCR compared well with the Elek immunodiffusion assay (59).

Pathological examination of infected tissues including membranes can often reveal suggestive microscopic changes and bacilli which are morphologically consistent with C. *diphtheriae* infection. However, definitive diagnosis rests on clinical and microbiological results (12, 50).

Treatment and Prevention

The mainstay of treatment of diphtheria is equine diphtheria antitoxin. Because diphtheria antitoxin only neutralizes toxin that is extracellular, it is important to administer it as early in the course of illness as possible. Delays in administering antitoxin beyond the first few days of illness are clearly associated with poorer outcomes (57, 79). A decision to administer antitoxin will often have to be made on clinical grounds, without waiting for laboratory confirmation. Patients should be asked about prior exposure to horse serum and tested for hypersensitivity prior to administration of antitoxin.

The recommended dose of antitoxin depends on the site and extent of local disease as well as the severity and duration of illness, and ranges from 10,000–20,000 U of diphtheria antitoxin for anterior nasal diphtheria to 80,000–120,000 U for extensive disease of 3 or more days duration with brawny swelling of the neck. The patient should be monitored carefully during administration for any signs of shock. Although no longer available commercially in the United States, diphtheria antitoxin is available through an investigational new drug protocol from the Centers for Disease Control and Prevention (CDC) (18).

Although antimicrobial therapy plays a secondary role in treatment of diphtheria, it will hasten clearing of the organism and may lessen the risk of transmission to others

Although antimicrobial therapy plays a secondary role in treatment of diphtheria, it will hasten clearing of the organism and may lessen the risk of transmission to others. Penicillin and erythromycin are both highly active against C. *diphtheriae* and are the agents of choice. Parenteral therapy is recommended initially with intramuscular procaine penicillin G (25,000 to 50,000 U/kg per day for children and 1.2 million U/day for adults in two divided doses) or parenteral erythromycin (40 to 50 mg/kg per day with maximum dosage of 2 g/day); once the patient can swallow easily, oral erythromycin or oral penicillin can be substituted to complete the 14-day course of therapy (26). Although newer macrolide antibiotics may be better tolerated than erythromycin and have been found to be highly active in vitro, clinical data on their use in treatment of diphtheria are limited (81). Bed rest and close clinical monitoring are essential. In one controlled trial, steroids were ineffective in preventing diphtheria myocarditis or neuritis (75).

To prevent transmission of disease to others, antimicrobial prophylaxis of close contacts of cases is recommended after nasal and pharyngeal cultures are obtained for isolation of C. *diphtheriae*. A single dose of intramuscular benzathine penicillin (600,000 U for children under 6 years of age and 1.2

million U for persons 6 years of age or over) or a 7- to 10-day course of erythromycin (40 mg/kg per day for children and 1 g/day for adults) is recommended. Although there is some evidence that erythromycin may be more effective than penicillin in elimination of the organism, penicillin may be preferred if compliance is in doubt (26).

Introduction of routine vaccination of infants and children with diphtheria toxoid (usually given in combination with tetanus toxoid and pertussis vaccine as DTP) has resulted in dramatic decreases in diphtheria incidence worldwide. Because immunity induced by diphtheria toxoid wanes over time, booster doses at school entry, in adolescents, and in adults are needed to prevent disease in older age groups. The occurrence of outbreaks among adolescents and young adults in several countries 5 to 10 years after implementation of childhood diphtheria vaccination programs highlights the risk that diphtheria continues to present, even with high vaccination coverage among children. Likewise, the extraordinary epidemic of diphtheria in the former Soviet Union potentially could have been prevented by routine vaccination of older children, adolescents, and adults and by maintaining high vaccination coverage among children. With the recent demonstration of continued endemic circulation of toxigenic C. *diphtheriae* in both the United States and Canada, as well the continued threat of importation from other countries, diphtheria must be considered a continued threat worldwide.

Figure 7.1 Typical membrane of respiratory diphtheria. (Courtesy of Peter Strebel, CDC.)

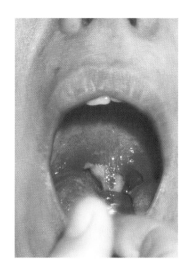

Figure 7.2 Diphtheritic membranes involving the tonsils and uvula, from a drawing in a classic work on diphtheria published in 1895 (12a).

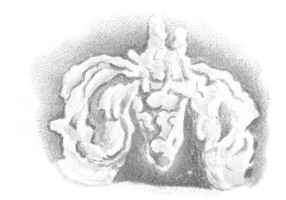

Fig. 37.

Figure 7.3 This Brazilian child has a "bull neck" appearance and cutaneous erythema as a result of pharyngeal diphtheria, resulting in difficulty in breathing. The hemorrhaging from the nose suggests nasal involvement as well. (Courtesy of Anastacio de Queiroz Sousa, Universidade Federal do Ceara, Fortaleza, Brazil, and Martin Cetron, CDC. From reference 72 with permission.)

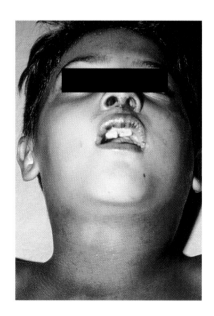

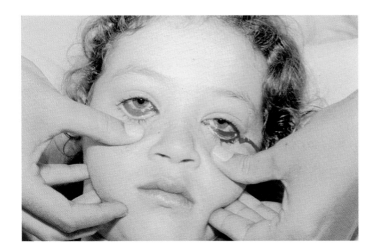

Figure 7.4   "Bloody tears" resulting from infection of this Brazilian girl's left eye with C. *diphtheriae*. Involvement of the eyes is an unusual manifestation of diphtherial infection. (Courtesy of Anastacio de Queiroz Sousa, Universidade Federal do Ceara, Fortaleza, Brazil, and Martin Cetron, CDC. From reference 72 with permission.)

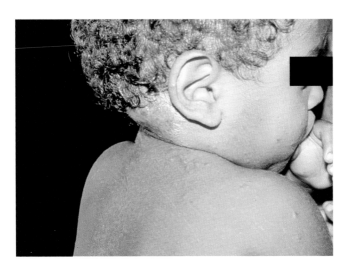

Figure 7.5   Cutaneous diphtherial ulcer at the hairline of the base of the neck in a Brazilian infant. The gross appearance of this lesion is not distinctive for C. *diphtheriae* infection. (Courtesy of Anastacio de Queiroz Sousa, Universidade Federal do Ceara, Fortaleza, Brazil, and Martin Cetron, CDC. From reference 72 with permission.)

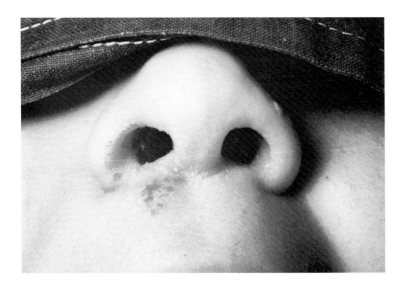

Figure 7.6   Nasal diphtheria, a rare clinical manifestation of C. *diphtheriae* infection.

Figure 7.7   Posterior view of the upper respiratory tract organs (tongue, larynx, trachea, bronchi) removed at autopsy of a child with laryngeal diphtheria. The diphtheritic pseudomembrane extends to involve the larynx and main bronchi. (From reference 72 with permission.)

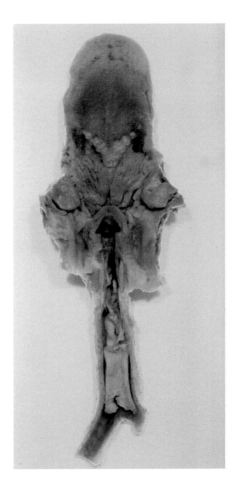

Figure 7.8   Ulcer from scalp of a 31-year-old soldier serving in the Pacific Theater during World War II. On 30 November 1943 he was admitted to the area Army Hospital for malaise, anuria, nausea, and fever, all of about 12 days duration. He had ulcers on face and scalp, treated with sulfadiazine by mouth and $KMNO_4$ soaks. Most of the ulcers healed, but one on the scalp persisted. On 23 December he complained of severe precordial pain. He had a rapid pulse, an enlarged heart with a "mitral configuration" by chest X-ray, and evidence of myocardial damage by electrocardiogram. He died a few hours later on 24 December. The clinical diagnosis was mitral stenosis and coronary occlusion, but an autopsy performed 5 h later by Capt. Victor M. Tompkins, M.C., U.S. Army (later Director of Laboratories for the State of New York), revealed fatal pulmonary edema, a severely degenerated heart, and, on the scalp, an ulcer covered by a "glassy membrane" from which Dr. Tompkins cultured a toxigenic strain of C. *diphtheriae*. This low-power micrograph shows the cutaneous pseudomembrane and underlying hair-bearing skin. Hematoxylin and eosin (H&E) stain; ×10. (Courtesy of Daniel H. Connor. From reference 72 with permission.)

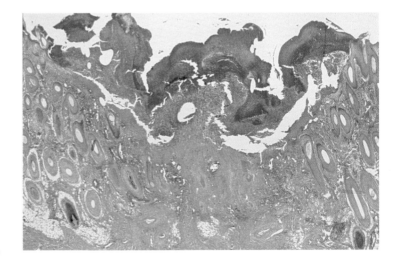

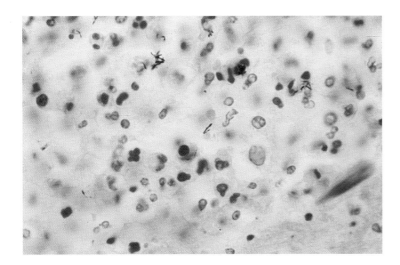

Figure 7.9 Clusters of gram-positive bacilli in the base of the ulcer shown in Fig. 7.8. Many of the bacilli are club shaped, e.g., the bacillus in the center of the picture. Brown and Hopps Gram stain; ×300. (Courtesy of Daniel H. Connor. From reference 72 with permission.)

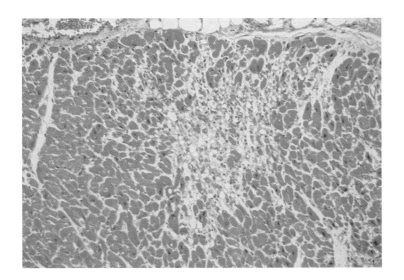

Figure 7.10 Section of myocardium from patient described in Fig. 7.8. There is myocardial necrosis and myocarditis. H&E stain; ×100. (Courtesy of Daniel H. Connor.)

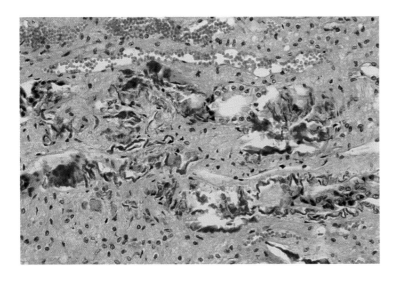

Figure 7.11 Kidney with interstitial inflammation and degenerative changes in renal tubules, from the patient described in Fig. 7.8. These changes are the result of circulating diphtheria exotoxin, not direct tissue invasion by the organisms. H&E stain; ×100. (Courtesy of Daniel H. Connor.)

References

1. **Afghani, B., and H. R. Stutman.** 1993. Bacterial arthritis caused by *Corynebacterium diphtheriae. Pediatr. Infect. Dis. J.* **12:**881–882.

2. **Agrifoglio, L.** 1961. Historical delineation of diphtheria. *Riv. Ital. Igiene* **21:**205.

3. **Barksdale, L., L. Garmise, and K. Horibata.** 1960. Virulence, toxigenicity, and lysogeny in *Corynebacterium diphtheriae. Ann. N.Y. Acad. Sci.* **88:**1093–1108.

4. **Belsey, M. A.** 1970. Isolation of *Corynebacterium diphtheriae* in the environment of skin carriers. *Am. J. Epidemiol.* **91:**294–299.

5. **Belsey, M. A., and D. R. LeBlanc.** 1975. Skin infections and the epidemiology of diphtheria: acquisition and persistence of *C. diphtheriae* infections. *Am. J. Epidemiol.* **102:**179–184.

6. **Belsey, M. A., M. Sinclair, M. R. Roder, and D. R. LeBlanc.** 1969. *Corynebacterium diphtheriae* skin infections in Alabama and Louisiana. *N. Engl. J. Med.* **280:**135–141.

7. **Bethell, D. B., N. M. Dung, H. T. Loan, L.T. N. Minh, N. Q. Dung, N. P. J. Day, and N. J. White.** 1995. Prognostic value of electrocardiographic monitoring of patients with severe diphtheria. *Clin. Infect. Dis.* **20:**1259–1265.

8. **Bezjack, V., and S. J. Farsey.** 1970. *Corynebacterium diphtheriae* in skin lesions in Ugandan children. *Bull. W.H.O.* **43:**643–650.

9. **Bisgard, K. M., I. R. Hardy, T. Popovic, P. M. Strebel, M. Wharton, R. T. Chen, and S. C. Hadler.** 1998. Respiratory diphtheria in the United States, 1980 through 1995. *Am. J. Public Health* **88:**787–791.

10. **Boyer, N. H., and L. Weinstein.** 1948. Diphtheric myocarditis. *N. Engl. J. Med.* **239:**913–919.

11. **Bray, J. P., E. G. Burt, E. V. Potter, T. Poon-King, and D. P. Earle.** 1972. Epidemic diphtheria and skin infections in Trinidad. *J. Infect. Dis.* **126:**34–40.

12. **Brooks, R., and D. H. M. Joynson.** 1990. Bacteriological diagnosis of diphtheria. *J. Clin. Pathol.* **43:**576–580.

12a. **Brown, L.** 1895. *Diphtheria and Its Associates.* Balliere, Tindall & Cox, London.

13. **Cahoon, F. E., S. Brown, and F. Jamieson.** 1997. *Corynebacterium diphtheriae:* toxigenic isolations from northeastern Ontario, abstr. K-171, p. 358. *In Abstracts of the 37th Interscience Conference on Antimicrobial Agents and Chemotherapy, 28 September–1 October 1997.*

14. **Caulfield, E.** 1939. A true history of the terrible epidemic vulgarly called the throat distemper: which occurred in His Majesty's New England colonies between the years 1735 and 1740. *Yale J. Biol. Med.* **11:**219–277.

15. **Centers for Disease Control and Prevention.** 1996. Update: diphtheria epidemic—new independent states of the former Soviet Union, January 1995–March 1996. *Morbid. Mortal. Weekly Rep.* **45:**693–697.

16. **Centers for Disease Control and Prevention.** 1997. Respiratory diphtheria caused by *Corynebacterium ulcerans*—Terre Haute, Indiana, 1996. *Morbid. Mortal. Weekly Rep.* **46:**330–332.

17. **Centers for Disease Control and Prevention.** 1997. Toxigenic *Corynebacterium diphtheriae*—Northern Plains Indian community, August–October 1996. *Morbid. Mortal. Weekly Rep.* **46:**506–510.

18. **Centers for Disease Control and Prevention.** 1997. Availability of diphtheria antitoxin through an investigational new drug protocol. *Morbid. Mortal. Weekly Rep.* **47:**380.

19. **Christenson, B., L. Hellström, and A. Aust-Kettis.** 1989. Diphtheria in Stockholm, with a theory concerning transmission. *J. Infect.* **19:**177–183.

20. **Crosbie, W. E., and H. D. Wright.** 1941. Diphtheria bacilli in floor dust. *Lancet* **i:**656–659.

21. **Dittman, S.** 1997. Epidemic diphtheria in the newly independent states of the former USSR—situation and lessons learned. *Biologicals* **25:**179–186.

22. **Edington, G. M., and H. M. Gilles.** 1976. *Pathology in the Tropics*, 2nd ed., p. 372. Edward Arnold, London.

23. **Edward, D. G., and V. D. Allison.** 1951. Diphtheria in the immunized with observations on a diphtheria-like disease associated with non-toxigenic strains of *Corynebacterium diphtheriae*. *J. Hyg.* **49:**205–219.

24. **Ehrlich, P.** 1897. Die Werthbemessung des Diphtherieheilserums und deren theoretische Grundlagen. *Klin. Jahrb.* **vi:**299–326.

25. **English, P. C.** 1985. Diphtheria and theories of infectious disease: centennial appreciation of the critical role of diphtheria in the history of medicine. *Pediatrics* **76:**1–9.

26. **Farizo, K. M., P. M. Strebel, R. T. Chen, A. Kimbler, T. J. Cleary, and S. L. Cochi.** 1993. Fatal respiratory disease due to *Corynebacterium diphtheriae*: case report and review of guidelines for management, investigation, and control. *Clin. Infect. Dis.* **16:**59–68.

27. **Funke, G., A. Efstratiou, D. Kuklinska, R. A. Hutson, A. De Zoysa, K. H. Engler, and M. D. Collins.** 1997. *Corynebacterium imitans* sp. nov. isolated from patients with suspected diphtheria. *J. Clin. Microbiol.* **35:**1978–1983.

28. **Galazka, A. M., and S. E. Robertson.** 1995. Diphtheria: changing patterns in the developing world. *Eur. J. Epidemiol.* **11:**107–117.

29. **Galazka, A. M., S. E. Robertson, and G. P. Oblapenko.** 1995. Resurgence of diphtheria. *Eur. J. Epidemiol.* **11:**95–105.

30. **Gaskill, H. S., and M. Korb.** 1946. Occurrence of multiple neuritis in cases of cutaneous diphtheria. *Arch. Neurol. Psychiat.* **55:**559–572.

31. **Ghanem, Q.** 1993. Serial measurements of nerve conduction velocity and F-wave latency in diphtheritic neuropathy. *Muscle Nerve* **16:**985–986.

32. **Godfrey, E. S.** 1932. Study in the epidemiology of diphtheria in relation to the active immunization of certain age groups. *Am. J. Public Health* **22:**237–256.

33. **Groman, N., J. Schiller, and J. Russell.** 1984. *Corynebacterium ulcerans* and *Corynebacterium pseudotuberculosis* responses to DNA probes derived from corynephage ß and *Corynebacterium diphtheriae*. *Infect. Immun.* **45:**511–517.

34. **Gruner, E., M. Opravil, M. Altwegg, and A. von Graevenitz.** 1994. Nontoxigenic *Corynebacterium diphtheriae* isolated from intravenous drug users. *Clin. Infect. Dis.* **18:**94–96.

35. **Hardy, I. R. B., S. Dittman, and R. W. Sutter.** 1996. Current situation and control strategies for resurgence of diphtheria in newly independent states of the former Soviet Union. *Lancet* **347:**1739–1744.

36. **Harnisch, J. P., E. Tronca, C. M. Nolan, M. Turck, and K. K. Holmes.** 1989. Diphtheria among alcoholic urban adults: a decade of experience in Seattle. *Ann. Intern. Med.* **111:**71–82.

37. **Hodes, H. L.** 1979. Diphtheria. *Pediatr. Clin. North Am.* **26:**445–459.

38. **Höfler, W.** 1991. Cutaneous diphtheria. *Int. J. Dermatol.* **30:**845–847.

39. **Hogan, M. J.** 1947. Conjunctivitis with membrane formation. *Am. J. Ophthamol.* **302:**1495–1513.

40. **Hoyne, A., and N. T. Welford.** 1934. Diphtheritic myocarditis: a review of 496 cases. *J. Pediatr.* **5:**642–653.

41. **Hust, M. H., B. Metzler, U. Schubert, A. Weidhase, and R. H. Seuffer.** 1994. Toxische Diphtherie durch *Corynebacterium ulcerans. Dtsch. Med. Wschr.* **119:**548–553.

42. **Idiaquez, J.** 1992. Autonomic dysfunction in diphtheritic neuropathy. *J. Neurol. Neurosurg. Psychiat.* **55:**159–161.

43. **Kadyrov, S. N., V. A. Tsinzerling, K. K. Amineva, and D. V. Komarova.** 1996. Cardiac involvement in diphtheria today in adults. *Terapevticheskii Arkhiv* **68:**7–11.

44. **Kalapothaki, V., T. Sapounas, E. Xirouchaki, G. Papoutsakis, and D. Trichopoulos.** 1984. Prevalence of diphtheria carriers in a population with disappearing clinical diphtheria. *Infection* **12:**387–389.

45. **Keller, W. F.** 1941. Diphtheria of the middle ear. *J. Okla. Med. Assn.* **34:**519–521.

46. **Khuri-Bulos, N., Y. Hamzah, S. M. Sammerrai, A. Shehabi, R. Hamed, M. A. Arnaout, J. Turk, and H. Qubain.** 1988. The changing epidemiology of diphtheria in Jordan. *Bull. W.H.O.* **66:**65–68.

47. **Leigh, A. D.** 1948. Diphtheritic polyneuritis in the Far East. *Lancet* **i:**277–280.

48. **Loeffler, F.** 1884. Untersuchugen über die Bedeutung der Mikroorganismen für die Entstehung der Diphtherie. *Mitt. Kaiserl. Ges.* **2:**421–499.

49. **Loevinsohn, B. P.** 1990. The changing age structure of diphtheria patients: evidence for the effectiveness of EPI in the Sudan. *Bull. W.H.O.* **68:**353–357.

50. **MacGregor, R. R.** 1995. *Corynebacterium diphtheriae,* p. 1865–1872. *In* G. L. Mandell, J. E. Bennett, and R. Dolin (ed.), *Principles and Practice of Infectious Diseases,* 4th ed. Churchill Livingstone, Inc., New York.

51. **Maximescu, P., A. Oprian, A. Pop, and E. Potorac.** 1974. Further studies on *Corynebacterium* species capable of producing diphtheria toxin (*C. diphtheriae, C. ulcerans, C. ovis*). *J. Gen. Microbiol.* **82:**49–56.

52. **Melby, E. L., J. Jacobsen, S. Olsnes, and K. Sandrig.** 1993. Entry of protein toxins in polarized epithelial cells. *Cancer Res.* **53:**1755–1760.

53. **Mencarelli, M., A. Zanchi, C. Cellesi, A. Rossolini, R. Rappuoli, and G. M. Rossolini.** 1992. Molecular epidemiology of nasopharyngeal corynebacteria in healthy adults from an area where diphtheria vaccination has been extensively practiced. *Eur. J. Epidemiol.* **8:**560–567.

54. **Montgomery, J.** 1984. Carriage of *Corynebacterium diphtheriae* in children of the Eastern Highlands Province. *Papua New Guinea Med. J.* **27:**20–23.

55. **Morgan, B. C.** 1963. Cardiac complications of diphtheria. *Pediatrics* **32:**549–557.

56. **Muyembe, J. J., F. Gatti, J. Spaepen, and J. Vandepitt.** 1972. L'epidemiologie de la diphtérie en République du Zaire: le rôle de l'infection cutanée. *Ann. Soc. Belge Med. Trop.* **52:**141–152.

57. **Naiditch, M. J., and A. G. Bower.** 1954. Diphtheria: a study of 1,433 cases observed during a ten-year period at the Los Angeles County Hospital. *Am. J. Med.* **17:**229–245.

58. **Nakao, H., I. K. Mazurova, T. Glushkevich, and T. Popovic.** 1997. Heterogeneity of diphtheria toxin gene, *tox*, and its regulatory element, *dtxR*, in *Corynebacterium diphtheriae* strains causing epidemic diphtheria in Russia and Ukraine. *Res. Microbiol.* **148:**45–54.

59. **Nakao, H., and T. Popovic.** 1997. Development of a direct PCR assay for detection of the diphtheria toxin gene. *J. Clin. Microbiol.* **35:**1651–1655.

60. **Pappenheimer, A. M.** 1984. The diphtheria bacillus and its toxin: a model system. *J. Hyg.* **93:**397–404.

61. **Pappenheimer, A. M., and D. M. Gill.** 1973. Diphtheria: recent studies have clarified the molecular mechanisms involved in its pathogenesis. *Science* **182:**353–358.

62. **Pappenheimer, A. M., and J. R. Murphy.** 1983. Studies in the molecular epidemiology of diphtheria. *Lancet* **ii:**923–926.

63. **Pascual, C., P. A. Lawson, J. A. E. Farrow, M. Navarro Gimenez, and M. D. Collins.** 1995. Analysis of the genus *Corynebacterium* based on 16S rRNA gene sequences. *Int. J. Syst. Bacteriol.* **45:**724–728.

64. **Patey, O., F. Bimet, P. Riegel, B. Halioua, J. P. Emond, E. Estrangin, S. Dellion, J. M. Alonso, M. Kiredjian, A. Dublanchet, C. Lafaix, and the Coryne Study Group.** 1997. Clinical and molecular study of *Corynebacterium diphtheriae* systemic infections in France. *J. Clin. Microbiol.* **35:**441–445.

65. **Popovic, T., S. Y. Kombarova, M. W. Reeves, H. Nakao, I. K. Mazurova, M. Wharton, I. K. Wachsmuth, and J. D. Wenger.** 1996. Molecular epidemiology of diphtheria in Russia, 1985–1994. *J. Infect. Dis.* **174:**1064–1072.

66. **Quick, L., I. Hardy, R. W. Sutter, P. Strebel, K. Kobaidze, and N. Malakmadze.** 1997. Risk factors for transmission of diphtheria among 219 cases in the Republic of Georgia, 1995–1996, abstr. K-168, p. 358. *In Abstracts of the 37th Interscience Conference on Antimicrobial Agents and Chemotherapy, 28 September–1 October, 1997.*

67. **Reidermann, M. I.** 1996. Herzkomplikationen der Erwachsenendiphtherie: Analyse von 212 Fallen. *Schweiz. Rundsch. Med. Praxis* **85:**1647–1651.

68. **Rolleston, J. D.** 1904. Clinical observations on diphtheritic paralysis. *Practitioner* **72:**597–623.

69. **Roux, E., and A. Yersin.** 1889. Contribution a l'étude de la diphtérie. *Ann. Inst. Pasteur* **iii:**273–288.

70. **Sayers, E. G.** 1958. Diphtheritic myocarditis with permanent heart damage. *Ann. Intern. Med.* **48:**146–157.

71. **Schwartz, D. A., and C. J. Herman.** 1996. The importance of the autopsy in emerging and reemerging infectious diseases. *Clin. Infect. Dis.* **23:**248–254.

72. **Schwartz, D. A., A. B. Jenson, and L. Y. Lim.** 1997. Corynebacterial infections, p. 533–542. *In* D. H. Connor, F. W. Chandler, D. A. Schwartz, H. J. Manz, and E. E. Lack (ed.), *Pathology of Infectious Diseases.* Appleton & Lange, Stamford, Conn.

73. **Stockins, B. A., F. T. Lanas, J. G. Saavedra, and J. A. Opazo.** 1994. Prognosis in patients with diphtheritic myocarditis and bradyarrhythmias: assessment of results of ventricular pacing. *Br. Heart J.* **72:**190–191.

74. **Thaung, U., T. Naung, K. S. Khine, and C. K. Ming.** 1978. Epidemiological features of skin diphtheria infection in Rangoon, Burma. *S. E. Asian J. Trop. Med. Public Health* **9:**4–10.

75. **Thisyakorn, U., J. Wongvanich, and V. Kumpeng.** 1984. Failure of corticosteroid therapy to prevent diphtheritic myocarditis or neuritis. *Pediatr. Infect. Dis. J.* **3:**126–128.

76. **Thomann, U., M. Gasser, J. Pietrzak, A. Tschopp, C. Bignens, and E. Stahel.** 1988. Importierte Hautdiphtherie aus tropischen Ländern. *Schweiz. Med. Wschr.* **118:**676–679.

77. **Trichopoulos, D., G. Politou, G. Papoutsakis, A. Kyriakidou, and P. Vassiliadis.** 1972. Diphtheria carriers among schoolchildren in Athens. *Scand. J. Infect. Dis.* **4:**197–201.

78. **Van Geldermalsen, A. A., and U. Wenning.** 1993. A diphtheria epidemic in Lesotho, 1989. Did vaccination increase the population's susceptibility? *Ann. Trop. Paediatr.* **13:**13–20.

79. **Welch, W. W.** 1895. The treatment of diphtheria by antitoxin. *Bull. Johns Hopkins Hosp.* **6:**97–120.

80. **Wesley, A. G., M. Pather, and V. Chrystal.** 1981. The haemorrhagic diathesis in diphtheria with special reference to disseminated intravascular coagulation. *Ann. Trop. Paediatr.* **1:**51–56.

81. **Wilson, A. P. R.** 1995. Treatment of infection caused by toxigenic and non-toxigenic strains of *Corynebacterium diphtheriae*. *J. Antimicrob. Chemother.* **35:**717–720.

82. **Wilson, A. P. R., A. Efstratiou, E. Weaver, E. Allason-Jones, J. Bingham, G. L. Ridgway, A. Robinson, D. Mercey, G. Colman, and B. D. Cookson.** 1992. Unusual non-toxigenic *Corynebacterium diphtheriae* in homosexual men. *Lancet* **339:**998.

83. **Wilson, C. R., R. I. Casson, B. Wherrett, and N. Fraser.** 1991. Toxigenic diphtheria in two isolated northern communities. *Arctic Med. Res.* **1991** (Suppl.):346–347.

84. **Wong, T. P., and N. Groman.** 1984. Production of diphtheria toxin by selected isolates of *Corynebacterium ulcerans* and *Corynebacterium pseudotuberculosis*. *Infect. Immun.* **43:**1114–1116.

85. **Youwang, Y., D. Jianming, X. Yong, and Z. Pong.** 1992. Epidemiological features of an outbreak of diphtheria and its control with diphtheria toxoid immunization. *Int. J. Epidemiol.* **21:**807–811.

86. **Zuber, P. L. F., E. Gruner, M. Altwegg, and A. von Graevenitz.** 1992. Invasive infection with non-toxigenic *Corynebacterium diphtheriae* among drug users. *Lancet* **339:**1359.

chapter 8

Tuberculosis

Henry M. Blumberg and Ann Marie Nelson

Events of the past decade have dramatically changed the nature and magnitude of the problem of tuberculosis. Much of what many physicians learned in training about this disease is no longer true. In many respects, tuberculosis has become a new entity. (72)

Mycobacterium tuberculosis is the causative agent of tuberculosis (or, TB) and a member of the *Mycobacterium tuberculosis* complex, a group of closely related organisms including M. *microti*, M. *africanum*, M. *bovis*, and M. *tuberculosis*. Tuberculosis is an ancient disease, with evidence of skeletal tuberculosis (Pott's disease) dating back to Neolithic times (5000 BCE), ancient Egypt, and, in the New World, the pre-Columbian era (47). Tuberculosis has been recognized by the medical profession since at least the time of Hippocrates, when it was known as "phthisis" for the wasting nature of the disease. Tuberculosis became widespread in the 17th century, and by the time of the Industrial Revolution in

Henry M. Blumberg, Division of Infectious Diseases, Department of Medicine, Emory University School of Medicine, 69 Butler Street, S.E., Atlanta, GA 30303. **Ann Marie Nelson,** Division of AIDS Pathology, Department of Infectious and Parasitic Disease Pathology, Armed Forces Institute of Pathology, Washington, DC 20306-6000.

Pathology of Emerging Infections 2
Edited by Ann Marie Nelson and C. Robert Horsburgh, Jr.
© 1998 American Society for Microbiology, Washington, D.C.

Europe it caused one-fourth of all deaths among adults (47). As recently as the early 20th century, tuberculosis was a leading cause of death in the United States. Tuberculosis case and mortality rates in Europe and the United States had been falling for some time due to improved living conditions (and perhaps natural selection) in the 19th and 20th centuries before the introduction of effective chemotherapy beginning with streptomycin in 1946. Tuberculosis is now endemic and devastating in much of Africa and parts of Asia. Over the past decade there has been a resurgence of disease in developed countries as well. Tuberculosis remains a unique disease, for unlike other disorders in which achieving cure is primarily the patient's concern, the responsibility for cure rests with the health care professional, the public health system, and ultimately society (65).

Epidemiology

Tuberculosis has become a public health problem of major proportions worldwide

Tuberculosis has become a public health problem of major proportions worldwide, and in 1993 the World Health Organization (WHO) declared the disease to be a "global emergency." Globally, tuberculosis is the leading cause of death due to infectious disease; each year it is estimated that there are more than 8 million new cases and more than 3 million deaths from the disease (62, 64). Tuberculosis now accounts for 6% of *all* deaths worldwide (6). One third of the world's population harbors M. *tuberculosis* (i.e., tuberculosis infection) and therefore is at risk for developing active disease.

Tuberculosis has been neglected as a public health issue for years by many countries (62). This has fostered a resurgence of disease in developed countries over the past decade and has led to inadequate control programs in many developing countries, where 95% of the cases occur. In a number of countries in Africa and Southeast Asia, infection with human immunodeficiency virus (HIV) has further increased tuberculosis-related morbidity and mortality (5, 20, 54). In several of the countries which had been part of the former Soviet Union, tuberculosis morbidity and mortality have increased because of deterioration of the public health infrastructure (63).

Between 1985 and 1992, there was a resurgence of tuberculosis in the United States (Fig. 8.1); the number of cases increased by 20% from 1985 to 1992, when 26,673 cases were reported in the United States, or 10.5 cases per 100,000 population (10, 13). This reversed a trend seen throughout the 20th century in the United States of cases declining at a rate of about 6% per year since 1953, when national data on the number of tuberculosis cases became available. Major factors responsible for the resurgence of tuberculosis in the United States include the HIV/AIDS epidemic and decay of the public health infrastructure (in large part due to underfunding) (32).

Other factors that contributed to the increasing numbers of tuberculosis cases in the United States include immigration from areas endemic for tuberculosis, homelessness and poverty, drug abuse, and noncompliance (which can lead to the development of drug resistance). The resurgence exposed fundamental weaknesses of local tuberculosis control programs. Consequently, many communities in the United States were not equipped to confront the increasing number of cases or the shifting epidemiological and clinical features of disease (32). Tuberculosis is not evenly distributed throughout the population. About half the counties in the United States have no tuberculosis cases reported each year. To a large extent, it has become an inner-city disease in the United States, with the majority of cases occurring in urban areas (49). In fact, in a number of inner-city areas case rates are 10 to 20 times higher than the national average.

Recent studies from the United States (San Francisco and New York) and Europe (Bern, Switzerland), employing molecular typing methods (IS6110-restriction fragment length polymorphism analysis) of M. *tuberculosis* isolates, indicate that many more cases are due to recent transmission than had been previously thought. These molecular epidemiologic studies suggest that a third or more of cases are due to recent person-to-person transmission, with the remainder due to reactivation of latent infection (1, 25, 69). Two-thirds of tuberculosis cases in HIV/AIDS patients appear to be due to recent transmission rather than reactivation of remote infection.

*M*any more cases are due to recent transmission than had been previously thought

During 1996, there were 21,337 cases of tuberculosis (8.0 cases per 100,000) in the United States. This represented the fourth consecutive year of decreases in the number of cases following the resurgence between 1985 and 1992. The continued decline in the number of cases reported annually in the United States since 1992 reflects improvement in the public health infrastructure due to marked increases in federal funding to states and cities for tuberculosis control (13). This has led to improved patient management and increased funding for directly observed therapy (DOT) programs, which have been demonstrated to improve completion-of-therapy rates. In addition, improvements in hospital tuberculosis infection control activities which have prevented nosocomial transmission have been important in "turning the tide" (8, 9).

Tuberculosis cases in the United States occur disproportionately among members of racial/ethnic minority groups. Currently, greater than 70% of all cases in the United States and 85% of those among children less than 15 years old occur among racial or ethnic minorities (13). The proportion of United States tuberculosis cases occurring among the foreign born has increased from about 22% in 1986 to 36.4% of all cases in 1996, reflecting the global nature of tuberculosis as a public health problem (13).

A nationwide survey by the Centers for Disease Control and Prevention (CDC) on drug susceptibility testing results of M. *tuberculosis* isolates from tuberculosis cases between 1993 and 1996 indicated that in the United States 13.5% of patients had some type of drug-resistant disease; 8.4% had isoniazid (INH)-resistant disease, and 2.2% had multidrug-resistant disease (MDR-TB) as defined by resistance to at least INH and rifampin (RIF) (50). Foreign-born patients had significantly higher rates of drug resistance (22.4% overall) than American-born patients, and those who had a history of prior tuberculosis also had higher rates of drug resistance. MDR-TB cases were reported from 42 different states; however, 38% of all MDR-TB cases occurred in New York City. Frieden and colleagues reported results from a 1-month survey (April 1991) on susceptibility testing of M. *tuberculosis* isolates from New York City hospitals: one-third of tuberculosis patients had isolates with resistance to at least one drug, and 19% had isolates that were multidrug resistant (i.e., resistant to at least INH and RIF) (24). A subsequent 47% decrease in MDR-TB cases in New York City over a 4-year period correlated with strong leadership in the tuberculosis control program and a massive infusion of funding, providing adequate resources leading to rebuilding of the public health infrastructure (23, 65). The cost of caring for a patient with MDR-TB is quite high, approximately $200,000 per patient (44, 45); this emphasizes the importance and cost-effectiveness of efforts to control the development and spread of MDR-TB.

The cost of caring for a patient with MDR-TB is quite high, approximately $200,000 per patient

Microbiology

Mycobacteria are aerobic, non-sporeforming, nonmotile, facultative intracellular bacilli measuring 0.2 to 0.5 by 2.0 to 4.0 μm. Their cell walls contain mycolic acid-rich long-chain glycolipids and/or phospholipoglycans (mycosides) which protect them from lysosomal attack. Mycosides avidly retain red basic fuchsin dye after acid rinsing; acid-fastness varies among species of mycobacteria. Although highly specific, these stains are not very sensitive, requiring concentrations of at least 10,000 bacilli per ml. The auramine-rhodamine fluorescence stain is more sensitive but less specific than the carbol-fuchsin stains; because of its increased sensitivity the fluorochrome is used by most clinical microbiology laboratories (52, 80, 84).

Routine culture techniques include a decontamination procedure and must be performed in a biological safety cabinet. A nonselective egg medium, such as Lowenstein-Jensen, and a Middlebrook medium (7H10 or 7H11, with or without antibiotics) can be used for primary isolation. Species can be identified by pigmentation, growth characteristics, the ability to produce disease in laboratory animals, and DNA probes (31, 39, 52). Growth of M. *tuberculosis* is favored in 5–10% CO_2 but inhibited by pH of <6.5 and by long-chain fatty acids. In vitro, bacilli grow at 35 to 37°C. Three weeks or more are required for routine culture (on solid media) because of the long doubling time of M. *tuberculosis* (22 h compared with less than 1 h for most bacteria). M. *tuberculosis* is niacin positive, reduces nitrate, hydrolyzes Tween, and will produce disease in guinea pigs (81, 82). Radiometric broth culture (BACTEC, Becton-Dickinson Laboratories, Towson, Md.) methods have been shown to significantly decrease the time to recovery of mycobacteria as compared with solid media. NAP (*p*-nitro-α-acetyl-amino-β-hydroxy-propriophenone) inhibition can be used to differentiate M. *tuberculosis* and M. *bovis* from other mycobacteria; most clinical microbiology laboratories use DNA probes specific to the rRNA of mycobacteria (e.g., GenProbe [Gen Probe, San Diego, Calif.]) to identify clinically significant organisms to the species level following recovery in culture (31, 67).

Gas-liquid chromatography can be used to identify organisms in clinical specimens (74) but is not widely available (except in research or large reference laboratory settings). PCR (polymerase chain reaction) techniques are able to detect very small numbers of specific mycobacteria in clinical specimens (22) or in tissue sections (30). Nucleic acid amplification procedures which can detect M. *tuberculosis* directly from clinical specimens are being introduced into the clinical microbiology laboratory. DNA fingerprinting using restriction fragment length polymorphism is a useful epidemiological tool and may provide a rapid method for identifying multidrug-resistant strains (28).

M. *bovis* causes tuberculosis in cattle and is highly virulent in humans. Prior to the use of pasteurization, milk from infected cows was an important source of primary gastrointestinal and oropharyngeal tuberculosis. M. *bovis* cannot necessarily be distinguished by disease manifestations nor by PPD (purified protein derivative) reaction, but does demonstrate different culture characteristics. It is slightly smaller than M. *tuberculosis* and is slower growing and uniformly resistant to pyrazinamide. It is niacin negative, does not reduce nitrates or hydrolyze Tween, and does not produce disease in guinea pigs. Attenuated strains of M. *bovis* are used to produce BCG (bacille Calmette-Guérin) vaccine (81, 84).

> M. *bovis* causes tuberculosis in cattle and is highly virulent in humans

Virulence

Genetic and phenotypic differences in virulence of mycobacteria have been described. The pathogenic laboratory M. *tuberculosis* strain is H37Rv (human, 37, rough, virulent). Repeated passage through subcultures, exposure to UV light, and air drying decrease the virulence of some mycobacteria. There are also geographic differences in the virulence of organisms (81, 84). The virulence appears to be inversely related to the capacity of the microorganisms to induce production of protective cytokines (e.g., tumor necrosis factor-α, gamma interferon) (78).

No exotoxins, endotoxins, or tissue-necrotizing enzymes of M. *tuberculosis* have been discovered in intact tubercle bacilli. Some toxic components (e.g., cord factor) may be released when the mycobacteria disintegrate. Glycolipids and peptides such as wax D and muramyl dipeptide enhance delayed-type hypersensitivity (DTH), one of the major causes of cell death. Another mechanism that allows mycobacteria to multiply within macrophages of the nonimmune host is their ability to block phago-lysosomal fusion. Sulfatides (polyanionic trehalose tuberculoglycolipids) modify lysosome membranes to prevent fusion with phagosomes (27, 77).

Though morphology is not consistently related to virulence, virulent strains tend to produce rough colonies. The formation of serpentine cords in either liquid or solid media is associated with increased virulence. Cord factor (6,6'-dimycolyltrehalose) inhibits neutrophil migration in vitro, is lethal to mice, is more abundant in virulent strains, and decreases with serial passage of the organism. Cord factor has been related to profound disturbances of microsomal enzymes, mitochondria, and lipid metabolism in livers of mice (21).

Pathogenesis

M. *tuberculosis* is transmitted by an airborne route. Infection with M. *tuberculosis* occurs following inhalation of droplet nuclei which are produced when a patient with pulmonary or laryngeal tuberculosis coughs, sneezes, speaks, or sings. Droplet nuclei are so small (1–5 μm) that air currents can keep them airborne for long periods of time. Transmission can occur only from a patient with active tuberculosis disease (e.g., laryngeal or pulmonary) and not from an individual with tuberculous infection alone (i.e., positive tuberculin skin test, normal chest radiograph, asymptomatic patient). Transmission is facilitated by prolonged exposure to an infectious environment (e.g., relatively small enclosed spaces with inadequate ventilation). Patients who are coughing and have bacilli detectable by microscopy are considered to be most infectious.

Data from Europe and the United States from the 1970s suggest that approximately 30 to 50% of household contacts of smear-positive pulmonary tuberculosis patients become infected (tuberculin skin test positive) (27). However, microepidemics have demonstrated much higher rates (e.g., 80% of sailors on a submarine who shared a room with a bunk mate who had active pulmonary tuberculosis converted their tuberculin skin test) (34).

Overall, there is about a 10% lifetime chance of developing active disease after tuberculosis infection (if no preventive therapy is given): 5% within the first 2 years of infection (greatest risk period) and an additional 5% lifetime risk. Risk and rates of progression from infection to active disease are greatest among individuals with HIV infection (e.g., 8 to 10% per year progression to active disease for tuberculin skin test-positive HIV-infected patients). Increased risk of active disease after infection is also seen among those with renal failure, diabetes, post-gastrectomy, malignancy, and other immunosuppressive diseases (or those on immunosuppressive medications) and among young children (less than 2 years of age).

The risk of developing active tuberculosis in an individual coinfected with HIV and tuberculosis (i.e., tuberculin skin test-positive patient with HIV infection) is about 8 to 10% per year (32). In addition, HIV-infected patients, especially those with severe immunosuppression (i.e., low CD4 counts), are likely to develop active disease rapidly after exposure to tuberculosis. This has been dramatically demonstrated by outbreaks of tuberculosis in hospitals, prisons, and AIDS residential centers. For example, at an AIDS residential center in San Francisco there was an outbreak of tuberculosis due to a resident with unsuspected tuberculosis; 37% of the exposed HIV-infected individuals developed *active* tuberculosis within 110 days after exposure (15). The overall attack rate was greater than 50%.

Because tuberculosis infection results in a specific cell-mediated immune response, further exposures to the tubercle bacillus are far less likely to cause new infections (in immunocompetent individuals). Thus, PPD-positive individuals (who are immunocompetent) are at much lower risk of acquiring a new tuberculous infection than are PPD-negative individuals. HIV-infected tuberculosis patients have been documented to have been rein-

> *Droplet nuclei are so small (1–5 μm) that air currents can keep them airborne for long periods of time*

fected with a different (i.e., second) strain of M. *tuberculosis* and developed active disease, either after successful treatment or during treatment (e.g., superinfection with a resistant strain) (71). This is relatively uncommon, however; recurrent disease is more likely to be due to relapse of previous disease rather than reinfection with a different strain of M. *tuberculosis*. Reactivation tuberculosis not uncommonly occurs with some alteration in the host's immune status such as illness, malnutrition, alcoholism, or corticosteroid therapy.

The host response to an infective dose of mycobacteria is determined by the immune status of the host and possibly by genetic factors (36). Lurie and Dannenberg have described four stages of infection and disease (17–19). Primary infection occurs in an immunologically naive host when inhaled or ingested viable mycobacteria are phagocytized by the resident alveolar macrophages. Whether the infection progresses or not depends on the microbicidal abilities of resident macrophages, the infective dose, and the virulence of the infecting agent. If the mycobacteria are able to survive and multiply, they destroy the macrophage and the infection passes to the second or symbiotic stage. The mycobacterial antigens along with complement component C5a and cytokines (e.g., monocyte chemotactic protein-1) induce chemotaxis, and macrophages (monocytes) are recruited from the peripheral blood. Bacilli are phagocytized and then multiply logarithmically within these immature macrophages.

Stage three, the onset of acquired cellular resistance (cell-mediated immunity [CMI]), occurs 4 to 8 weeks after the initial infection. Stage three is characterized by local accumulation of large numbers of macrophages and lymphocytes and a local activation of these cells. Presentation of antigen fragments in combination with class II major histocompatibility complex is essential in activation of CD4$^+$ T lymphocytes and the development of CMI. Dendritic cells and macrophages are important antigen-presenting cells which stimulate specific clonal proliferation of T cells, resulting in the activation of macrophages and enhanced intracellular killing of mycobacteria (55). With the development of CMI, there is an indurated reaction to the intradermal injection of purified tuberculin (PPD).

The second arm of the cellular immune response is DTH. This response is directly or indirectly responsible for most cell death. It is mediated by toxic effects of lymphokines and mycobacterial degradation products, ischemic necrosis, complement-mediated injury, hydrolytic enzymes from phagocytes, and reactive superoxides. DTH results in the formation of acellular, caseous "cheesy" necrosis. Mycobacterial growth is inhibited by high concentrations of fatty acids, low pH, and low oxygen tension in these caseous centers (17–19).

The fourth stage refers primarily to pulmonary tuberculosis and the formation of cavities. If cavities form adjacent to bronchi, increased DTH-stimulated tissue destruction may cause erosion into the bronchi, allowing mycobacteria to spread in the airways or be exhaled into the environment. This is the most infective stage of the disease.

CMI-DTH interactions vary with changes in host immunity and mycobacterial concentration. CMI predominates when antigen levels are

The host response to an infective dose of mycobacteria is determined by the immune status of the host

low, and DTH occurs when large concentrations of bacilli are present or macrophage activation is impaired. In the immunocompromised host, bacilli which escape from the caseous centers are phagocytized by poorly activated macrophages which are in turn destroyed by cytotoxic lymphocytes and other DTH mechanisms (18, 56).

In the HIV-infected patient, Dannenberg's stages regress as immunosuppression advances. The loss of CMI is directly related to the loss of CD4$^+$ T cells. T lymphocytes have a helper/inducer function (CD4$^+$, Th) which enhances immune response or cytotoxic function (CD8$^+$). Two subsets of T-helper cells (Th1 and Th2) have been described. Th1 cells secrete interleukin-2 and gamma interferon and are thought to be responsible for macrophage activation in response to various antigens in the tubercle bacillus. Th2 cells secrete interleukins 4, 5, and 10, which stimulate B cells. These two T-cell subsets seem negatively to regulate each other (51). Recent studies of HIV-infected individuals show that Th1 cells are progressively lost, shifting the ratio to a Th2-dominant population (14, 41).

There clearly is an important HIV-tuberculosis interaction and, as noted, HIV infection greatly increases the risk of developing active disease after infection with M. tuberculosis. M. tuberculosis is a virulent pathogen, and control of latent infection depends on constant vigilance by the cellular immune system. Loss of immune function, especially the cellular component, is the hallmark of HIV disease. Loss of T-helper cells leads to decreased production of gamma interferon and macrophage-activating lymphokines, two of the most important immune modulators in tuberculosis. M. tuberculosis also has been shown to up-regulate HIV expression. Wallis reported a 3- to 10-fold increase in levels of tumor necrosis factor-α (a product of activated macrophages) in patients with HIV/tuberculosis coinfection (79). This immune activation may promote the increased expression of HIV (46) in both macrophages and lymphocytes and lead to more rapid progression to AIDS (83). The presence of tuberculous disease causes increased HIV viral load, and treatment of tuberculosis can result in decreased HIV plasma viral levels (26).

There clearly is an important HIV-tuberculosis interaction

Pathology

The word "tuberculosis" is Latin for a disease of small nodules. "Tubercle" refers to the classic lesion associated with this disease, the epithelioid granuloma with central caseous necrosis. The most common site of the primary lesion is within the alveolar macrophage in a subpleural area of the lung (the "Gohn focus"). During the initial phase of the infection, bacilli proliferate locally and spread via the lymphatics to a hilar node, thus forming the Gohn complex. The early tubercles that form within the lung or other sites of infection are small and usually spherical and vary in size from 0.5 to 3.0 mm in diameter. There are three or four zones: the central area of caseous necrosis; the cellular zone of epithelioid macrophages, Langhans giant cells, and a few interspersed lymphocytes; an outer zone of lymphocytes, plasma cells, and immature macrophages; and, in healing lesions, a rim of fibrosis (19, 42, 77).

The initial lesion may heal and become latent before any symptomatic illness occurs. The smallest tubercles are completely eliminated by the phagocytic activity of the macrophages. Fibrosis occurs when hydrolytic enzymes dissolve mid-sized tubercles (2 to 8 mm). Larger caseous lesions are surrounded by a fibrous capsule. These fibrocaseous nodules usually contain small numbers of viable mycobacteria and are potential foci of reactivation or cavitation. Some nodules calcify or ossify and are easily seen on chest X-rays.

If the host is unable to arrest the infection in the initial stage, the patient develops progressive primary tuberculosis. Primary tuberculous pneumonia classically involves the lower and middle lobes of the lung and is often purulent with large numbers of acid-fast bacilli (AFB) found in sputum and tissue. Serosal disease, pleuritis or pericarditis, can occur at this period if subserosal granulomas rupture into the pleural or pericardial space and cause local serous inflammation. AFB can usually be found in tissue but are less commonly recovered from effusions. Pleuritis may be an isolated finding, without concomitant pulmonary parenchymal lesions. Some patients manifest severe systemic immune abnormalities such as erythema nodosa or Poncet disease (tuberculous rheumatism) (16). Simultaneous development of pulmonary, mediastinal, and meningeal tuberculosis is a well-described manifestation in young children.

With the onset of the cellular immune response, the lesions which develop around foci of mycobacteria can be either proliferative or exudative. Both types of lesions are usually present within the same host, since infective doses and local immunity vary from site to site. Proliferative lesions are most common when the bacillary load is small and CMI predominates. The resultant nodules are "hard" and compact and are composed of activated macrophages with palisading lymphocytes and plasma cells and an outer rim of fibrosis. There is effective intracellular killing of mycobacteria, and the bacillary load remains low. If local immunity wanes, the lesions may progress, form satellites, or coalesce with neighboring lesions.

Exudative lesions predominate if large numbers of bacilli are present and/or host defenses are weak. The loose aggregates of immature macrophages, neutrophils, fibrin, and caseous necrosis are sites of mycobacterial growth. Without therapy, these lesions usually progress and the infection spreads.

Although bacilli are often carried via the bloodstream to other parts of the body at the time of initial infection, primary extrapulmonary disease is rare except in severely immunocompromised hosts. Resistant hosts are able to control mycobacterial growth in these distant foci before active disease develops. Many organisms do remain viable and are potential sites of extrapulmonary disease in the immunosuppressed host. A sudden release of large numbers of mycobacteria into the circulation causes hematogenous seeding of multiple organs. Infants, the elderly, or otherwise immunosuppressed hosts are unable to control the infection and develop disseminated (primary

The initial lesion may heal and become latent before any symptomatic illness occurs

miliary) tuberculosis; the lesions are typically small (2 to 4 mm) and resemble millet seeds. Patients who become immunosuppressed months to years following the primary infection can develop late generalized disease (68).

Progressive granulomatous or cavitary disease of the upper lobes can occur as a late complication of primary disease, but the majority of cases are post-primary or reactivation. Mycobacteria, previously latent within fibrocaseous nodules, are able to overcome weakened host defenses in patients with impaired cellular immunity. Lesions expand and often cavitate, or old lesions may also undergo spontaneous liquefaction with cavity formation. Most cavitary disease does not regress without treatment.

Erosion of blood vessels may occur as a complication of cavitary disease. Hemoptysis is one of the most frightening clinical manifestations of the disease and historically was an important cause of mortality. Tuberculous empyema and bronchopleural fistulas also occurred more commonly before the introduction of antituberculous drugs.

Extrapulmonary tuberculosis can occur as part of a primary or late generalized infection or as a reactivation site that may or may not coexist with pulmonary reactivation. The most common sites of extrapulmonary disease are mediastinal, retroperitoneal, and cervical (scrofula) lymph nodes; apex of the kidneys; vertebral bodies (Pott's disease); adrenals; meninges; and gastrointestinal tract. The lesions themselves are similar to those described in the lung. Isolated involvement of lymph nodes is a common site of reactivation tuberculosis, especially in HIV-infected patients (20), and is also seen with primary disease.

"Hyporeactive" tuberculosis is a term first used by Lucas and his coworkers to describe the histologic patterns found in lymph nodes from HIV-infected Ugandans (53). He described a spectrum of cellular immune response that was similar to that seen in leprosy. Further studies have shown a regression of the host response over the course of HIV disease and AIDS (44).

Patients whose cellular immunity is still relatively intact will have the typical granulomatous response (Fig. 8.2A, B, and C). The necrotic center is often large, epithelioid macrophages and Langhans giant cells are abundant, and numbers of mycobacteria are low. As the CD4$^+$ lymphocyte count drops, cellular immunity decreases. The first obvious change is the loss of Langhans giant cells, followed by a decrease in epithelioid macrophages. With poor intracellular killing of mycobacteria, the lesions expand, form satellites, and eventually disseminate. Histologically there is breakdown of the fibrous capsule and small clusters of epithelioid macrophages outside the lesion. Lesions may have a thin rim of macrophages and fibrosis; necrosis is mixed suppurative and caseous. AFB are numerous, both in the areas of necrosis and within macrophages (Fig. 8.3A, B, and C).

In the final stages, a diffuse inflammatory response composed of immature macrophages, neutrophils, and coagulative necrosis replaces the typical granulomatous response. Miliary or disseminated anergic disease is present in almost all patients at this stage. AFB are myriad within the necrosis. The large numbers of AFB within macrophages are reminiscent of proliferation in the naive host.

Hemoptysis is one of the most frightening clinical manifestations of the disease and historically was an important cause of mortality

In the dual-infected patient, pulmonary tuberculosis is still the most common site, but the lesions are often atypical. Pulmonary disease is diffuse and often noncavitary and affects the middle or lower lobes; sputum exams are often negative. Pleural and pericardial effusions (as seen in primary tuberculous pneumonia) are common.

Tuberculosis must be differentiated from other granulomatous diseases such as histoplasmosis, coccidioidomycosis, or nocardiosis (40, 42). Cultures and biopsy are both adequate for identification. With loss of the granulomatous response, the list of possible etiologies for infection increases. Special stains for microorganisms and culture are essential to establish the diagnosis and to rule out the possibility of multiple infections. A silver impregnation technique (such as Gomori methenamine silver [GMS]) will readily demonstrate the fungal forms and the branching bacterial filaments of *Nocardia* sp. These can then be identified by their partial acid-fast staining characteristics with the Coates-Fite modification of the carbol fuchsin stain.

In the dual-infected patient, pulmonary tuberculosis is still the most common site, but the lesions are often atypical

Tuberculosis Disease

Diagnosis

A definitive diagnosis (culture proven) is very important, especially in the present era of multidrug-resistant tuberculosis. Efforts should be made to establish a definitive diagnosis through culture of appropriate specimens. All *M. tuberculosis* isolates should be sent for drug susceptibility testing, the results of which are essential for appropriate treatment. All patients with tuberculosis should be offered HIV testing, as tuberculosis can be the initial AIDS-defining diagnosis.

A positive tuberculin skin test (discussed in further detail below) in conjunction with the proper clinical syndrome can be highly suggestive of the diagnosis of tuberculous disease. As noted below, however, anergy is not uncommon in the setting of active disease. A positive AFB smear generally indicates mycobacterial disease and can be used to make a presumptive diagnosis; culture results are required for species identification (e.g., M. *tuberculosis* versus M. *avium* complex versus other mycobacterial species). The positive predictive value of an AFB smear for M. *tuberculosis* is in large part dependent upon the patient's HIV serological status. HIV-seronegative patients with a positive AFB smear have a greater than 90% likelihood of having a positive culture for M. *tuberculosis*, whereas an HIV-infected patient may only have a 50% likelihood, given the high prevalence of other mycobacteria such as M. *avium* complex (8). As noted above, the radiometric broth method (BACTEC system) for culturing mycobacteria can reduce the time to detection of growth by 2 weeks (compared to solid media) (67) and is considered optimal.

Nucleic acid amplification (e.g., PCR) tests for rapid identification of M. *tuberculosis*, performed directly in clinical specimens (e.g., sputum), have recently been FDA approved for use in clinical microbiology laboratories (on AFB smear-positive respiratory specimens). These tests appear to be highly sensitive for smear-positive sputum specimens but significantly less sensitive for smear-negative, culture-positive specimens (2). PCR has also been used to detect the presence of M. *tuberculosis* in other specimens (e.g., cerebrospinal fluid). The utility and most effective use of these rapid tests in the clinical microbiology laboratory are still being defined, but these tests will probably be most useful for HIV-infected patients with AFB smear-positive sputum specimens, where the positive predictive value for M. *tuberculosis* may only be 50%.

Clinical Manifestations

Approximately 80% of tuberculosis cases present as pulmonary disease (10). Early pulmonary tuberculosis can be asymptomatic and discovered by a chance chest X-ray or during tuberculin skin test screening. Most patients with active disease have nonspecific constitutional symptoms such as anorexia, fatigue, weight loss, chills, fever, and night sweats. Cough, which is usually productive, is often present. Hemoptysis may occur. The onset of symptoms is often very insidious, and both cough and sputum production may be ignored by patients with chronic bronchitis (3).

Manifestations of clinical disease in HIV-infected patients are often related to the degree of immunosuppression (as assessed by CD4 counts). At a number of centers, diagnosis of tuberculosis in HIV-infected patients has been delayed due to "atypical" manifestations of disease (32). Therefore there needs to be a high suspicion for disease in any HIV-infected patient with respiratory symptoms and/or abnormal chest X-ray, as well as recognition that HIV-infected patients may present very differently from the classic patient with an upper lobe cavitary infiltrate. This is most likely related to presentation with primary disease rather than reactivation of latent disease among those HIV-infected patients with low CD4 counts (Fig. 8.4).

HIV-infected patients with tuberculosis are more likely to have disseminated or extrapulmonary disease (e.g., blood, bone, gastric, pleural, or lymph node involvement, peritonitis, pericarditis, meningitis, etc.) than are HIV-seronegative tuberculosis patients (32). Pulmonary and extrapulmonary disease are frequently present in HIV-infected patients. HIV-infected patients (especially those with low CD4 counts) may have "unusual" radiographic findings; often they will not have classic findings of upper lobe infiltrate with cavitation, but rather middle or lower lung (lobar) infiltrates, diffuse infiltrates, interstitial infiltrates, or even pulmonary disease (including AFB smear-positive disease) with no obvious infiltrates on chest X-ray. Lymphadenopathy (peripheral or intrathoracic) is common among tuberculosis patients with HIV infection but not among HIV-seronegative patients. Clinical features of tuberculosis in HIV-infected patients are summarized in Table 8.1.

Common chest radiographic findings for patients with tuberculous disease due to reactivation of latent infection include upper lobe predominance, cavitation, pleural thickening or scarring, hilar retraction, and volume loss (43). Examples are shown in Fig. 8.5. Examples of chest X-ray findings from HIV-infected patients are shown in Fig. 8.6 and are generally those of primary disease (parenchymal infiltrates, lymphadenopathy, pleural effusion, miliary disease). In addition, 10 to 15% of HIV-infected patients with positive sputum cultures for M. *tuberculosis* may have normal chest radiographs (57).

Early pulmonary tuberculosis can be asymptomatic and discovered by a chance chest X-ray or during tuberculin skin test screening

Table 8.1 Clinical features of tuberculosis in HIV-infected patients

- Diagnosis delayed; frequently atypical manifestations
- Disseminated/extrapulmonary disease is common; often coexists with pulmonary disease
- Chest X-ray findings are frequently "atypical": lower lobe and interstitial infiltrates; adenopathy
- Granulomatous disease is less likely, poorly formed
- PPD negative/anergy are common findings
- Treatment: response is good if organism is drug sensitive and patient adheres to therapy

Treatment

It is important that drug susceptibility studies be performed for M. *tuberculosis* isolates to ensure that appropriate therapy is selected. For fully susceptible isolates, cure rates are >95% and can approach 100% with adherence to therapy. For single-drug resistance, cure rates are ~95%. Isoniazid (INH) and rifampin (RIF) are the cornerstones of therapy; when there is resistance to both drugs, treatment and potential for cure become much more difficult (37).

In most areas (i.e., where single-drug resistance is >4%) it is recommended that antituberculosis therapy be initiated with a four-drug therapy (INH, RIF, pyrazinamide [PZA], and ethambutol [EMB]) (7). Recommended treatment regimens and programs for monitoring adverse reactions are published by the American Thoracic Society and CDC (7).

Short-course therapy (for drug-susceptible strains in HIV-seronegative patients) consists of a total of 6 months of therapy: INH/RIF/PZA/EMB for 2 months *plus* INH/RIF for an additional 4 months (4, 7). This regimen can be given twice weekly (by DOT) after 2 to 8 weeks of daily therapy. Because of a somewhat higher risk of relapse among HIV-infected patients after 6 months of therapy (58, 61), many authorities recommend a total of 9 to 12 months of therapy for HIV-infected patients with drug-susceptible isolates. HIV-infected patients with active tuberculosis will respond quite well to therapy if the isolate is drug susceptible and the patient is adherent to therapy (70).

Directly observed therapy (DOT) should be considered for all patients with active disease (7). DOT has been demonstrated to improve adherence and cure rates. Significant resources are needed to implement this program for all patients, but DOT is clearly cost-effective because it enhances cure rates, decreases transmission of disease, and prevents emergence of MDR-TB (82). DOT can be given twice or three times weekly to patients with susceptible isolates. Daily therapy is required for treatment of drug-resistant disease.

The treatment of drug-resistant strains, especially MDR-TB, should be carried out in consultation with a physician with expertise in this area. For single-drug INH resistance, a three-drug regimen can be given (RIF, EMB, PZA) for a total of 6 months (7). For RIF-resistant strains, a total of 12 months of INH, EMB, and PZA, or 18 months of INH plus EMB, can be given. For treatment of those with MDR-TB strains (e.g., resistance to INH and RIF), at least two and preferably three or more drugs to which the isolate is susceptible are generally given for 18 to 24 months (37). Daily DOT is recommended for all patients with MDR-TB. Second-line

It is important that drug susceptibility studies be performed for M. tuberculosis isolates to ensure that appropriate therapy is selected

drugs are generally more toxic and have much less antituberculous activity than the first-line drugs (INH, RIF, EMB, PZA, and streptomycin).

Secondary resistance is defined as emergence of resistance in a patient with a previously susceptible strain. Noncompliance as well as treatment errors can lead to secondary drug resistance. For all patients with tuberculous disease, a single drug should NEVER be added to a failing regimen. A minimum of two drugs to which the organism is susceptible should be used at all times. Primary resistance indicates that a patient was infected with a drug-resistant strain initially. Primary resistance is seen most often among immigrants from areas where tuberculosis is endemic and drug resistance is common (e.g., Southeast Asia, India, or Mexico, where up to 30% of strains may be INH resistant); other risk factors include prolonged contact with patients with drug-resistant strains, HIV-infected patients, and outbreaks (prisons, hospitals, shelters) (32).

Diagnosis of Tuberculosis Infection

Tuberculin skin testing is the only currently available method for detecting tuberculosis infection but is neither 100% specific nor sensitive

Tuberculin skin testing is the only currently available method for detecting tuberculosis infection but is neither 100% specific nor sensitive. PPD is a standardized preparation that contains a number of antigenic components; 5 tuberculin units (TU) is the usual dose given intradermally. Tuberculin skin testing is a DTH reaction which is read at 48 to 72 h (induration, not erythema) (35).

A reaction of 5 mm of induration should be considered positive in HIV-infected patients and contacts of active cases (e.g., family members); 10 mm often is considered positive in most other individuals, and 15 mm of induration is considered positive in low-risk individuals (Table 8.2). It is estimated that 90% of those with 10 mm of induration and virtually everyone with a 20-mm reaction will be infected with M. *tuberculosis*. Repeated tuberculin skin testing cannot sensitize a noninfected person, but it can restimulate or enhance remotely established weakened hypersensitivity (booster effect) (35).

Table 8.2 Recommendations for preventive therapy

Induration size	Length of therapy
≥5 mm	
• HIV positive	12 months
• Close contact of active tuberculosis	6 months
• Abnormal chest X-ray; fibrotic lesion	12 months
≥10 mm	
• Recent PPD conversion	6 months
• Drug injector (HIV negative)	6 months
• Medical conditions that increase risk	6 months
• <35 years old in high-incidence groups including immigrants, medically underserved racial and ethnic minorities, correctional institution inmates, etc.	6 months
≥15 mm	
• <35 years old in low-incidence group (HIV-seronegative children should receive 9 months of therapy)	6 months

Limitations of tuberculin skin testing exist because of nonspecificity (e.g., positive reaction due to nontuberculous mycobacteria) and, even more importantly, due to insensitivity (e.g., anergy). In the pre-HIV era 15 to 25% of patients with active tuberculous disease had a negative PPD test. This rate is now even higher, given diagnosis of active tuberculosis in many anergic HIV-infected patients. The presence of a positive PPD reaction strongly suggests the diagnosis of active disease in a patient with a consistent clinical syndrome. All individuals screened by tuberculin skin testing who have a positive test should have a chest radiograph performed.

Preventive Therapy for Tuberculosis Infection

INH is the drug of choice for preventive therapy and has an efficacy of 65 to 98% (66). In adults, INH is generally given daily at a dose of 300 mg/day for 6 months (12 months in HIV-infected patients). Pyridoxine (vitamin B_6) is given with INH to prevent peripheral neuropathy. Directly observed preventive therapy is a consideration (900 mg of INH twice a week) in certain high-risk situations. Recent data suggest that RIF is also efficacious when used for preventive therapy (59, 76). RIF is indicated for preventive therapy when an individual is thought to be infected with an INH-resistant strain of M. tuberculosis. The combination of a fluoroquinolone (e.g., ofloxacin or ciprofloxacin) plus PZA has been recommended for preventive therapy following exposure and presumed infection due to a multidrug-resistant strain (11), although there are no data on the efficacy of this regimen and it is often poorly tolerated (33). New short-course preventive therapy regimens (e.g., RIF plus PZA) are under investigation and appear promising.

American Thoracic Society/CDC guidelines for preventive therapy (including indications and management recommendations) have been published (7); a summary of the indications based on results of tuberculin skin test (amount of induration) and underlying risk factors is listed in Tables 8.2 and 8.3.

Control of Tuberculosis Transmission

The resurgence of tuberculosis in the United States has been accompanied by outbreaks of institutional transmission; many reported episodes have been due to MDR-TB. Most of the outbreaks have involved patient-to-patient transmission as well as patient-to-health care worker transmission.

The resurgence of tuberculosis in the United States has been accompanied by outbreaks of institutional transmission

Table 8.3   Medical conditions which increase risk of tuberculosis

- HIV
- Diabetes mellitus
- Steroids/immunosuppressive therapy
- Intravenous drug use
- Malignancy
- End-stage renal disease
- Malnutrition

In outbreaks investigated by CDC, >80% of the patients with MDR-TB were HIV infected and MDR-TB was associated with a high mortality (70–90%); the interval from tuberculosis diagnosis to death was between 4 and 16 weeks (38). In fact, in a number of outbreaks, AIDS patients with MDR-TB died before susceptibility results were received.

Factors which have contributed to recent outbreaks of tuberculosis including MDR strains include (12): (i) increases in the number of patients coinfected with M. *tuberculosis* and HIV; (ii) inefficient infection control procedures and facilities (e.g., clustering of patients with unsuspected tuberculosis with susceptible immunocompromised patients on AIDS wards of large urban hospitals; delayed recognition of tuberculosis in HIV-infected patients because of "atypical" presentation or low clinical suspicion leading to misdiagnosis; failure to isolate patients with active pulmonary disease); (iii) laboratory delays in identification and susceptibility testing of M. *tuberculosis* isolates; and (iv) failure to recognize ongoing infectiousness of patients (in addition to delayed institution of isolation, there has been inadequate duration of and/or inadequate facilities for AFB isolation).

In outbreaks in New York City and New York State facilities, 17 health care workers developed active disease due to MDR-TB and 7 of these died (most were HIV infected) (75). A subsequent study has suggested that with earlier diagnosis and appropriate therapy clinical outcome can be improved in patients with MDR-TB (73).

The key to infection control efforts is to prioritize strategies, establishing a hierarchy (12, 48, 60). "Administrative controls" are most important (9) and include measures to reduce the risk of exposure to persons with infectious tuberculosis. This includes careful screening and early identification of patients with or at risk for tuberculosis. A high index of suspicion is critical; patients with or at risk for tuberculosis need to be isolated upon admission, a diagnosis must be made expeditiously, and therapy should be initiated promptly. Prevention of nosocomial transmission of tuberculosis has been accomplished at a number of institutions by the introduction of an expanded respiratory isolation policy (8, 9). A comprehensive and mandatory periodic tuberculin skin testing program for all health care workers to evaluate transmission is important. Testing should be done at least annually, and considered more frequently (e.g., every 6 months) in high-incidence areas. Surveillance for health care worker conversions is essential in order to evaluate whether nosocomial transmission is occurring in an institution, and at what level, and to assess the efficacy of an institution's tuberculosis infection control efforts. In addition, it is important for the individual health care worker who has a positive tuberculin skin test so that preventive therapy can be offered.

Surveillance for health care worker conversions is essential in order to evaluate whether nosocomial transmission is occurring in an institution.

The second level of controls consists of engineering controls for tuberculosis isolation to reduce or eliminate tuberculosis droplet nuclei in the air. Hospitals should have an adequate number of isolation rooms to meet their needs (negative-pressure room so that air flows from the hall into the isolation room, 6 to 12 air exchanges per hour, air exhausted directly to the outside or through a HEPA filter before being recirculated) (12).

Personal respiratory protection (i.e., respirator masks) is the final or third level of control and has been the most controversial, given federal mandates in this area (8). The minimum level of respiratory protection mandated by the Occupational Safety and Health Administration (OSHA) is the National Institute for Occupational Safety and Health (NIOSH)-certified N-95 respirator. A respiratory protection program that includes medical evaluation, training, and individual fit testing of health care workers is required by OSHA. Developing a respiratory protection program including fit testing can be time-consuming, expensive, and logistically difficult, and published data suggest that the impact of formal fit testing on proper mask use is small (29, 60). It is important to note that men with beards cannot be certified for fit testing under the current OSHA regulations.

Figure 8.1 Number of reported tuberculosis cases in the United States, 1975–1996. (From reference 13.)

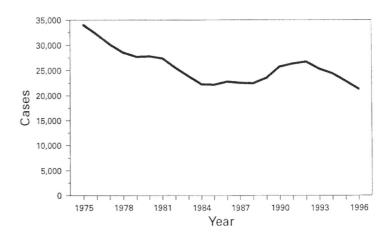

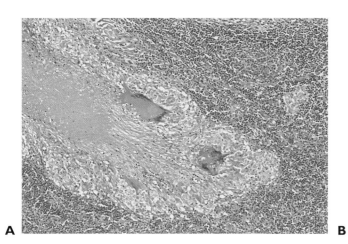

A

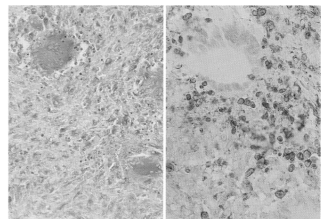

B

Figure 8.2 (A) Lymph node, caseating granulomas with giant cells. Hematoxylin and eosin (H&E) stain; ×10. (B, left) Granulomatous inflammation; KP-1 (CD68) macrophage immunostain is intensely reactive. ×50. (B, right) Granulomatous inflammation; OPD4 (CD4) immunostain is intensely reactive in T cells in the granuloma and surrounding a giant cell. ×100. (C) Granulomatous inflammation; rare acid-fast bacilli in a giant cell. Ziehl-Neelson stain; ×330.

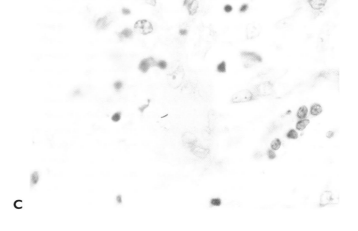

C

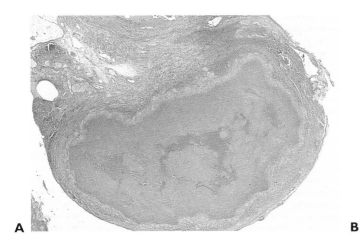

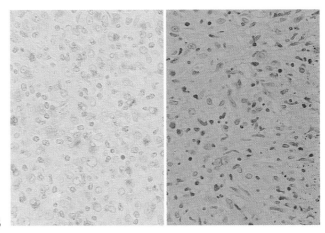

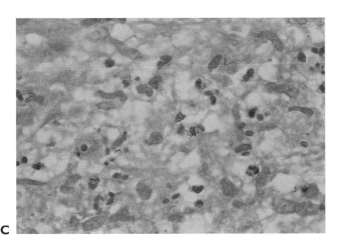

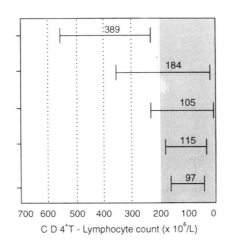

Figure 8.3 (A) Lymph node, extensive mixed caseous and suppurative necrosis; a thin rim of granulomatous inflammation and no giant cells. H&E stain; ×2.5. (B, left) Hyporeactive granulomatous inflammation; KP-1 (CD68) macrophage immunostain is only weakly reactive. ×50. (B, right) Hyporeactive granulomatous inflammation; OPD4 (CD4) immunostain is weakly reactive and CD4⁺ T cells are scarce. ×100. (C) Hyporeactive granuloma/anergic tuberculosis; many acid-fast bacilli are in areas of suppuration. Ziehl-Neelson stain; ×250.

A TYPICAL
  n = 18

B PLEURAL EFFUSION
  n = 32

C ATYPICAL INFILTRATE
  n = 51

D RETICULO - NODULAR
  n = 29

E ADENOPATHY
  n = 46

:389

184

105

115

97

700 600 500 400 300 200 100 0
C D 4⁺T - Lymphocyte count (x 10⁶/L)

Figure 8.4 CD counts associated with pulmonary tuberculosis radiographic patterns in 150 HIV-infected patients. CD4 counts are shown as mean ± standard deviation. Pattern A is defined by upper zone infiltrate with or without cavitation, and pattern C is defined by parenchymal infiltrate in mid or lower zone. Pattern A is associated with early HIV disease, and patterns C, D, and E are associated with advanced HIV infection. Patients may be included in one or more of categories B through E. (From reference 43 with permission.)

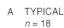

Figure 8.5 Chest radiographic manifestations of reactivation disease. (A) Evidence of a right upper lobe infiltrate, volume loss, and cavitation. (B) Bilateral upper lobe infiltrates and fibronodular disease.

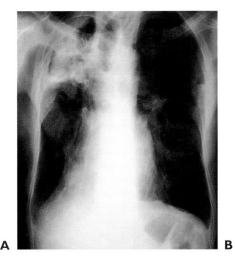
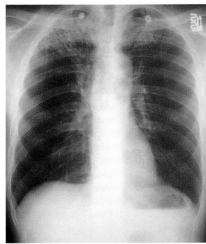

A B

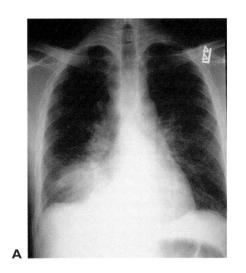
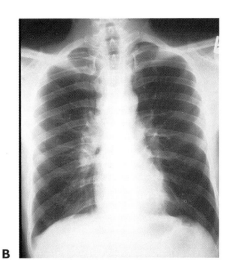
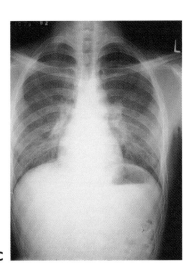

A B C

Figure 8.6 Chest radiographs from HIV-infected patients resembling primary pulmonary tuberculosis. (A) Right middle lobe infiltrate. (B) Right hilar adenopathy. (C) Bilateral interstitial infiltrates.

References

1. **Alland, D., G. E. Kalkut, A. R. Moss, R. A. McAdam, J. A. Hahn, W. Bosworth, E. Drucker, and B. R. Bloom.** 1994. Transmission of tuberculosis in New York City. An analysis by DNA fingerprinting and conventional epidemiologic methods. *N. Engl. J. Med.* **330**(24):1710–1716.

2. **American Thoracic Society.** 1997. Rapid diagnostic tests for tuberculosis: what is appropriate use? *Am. J. Respir. Crit. Care Med.* **155:**1804–1814.

3. **Anonymous.** 1990. Diagnosis and treatment of disease caused by nontuberculous mycobacteria. *Am. Rev. Respir. Dis.* **142:**940–953.

4. **Anonymous.** 1995. Drugs for tuberculosis. *Med. Lett. Drugs Therapeut.* **37:**67–70.

5. **Barnes, P. F., A. B. Bloch, P. T. Davidson, and D. E. Snider.** 1991. Tuberculosis in patients with human immunodeficiency virus infection. *N. Engl. J. Med.* **324:**1644–1650.

6. **Bartlett, J. G.** 1997. Update in infectious diseases. *Ann. Intern. Med.* **126:**48–56.

7. **Bass, J. B., Jr., L. S. Farer, P. C. Hopewell, R. O'Brien, R. F. Jacobs, F. Ruben, D. E. Snider, Jr., and G. Thornton.** 1994. Treatment of tuberculosis and tuberculosis infection in adults and children. American Thoracic Society and The Centers for Disease Control and Prevention. *Am. J. Respir. Crit. Care Med.* **149:**1359–1374.

8. **Blumberg, H. M.** 1997. Tuberculosis and infection control: what now? *Infect. Control Hosp. Epidemiol.* **18:**538–541. (Editorial.)

9. **Blumberg, H. M., D. L. Watkins, J. D. Berschling, A. Antle, P. Moore, N. White, M. Hunter, B. Green, S. M. Ray, and J. E. McGowan, Jr.** 1995. Preventing the nosocomial transmission of tuberculosis. *Ann. Intern. Med.* **122:**658–663.

10. **Cantwell, M. F., D. E. Snider, Jr., G. M. Cauthen, and I. M. Onorato.** 1994. Epidemiology of tuberculosis in the United States. *JAMA* **272:**535–539.

11. **Centers for Disease Control and Prevention.** 1992. Management of persons exposed to multidrug-resistant tuberculosis. *Morbid. Mortal. Weekly Rep.* **41**(RR-11):61–71.

12. **Centers for Disease Control and Prevention.** 1994. Guidelines for preventing the transmission of *Mycobacterium tuberculosis* in health-care facilities, 1994. *Morbid. Mortal. Weekly Rep.* **43**(RR-13):1–132.

13. **Centers for Disease Control and Prevention.** 1997. Tuberculosis morbidity. *Morbid. Mortal. Weekly Rep.* **46:**695–700.

14. **Clerici, M., and G. M. Shearer.** 1993. A TH1-TH2 switch is a critical step in the etiology of HIV infection. *Immunol. Today* **14:**107–111.

15. **Daley, C. L., P. M. Small, G. F. Schecter, G. K. Schoolnik, R. A. McAdam, W. R. Jacobs, Jr., and P. C. Hopewell.** 1992. An outbreak of tuberculosis with accelerated progression among persons infected with the human immunodeficiency virus. An analysis using restriction-fragment-length polymorphisms. *N. Engl. J. Med.* **326:**231–235.

16. **Dall, L., L. Long, and J. Stanford.** 1989. Poncet's disease: tuberculous rheumatism. *Rev. Infect. Dis.* **11:**105–107.

17. **Dannenberg, A. M., Jr.** 1993. Immunopathogenesis of pulmonary tuberculosis. *Immunol. Today* **12:**228–231.

18. **Dannenberg, A. M., Jr., and G. A. W. Rook.** 1994. Pathogenesis of pulmonary tuberculosis: an interplay of tissue-damaging and macrophage-activating immune responses. B. Dual mechanisms that control bacillary multiplication, p. 459–483. *In* B. R. Bloom (ed.), *Tuberculosis: Pathogenesis, Protection, and Control.* American Society for Microbiology, Washington, D.C.

19. **Dannenberg, A. M., Jr., and J. K. Tomashefski, Jr.** 1988. Pathogenesis of pulmonary tuberculosis, p. 1821–1842. *In* A. P. Fishman (ed.), *Pulmonary Diseases and Disorders,* 2nd ed., vol. 3. McGraw-Hill, New York.

20. **De Cock, K. M., B. Soro, I. M. Coulibaly, and S. B. Lucas.** 1992. Tuberculosis and HIV infection in sub-Saharan Africa. *JAMA* **268:**1581–1587.

21. **Edwards, D., and C. H. Kirkpatrick.** 1986. The immunology of mycobacterial diseases. *Am. Rev. Respir. Dis.* **134:**1062–1071.

22. **Eisenbach, K. D., M. D. Sifford, M. D. Cave, J. H. Bates, and J. T. Crawford.** 1991. Detection of *Mycobacterium tuberculosis* in sputum samples using a polymerase chain reaction. *Am. Rev. Respir. Dis.* **144:**1160–1163.

23. **Frieden, T. R., P. I. Fujiwara, R. M. Washko, and M. Hamburg.** 1995. Tuberculosis in New York City—turning the tide. *N. Engl. J. Med.* **333:**229–233.

24. **Frieden, T. R., T. Sterling, A. Pablos-Mendez, J. O. Kilburn, G. M. Cauthen, and S. W. Dooley.** 1993. The emergence of drug-resistant tuberculosis in New York City. *N. Engl. J. Med.* **328:**521–526.

25. **Genewein, A., A. Telenti, C. Bernasconi, C. Mordasini, S. Weiss, A. M. Maurer, H. L. Rieder, K. Schopfer, and T. Bodmer.** 1993. Molecular approach to identifying route of transmission of tuberculosis in the community. *Lancet* **342:**841–844.

26. **Goletti, D., D. Weissman, R. W. Jackson, N. M. Graham, D. Vlahov, R. S. Klein, S. S. Munsiff, L. Ortona, R. Cauda, and A. S. Fauci.** 1996. Effect of *Mycobacterium tuberculosis* on HIV replication. Role of immune activation. *J. Immunol.* **157:**1271–1278.

27. **Haas, D. W., and R. M. Des Prez.** 1995. *Mycobacterium tuberculosis,* p. 2213–2242. *In* G. L. Mandell, J. E. Bennett, and R. Dolin (ed.), *Principles and Practice of Infectious Diseases.* Churchill Livingstone, New York.

28. **Haas, W. H., W. R. Butler, C. L. Woodley, and J. T. Crawford.** 1993. Mixed-linker polymerase chain reaction: a new method for rapid fingerprinting of isolates of the *Mycobacterium tuberculosis* complex. *J. Clin. Microbiol.* **31:**1293–1298.

29. **Hannum, D., K. Cycan, L. Jones, M. Stewart, S. Morris, S. M. Markowitz, and E. S. Wong.** 1996. The effect of respirator training on the ability of health-care workers to pass a qualitative fit test. *Infect. Control Hosp. Epidemiol.* **17:**636–640.

30. **Hardman, W. J., G. M. Benian, T. Howard, J. E. McGowan, Jr., B. Metchcock, and J. Murtag.** 1996. Rapid detection of mycobacteria in inflammatory necrotizing granulomas from formalin-fixed, paraffin-embedded tissue by PCR in clinically high-risk patients with acid-fast stain and culture-negative tissue biopsies. *Am. J. Clin. Pathol.* **106:**384–389.

31. **Heifets, L. B., and R. C. Good.** 1994. Current laboratory methods for the diagnosis of tuberculosis, p. 85–110. *In* B. R. Bloom (ed.), *Tuberculosis: Pathogenesis, Protection, and Control.* American Society for Microbiology, Washington, D.C.

32. **Hopewell, P. C.** 1992. Impact of HIV infection on the epidemiology, clinical features, management and control of tuberculosis. *Clin. Infect. Dis.* **15:**540–547.

33. **Horn, D. L., D. Hewlett, Jr., C. Alfalla, S. Peterson, and S. M. Opal.** 1994. Limited tolerance of ofloxacin and pyrazinamide prophylaxis against tuberculosis. *N. Engl. J. Med.* **330:**1241.

34. **Houk, V. H., D. C. Kent, J. H. Baker, K. Sorenson, and G. D. Hanzel.** 1968. The Byrd study: in-depth analysis of a micro-outbreak of tuberculosis in a closed environment. *Arch. Environ. Health* **16:**4–6.

35. **Huebner, R. E., M. F. Schein, and J. B. Bass, Jr.** 1993. The tuberculin skin test. *Clin. Infect. Dis.* **17:**968–975.

36. **Hwang, C.-H., S. Kahn, N. Ende, B. T. Mangura, L. B. Reichman, and J. Chou.** 1985. The HLA-1,-B, and BDR phenotypes and tuberculosis. *Am. Rev. Respir. Dis.* **132:**382–385.

37. **Iseman, M. D.** 1993. Multidrug-resistant tuberculosis. *N. Engl. J. Med.* **329:**784–791.

38. **Jarvis, W. R.** 1993. Nosocomial transmission of multidrug-resistant *Mycobacterium tuberculosis. Res. Microbiol.* **144:**117–122.

39. **Jost, K. C., Jr., D. F. Dunbar, S. S. Barth, V. L. Headley, and L. B. Elliott.** 1995. Identification of *Mycobacterium tuberculosis* and M. *avium* complex directly from smear-positive sputum specimens and BACTEC 12B cultures by high-performance liquid chromatography with fluorescence detection and computer-driven pattern recognition models. *J. Clin. Microbiol.* **33:**1270–1277.

40. **Kim, J., G. Y. Minamoto, and M. H. Grieco.** 1991. Nocardial infection as a complication of AIDS: report of six cases and review. *Rev. Infect. Dis.* **13:**624–629.

41. **Klein, S. A., J. M. Dobmeyer, T. S. Dobmeyer, M. Pape, O. G. Ottman, E. B. Helm, D. Hoelzer, and R. Rossol.** 1997. Demonstration of the Th1 to Th2 cytokine shift during the course of HIV-1 infection using cytoplasmic cytokine detection on single cell flow cytometry. *AIDS* **11:**1111–1118.

42. **Lack, E. E., and D. H. Connor.** 1997. Tuberculosis, p. 857–868. *In* D. H. Connor, F. W. Chandler, D. A. Schwartz, H. J. Manz, and E. E. Lack (ed.), *Pathology of Infectious Diseases*, vol. 1. Appleton and Lange, Stamford, Conn.

43. **LoBue, P. A., A. Catanzaro, A. K. Dutt, and W. Stead.** 1997. Tuberculosis. Part II. *Disease-A-Month* **43:**181–274.

44. **Lucas, S. B., and A. M. Nelson.** 1994. Pathogenesis of tuberculosis in human immunodeficiency virus-infected people, p. 503–513. *In* B. R. Bloom (ed.), *Tuberculosis: Pathogenesis, Protection, and Control.* American Society for Microbiology, Washington, D.C.

45. **Mahmoudi, A., and M. D. Iseman.** 1993. Pitfalls in the care of patients with tuberculosis. Common errors and their association with the acquisition of drug resistance [see comments]. *JAMA* **270:**65–68.

46. **Matsuyama, T., N. Kobayashi, and N. Yamamoto.** 1991. Cytokines and HIV infection: is AIDS a tumour necrosis factor disease? *AIDS* **5:**1405–1417.

47. **McDermott, L. J., J. Glassroth, J. B. Mehta, and A. K. Dutt.** 1997. Tuberculosis. Part 1. *Disease-A-Month* **43:**115–180.

48. **McGowan, J. E., Jr.** 1995. Nosocomial tuberculosis: new progress in control and prevention. *Clin. Infect. Dis.* **21:**489–505.

49. **McGowan, J. E., Jr., and H. M. Blumberg.** 1995. Inner-city tuberculosis in the USA. *J. Hosp. Infect.* **30**(Suppl.)**:**282–295.

50. **Moore, M., I. Onorato, E. McCray, and K. G. Castro.** 1997. Trends in drug-resistant tuberculosis in the United States, 1993–1996. *JAMA* **278:**833–837.

51. **Mosmann, T. R., and R. L. Coffman.** 1989. TH1 and TH2 cells: different kinds of lymphokine secretion lead to different functional properties. *Annu. Rev. Immunol.* **7:**145–173.

52. **Musial, C. E., and G. D. Roberts.** 1987. Tuberculosis and other mycobacteria, p. 539-580. *In* B. B. Wentworth (ed.), *Diagnostic Procedures for Bacterial Infections,* 7th ed. American Public Health Association, Washington, D.C.

53. **Nambuya, A., N. Sewankambo, J. Mugerwa, R. W. Goodgame, and S. B. Lucas.** 1988. Tuberculous lymphadenitis associated with human immunodeficiency virus (HIV) in Uganda. *J. Clin. Pathol.* **41:**93–96.

54. **Narain, J. P., M. C. Raviglione, and A. Kochi.** 1992. HIV-associated tuberculosis in developing countries: epidemiology and strategies for prevention. *Tuberc. Lung Dis.* **73:**311–321.

55. **Pancholi, P., R. M. Steinman, and N. Bhardwaj.** 1992. Dendritic cells efficiently immunoselect mycobacterial-reactive cells in human blood, including antigen-reactive precursors. *Immunology* **76:**217–224.

56. **Placido, R., G. Mancino, A. Amendola, F. Mariani, S. Vendetti, M. Placentini, A. Sanduzzi, M. L. Bocchino, M. Zembala, and V. Colizzi.** 1997. Apoptosis of human monocytes/macrophages in *Mycobacterium tuberculosis* infection. *J. Pathol.* **181:**31–38.

57. **Perlman, D. C., W. M. El-Sadr, E. T. Nelson, J. P. Matts, E. E. Telzak, N. Salomon, K. Chirgwin, and R. Hafner.** 1997. Variation of chest radiograph patterns in pulmonary tuberculosis by degree of human immunodeficiency virus-related immunosuppression. *Clin. Infect. Dis.* **25:**242–246.

58. **Perriens, J. H., M. E. St. Louis, Y. B. Mukadi, C. Brown, J. Prignot, F. Pouthier, J. C. Willame, J. K. Mandala, M. Kaboto, R. W. Ryder, G. Roscigno, and P. Piot.** 1995. Pulmonary tuberculosis in HIV-infected patients in Zaire: a controlled trial of treatment for 6 or 12 months. *N. Engl. J. Med.* **332:**779–784.

59. **Polesky, A., H. W. Farber, D. J. Gottlieb, H. Park, S. Levinson, J. J. O'Connell, B. McInnis, R. L. Nieves, and J. Bernardo.** 1996. Rifampin preventive therapy for tuberculosis in Boston's homeless. *Am. J. Respir. Crit. Care Med.* **154:**1473–1477.

60. **Pugliese, G., and M. L. Tapper.** 1996. Tuberculosis control in health care. *Infect. Control Hosp. Epidemiol.* **17:**819–827.

61. **Pulido, F., J. M. Pena, R. Rubio, S. Moreno, J. Gonzalez, C. Guijarro, J. R. Costa, and J. J. Vazquez.** 1997. Relapse of tuberculosis after treatment in human immunodeficiency virus-infected patients. *Arch. Intern. Med.* **157:**227–232.

62. **Raviglione, M. C., C. Dye, S. Schmidt, and A. Kochi.** 1997. Assessment of worldwide tuberculosis control. *Lancet* **350:**624–629.

63. **Raviglione, M. C., H. L. Rieder, K. Styblo, A. G. Khomenko, K. Esteves, and A. Kochi.** 1994. Tuberculosis trends in eastern Europe and the former USSR. *Tubercle Lung Dis.* **75**(6):400–416.

64. **Raviglione, M. C., D. E. Snider, Jr., and A. Kochi.** 1995. Global epidemiology of tuberculosis: morbidity and mortality of a worldwide epidemic. *JAMA* **273:**220–226.

65. **Reichman, L. B.** 1997. Defending the public's health against tuberculosis. *JAMA* **278:**865–867.

66. **Salpeter, S.** 1992. Tuberculosis chemoprophylaxis. *West. J. Med.* **157:**421–424.

67. **Sewell, D. L., A. L. Rashad, W. J. Rourke, Jr., S. L. Poor, J. A. McCarthy, and M. A. Pfaller.** 1993. Comparison of the Septi-Chek AFB and BACTEC systems and conventional culture for recovery of mycobacteria. *J. Clin. Microbiol.* **31:**2689–2691.

68. **Slavin, R. E., T. J. Walsh, and A. D. Pollack.** 1980. Late generalized tuberculosis: a clinical pathological analysis and comparison of 100 cases in the pre-antibiotic eras. *Medicine* **59:**352–366.

69. **Small, P. M., P. C. Hopewell, S. P. Singh, A. Paz, J. Parsonnet, D. C. Ruston, G. F. Schecter, C. L. Daley, and G. K. Schoolnik.** 1994. The epidemiology of tuberculosis in San Francisco. A population-based study using conventional and molecular methods. *N. Engl. J. Med.* **330(24):**1703–1709.

70. **Small, P. M., G. F. Schecter, P. C. Goodman, M. A. Sande, R. E. Chaisson, and P. C. Hopewell.** 1991. Treatment of tuberculosis in patients with advanced human immunodeficiency virus infection. *N. Engl. J. Med.* **324:**289–294.

71. **Small, P. M., R. W. Shafer, P. C. Hopewell, S. P. Singh, M. J. Murphy, E. Desmond, M. F. Sierra, and G. K. Schoolnik.** 1993. Exogenous reinfection with multidrug-resistant *Mycobacterium tuberculosis* in patients with advanced HIV infection. *N. Engl. J. Med.* **328:**1137–1144.

72. **Snider, D. E., and W. L. Roper.** 1992. The new tuberculosis. *N. Engl. J. Med.* **326:**703–705.

73. **Telzak, E. E., K. Sepkowitz, P. Alpert, S. Mannheimer, F. Medard, W. el-Sadr, S. Blum, A. Gagliardi, N. Salomon, and G. Turett.** 1995. Multidrug-resistant tuberculosis in patients without HIV infection. *N. Engl. J. Med.* **333:**907–911.

74. **Tisdall, P. A., D. R. DeYoung, G. D. Roberts, and J. P. Anhalt.** 1982. Identification of clinical isolates of mycobacteria with gas-liquid chromatography: a 10-month follow-up study. *J. Clin. Microbiol.* **16:**400–402.

75. **Valway, S. E., M. L. Pearson, R. Ikeda, and B. R. Edlin.** 1993. HIV infected healthcare workers with multidrug resistant tuberculosis (MDR-TB), 1990–1992, p. 231. *In Programs and Abstracts of the 33rd Interscience Conference on Antimicrobial Agents and Chemotherapy, 1993.* New Orleans, La.

76. **Villarino, M. E., R. Ridzon, P. C. Weismuller, M. Elcock, R. M. Maxwell, J. Meador, P. J. Smith, M. L. Carson, and L. J. Geiter.** 1997. Rifampin preventive therapy for tuberculosis infection: experience with 157 adolescents. *Am. J. Respir. Crit. Care Med.* **155:**1735–1738.

77. **von Lichtenberg, F.** 1991. Mycobacterial diseases, p. 173–187. *In Pathology of Infectious Diseases.* Raven Press, New York.

78. **Wallis, R. S., J. J. Ellner, and H. Shiratsuchi.** 1992. Macrophages, mycobacteria and HIV: the role of cytokines in determining mycobacterial virulence and regulating viral replication. *Res. Microbiol.* **143:**398–405.

79. **Wallis, R. S., M. Vjecha, M. Amir-Tahmasseb, A. Okwera, F. Byekwaso, S. Nyole, S. Kabengera, R. D. Mugerwa, and J. J. Ellner.** 1993. Influence of tuberculosis on human immunodeficiency virus (HIV-1): enhanced cytokine expression and elevated ß2-microglobulin in HIV-1 associated tuberculosis. *J. Infect. Dis.* **167:**43–48.

80. **Warren, J.** 1992. Mycobacterial infections, p. 190–207. *In* S. T. Shulman, J. P. Phair, and H. M. Sommers (ed.), *The Biological and Clinical Basis of Infectious Diseases,* 4th ed. Saunders, Philadelphia.

81. **Wayne, L. G., and H. P. Willet.** 1986. Mycobacteria, p. 1435–1457. *In* P. H. A. Sneath (ed.), *Bergeys Manual of Systemic Bacteriology*, vol. 2. The Williams and Wilkins Co., Baltimore.

82. **Weis, S. E., P. C. Slocum, F. X. Blais, B. N. M. King, G. B. Matney, E. Gomez, and B. H. Foresman.** 1994. The effect of directly observed therapy on the rates of drug resistance and relapse in tuberculosis. *N. Engl. J. Med.* **330:**1179–1184.

83. **Whalen, C., A. Okwera, J. Johnson, M. Vjecha, D. Hom, R. Wallis, R. Huebner, R. Mugerwa, and J. Ellner.** 1996. Predictors of survival in human immunodeficiency virus-infected patients with pulmonary tuberculosis. The Makerere University-Case Western Reserve University Research Collaboration. *Am. J. Respir. Crit. Care Med.* **153:**1977–1981.

84. **Willet, H. P.** 1992. Mycobacteria, p. 344–354. *In* W. K. Joklik, H. P. Willet, D. B. Amos, and C. M. Wilfert (ed.), *Zinsser Microbiology*, 20th ed. Appleton and Lange, Norwalk, Conn.

chapter 9

Mycobacterium avium

C. Robert Horsburgh, Jr., and Ann Marie Nelson

The term "*Mycobacterium avium* complex" (MAC) describes two closely related organisms, M. *avium* and M. *intracellulare*. Three major disease syndromes are produced by MAC in humans: disseminated disease, usually in persons with advanced human immunodeficiency virus (HIV) infection; pulmonary disease, in adults whose systemic immunity is intact; and cervical lymphadenitis, in children with normal immunity. In addition, MAC infection can infrequently present as localized disease such as appendicitis, arthritis, tenosynovitis, and skin infection.

Reservoir and Mode of Transmission

MAC organisms are common in many environmental sites, including water, soil, and animals (41); MAC have also been found as colonizers of hot water systems (15, 115), dental devices (98), and cigarettes (16). Exposure to

> MAC *organisms are common in many environmental sites, including water, soil, and animals*

C. Robert Horsburgh, Jr., Emory University School of Medicine, 69 Butler Street, S.E., Atlanta, GA 30303. **Ann Marie Nelson,** Division of AIDS Pathology, Department of Infectious and Parasitic Disease Pathology, Armed Forces Institute of Pathology, Washington, DC 20306-6000.

Pathology of Emerging Infections 2
Edited by Ann Marie Nelson and C. Robert Horsburgh, Jr.
© 1998 American Society for Microbiology, Washington, D.C.

water, particularly contaminated recirculating hot water systems, has been identified as one route of acquisition of MAC in persons with AIDS (115). However, less than 15% of cases could be traced to this source, suggesting that other environmental reservoirs may also be important. An epidemiologic study observed increased risk for MAC in persons with AIDS who ate hard cheeses (such as cheddar, Swiss, and Monterey jack) (45), but intensive study of cheeses failed to recover MAC organisms (127), and the importance of the epidemiologic association is unclear. A recent study by von Reyn and colleagues noted increased risk for disseminated MAC in persons with AIDS with exposure to swimming pools and other water sources (114). In contrast, frequent showering was protective in another study (45), leaving doubt as to the importance of water exposures as a risk factor for disseminated disease. The recent identification of MAC in cigarettes appears to support the possibility that smoking may be associated with acquisition of MAC pulmonary disease, but the relationship of such exposures to disease has not been demonstrated. Aerosols of fresh and salt water may contain MAC, and these have also been proposed as vehicles leading to transmission of MAC respiratory disease (31, 83). The frequent occurrence of MAC in milk (even after pasteurization) and the preponderance of cases of cervical lymphadenitis in children under 3 years of age have led some investigators to speculate that oral exposure to organisms in milk is the route of infection for this clinical presentation (7).

Epidemiology

Disseminated Disease

Disseminated MAC disease was extremely rare before 1980 (48). However, the heightened susceptibility of AIDS patients to this disease has led to a marked increase in the number of cases of disseminated MAC disease in patients with AIDS (41). A recent study with careful follow-up identified a prevalence of disseminated MAC in 22% of AIDS patients (59); such follow-up is important in determining the true prevalence of MAC, because over 80% of cases occur after another AIDS-indicating condition and may be missed if only the initial condition is reported. In 1994, when there were approximately 171,000 persons living with AIDS in the United States, it can be estimated that there were 37,000 cases of disseminated MAC disease, making this the most common clinical manifestation of MAC and also the most common bacterial disease among persons with AIDS. Incidence of disseminated MAC has been observed in prospective cohort studies to be 20 to 35% per year (78, 79, 86).

The greatest risk for MAC in persons with AIDS is severe depression of the CD4$^+$ cell count

The greatest risk for MAC in persons with AIDS is severe depression of the CD4$^+$ cell count; disseminated MAC is rarely seen in persons with greater than 100 CD4$^+$ cells/µl, and the median CD4$^+$ cell count among persons with MAC is 10 cells/µl (41). The risk for MAC increases exponentially as the CD4$^+$ count declines (78). The prior occurrence of another opportunistic condition (other than tuberculosis) (46) increases the risk for MAC at a given CD4$^+$ cell level (22). Among HIV-infected persons, similar risks for MAC are seen when patients are compared by age, race, sex, or HIV transmission risk (52). Children with AIDS have a risk for MAC that is similar to that of adults, although children with AIDS whose exposure to HIV occurred through blood or blood products have a higher risk than children with perinatally acquired HIV infection (44); this difference is likely to be the result of lower CD4$^+$ cell levels in the children with blood or blood product exposure.

A recent report has identified higher rates of disseminated MAC disease in the southern United States as compared with persons in the northern United States or Canada; these differences may be due to decreased environmental exposure to MAC in the north during the winter (51). Disseminated MAC has been reported with a frequency of 10 to 25% of AIDS patients in Europe, North America, and Australia, but the disease is less common in developing countries, particularly in Africa, where less than 1% of persons with AIDS are affected (25, 30, 42, 81). These differences may be due to one or a combination of several factors: a smaller proportion of AIDS patients with extremely low CD4 cell counts; protection from MAC by prior exposure to M. *tuberculosis*; or decreased exposure to MAC in reservoirs such as recirculating water systems.

Beginning in 1987, disseminated MAC in the United States increased faster than the AIDS epidemic itself. The percentage of AIDS patients with disseminated MAC has continued to climb as the AIDS epidemic has matured. Such trends have been seen in both children and adults (23, 41). These increases were likely the result of an increasing proportion of AIDS patients having the low CD4$^+$ cell levels that put them at risk for MAC. Since more active antiretroviral agents and MAC prophylaxis regimens have become available, reported numbers of cases of disseminated MAC disease have stabilized or decreased in many areas.

Pulmonary Disease

MAC pulmonary disease is seen worldwide. In the United States (80) and in Japan (111), there are approximately 1.3 cases per 100,000 persons. In Switzerland, there are 0.9 cases per 100,000 persons (11). Although systematic surveillance for MAC pulmonary disease is not performed, the disease appears to be increasing in frequency as tuberculosis declines in both Europe and North America (11, 42, 80, 88, 122). An estimated 3,500 cases of MAC pulmonary disease are seen annually in the United States (42).

MAC pulmonary disease is uncommon under the age of 45, although some authors feel that there is a subgroup of young women in the 30- to 45-year age group that is particularly susceptible (56). The average age of persons with pulmonary MAC disease reported to the Centers for Disease Control and Prevention was 58 years, and the majority of cases were men (56%) (80). No specific risk factors for MAC pulmonary disease have been identified. Many of the reported cases have been in persons with a history of prior tuberculosis or heavy smoking, giving rise to the hypothesis that impaired pulmonary clearance mechanisms may predispose to this condition. However, many patients have no predisposing factor and tests of immunologic function are routinely normal.

*M*AC *pulmonary disease appears to be increasing in frequency as tuberculosis declines in both Europe and North America*

Recent reports have identified MAC in the sputum of persons with cystic fibrosis, and a causal role for this organism in the destruction of pulmonary tissue seen in such persons has been proposed (65, 108, 121). The prevalence of positive skin MAC tests in persons with cystic fibrosis supports the pathogenic role of MAC in this disease (87). In addition, MAC may cause pulmonary disease in patients with pulmonary alveolar proteinosis (124). These observations add to the likelihood that defective pulmonary clearance mechanisms may be a risk factor for MAC pulmonary disease.

Lymphadenitis

MAC cervical adenitis is almost entirely a disease of children, with most cases occurring in those under the age of 3 years. There is a modest female predominance, and nearly all reported cases are in Caucasians (80). MAC cervical lymphadenitis in children has been reported from Europe, North America, and Australia (27, 70, 125). The decline of tuberculosis as a cause of lymphadenitis in the United States has been accompanied by increased recognition of nontuberculous lymphadenitis (80), but it is unclear whether these increases are relative or absolute. A recent review has documented that, prior to 1980, most nontuberculous lymphadenitis in the United States was due to M. *scrofulaceum*, but in subsequent years MAC has been the cause of the majority of cases (125). In 1983, there were an estimated 300 cases of lymphadenitis in the United States in which MAC was confirmed by culture (80). However, this number is likely to be an underestimate, since many cases of lymphadenitis either are not cultured or fail to grow an organism.

Skin Disease

Various cutaneous lesions have also been described in immunocompetent patients

Various cutaneous lesions have also been described in immunocompetent patients, including prurigo nodularis (74), a lupus vulgaris-type lesion in a Thai woman (67), and several reports from Japan of ulceration, subcutaneous nodules, and fistulation (39), often in children (54).

Microbiology

General

Mycobacteria (order *Actinomycetales*) are slender, sometimes curved, aerobic, non-sporeforming, nonmotile bacilli. Their cell walls contain mycosides, i.e., mycolic acid-containing long-chain glycolipids and/or phospholipoglycans that protect these facultative intracellular parasites from lysosomal attack. Mycosides avidly retain red basic fuchsin dye after acid rinsing; acid-fastness can be strong or weak, and organisms often appear beaded. MAC organisms are weakly gram positive and periodic acid-Schiff positive and are easily seen with the methenamine silver impregnations (113, 119, 120).

M. *avium* causes disease similar to tuberculosis in chickens, birds, and swine. M. *intracellulare*, previously known as the Battey bacillus, is usually not pathogenic for humans or animals. These two organisms have similar characteristics and are grouped in the *Mycobacterium avium-intracellulare* complex (MAC). In culture they are thermophilic (can grow at 41°C), and some strains develop a pale yellow pigment with age (Runyon group III, non-chromogens). In contrast to M. *tuberculosis*, MAC organisms are niacin negative, do not reduce nitrates, are unable to hydrolyze Tween, and do not produce disease in guinea pigs (20, 120). M. *malmoense* is the other species in this group known to cause disease in humans (19). M. *scrofulaceum* is a common cause of lymphadenitis in children; it is classified as a scotochromogen (Runyon group II) because of the yellow-orange pigment produced, even in the dark. The organisms are not thermophilic, but have other characteristics similar to those of MAC (77, 120). However, on the basis of DNA homology, some authors include this organism with MAC, which then becomes "MAIS" (M. *avium-intracellulare-scrofulaceum*).

Glycolipid typing has divided MAC into 28 serovars; those designated 1 through 6, 8 through 11, and 21 are M. *avium*, and serovars 7, 12 through 20, and 25 are M. *intracellulare* (110). Restriction fragment length polymorphism studies detected two groups of MAC. One type predominates in AIDS patients but not in non-AIDS-associated infections (35). Pulsed-field gel electrophoresis has been able to resolve greater differences in these isolates, indicating there is considerable diversity in strains of MAC infecting AIDS patients (3).

Virulence Factors

MAC is relatively avirulent in the normal host. Serovars 1, 4, and 8 are uncommon in the environment, yet cause most cases of disseminated disease in AIDS patients (41, 110). These serovars are likely to be associated with virulence factors or to be able to overcome host defenses more easily than other serovars. Possible virulence factors such as differing abilities to adhere to intestinal epithelial cells or to produce catalase have been described and linked to invasiveness (71, 84). Clinical isolates from patients with disseminated disease are always of the smooth, transparent colony type, rather than the domed or opaque type. Colonies that are smooth and transparent are more likely to replicate in vivo and are also more likely to induce the cytokines tumor necrosis factor-alpha (TNF-α) and interleukin-1 (IL-1); they usually have decreased susceptibility to antimycobacterial agents in vitro (102). The relationship between these two phenotypes is complicated by the ability of isolates to transform from one to the other and back, depending on culture conditions (100).

> MAC *is relatively avirulent in the normal host*

Diagnosis

Cultures of specimens from normally sterile sites (blood, bone marrow, lymph node, or liver biopsies) that are positive for MAC are diagnostic of disseminated disease. Blood is the preferred specimen, and over 90% of cases of disseminated disease are diagnosed by blood culture. Lysis centrifugation technique to liberate intracellular organisms is essential for recovery from blood cultures. Cultures from nonsterile sites (sputum, bronchial washings, gastrointestinal biopsies, or stool) can represent colonization or localized disease; in such cases, either repeatedly positive cultures or smears or biopsy are required to establish a diagnosis of localized disease (76, 118). In the absence of a biopsy, diagnosis of MAC pulmonary disease requires an abnormal chest radiograph and either two culture-positive sputum specimens (if one is smear positive) or three culture-positive sputum specimens (if none is smear positive) (2). Computed tomographic scans of the chest can be helpful, especially when multiple small lung nodules or bronchiectasis are seen (104, 105). Diagnosis of MAC lymphadenitis requires growth of MAC from the excised node. However, in the HIV-uninfected host, cultures are likely to yield no growth when excision is performed more than 1 month after the appearance of the node. In such cases, or when excision is not performed, skin testing with specific antigens for MAC is very helpful; unfortunately, such reagents are not licensed for use in the United States at present (12).

When cultures are positive for mycobacteria, specific probes can be used to identify MAC

When cultures are positive for mycobacteria, specific probes can be used to identify MAC (85). Routine culture techniques include a decontamination procedure and must be done using a biological safety cabinet. A nonselective egg medium, such as Lowenstein-Jensen or Middlebrook (7H10 or 7H11, with or without antibiotics), can be used for primary recovery. Species are identified by pigmentation, growth characteristics, biochemical tests, and ability to produce disease in laboratory animals (77).

Radiometric and other rapid detection methods have been developed to reduce the long incubation period of culture-based techniques. The BACTEC (Becton Dickinson Laboratories, Towson, Md.) and Isolator (DuPont, Wilmington, Del.) systems can detect nontuberculous mycobacteria in as little as 5 days (85). NAP (p-nitro-α-acetyl-amino-β-hydroxy-propriophenone) inhibition can be used to differentiate *M. tuberculosis* and *M. bovis* from other mycobacteria. Gas-liquid chromatography can be used to identify organisms in clinical specimens (107) but is not widely available. GenProbe (GenProbe Corp., San Diego, Calif.) uses specific DNA probes to the rRNA of mycobacteria to identify clinically significant organisms to the species level (85). PCR (polymerase chain reaction) techniques are able to detect very small numbers of specific mycobacteria in clinical specimens (17) or in tissue sections, but there is little experience with detection of MAC. Direct detection of MAC in blood by PCR has recently been reported and may prove useful in shortening the time to definitive diagnosis (24). A new method using immunomagnetic PCR may increase sensitivity and specificity of this rapid technique (68). DNA fingerprinting using restriction fragment length polymorphism is a useful epidemiological tool and may provide a rapid method for identifying strains of MAC as well as *M. tuberculosis* (33). However, cost and availability limit the use of these techniques to research and reference laboratories.

Immunohistochemical procedures are available for detection of mycobacterial antigens in tissue sections. They have the advantage that killed mycobacteria stain even when acid-fastness has been lost. Cross-reactivity with other mycobacteria makes species identification difficult, but the technique may be useful for the differential diagnosis of granulomatous disease in any organ (53, 123).

Pathogenesis

Disseminated MAC disease is reported primarily in patients with advanced HIV disease and severe immunosuppression. Infection is acquired through ingestion or inhalation of MAC from the environment. The gastrointestinal tract is the most common portal of entry, with colonization followed by localized disease prior to dissemination (9, 58). The organisms penetrate the gut wall, possibly through Peyer's patches, and subsequently are phagocytized by macrophages and other reticuloendothelial cells. In AIDS patients, an undefined defect leads to an inability of these cells to kill the organisms. Recent evidence indicates that some cytokines inhibit intracellular growth of MAC (e.g., TNF-α and granulocyte-macrophage colony-stimulating factor), while other cytokines (IL-1, IL-6) and possibly the gp120 envelope protein of HIV may enhance replication (101). Imbalances of these cytokines may contribute to the inability of the host to control MAC infection; indeed, patients with disseminated MAC have markedly elevated TNF-α and soluble TNF receptor levels and decreased levels of 1,25-dihydroxyvitamin D (37). Moreover, MAC-infected macrophages demonstrate increased HIV production (82).

Humoral factors may also play a role. Antibodies against MAC are produced in response to MAC infection in normal hosts, but not in AIDS patients (41). While these antibodies are not known to have a role in protection against MAC disease, they have been shown to increase MAC killing in vitro (97). Lactoferrin deficiency has been observed to enhance growth of MAC by increasing the availability of iron, an essential nutrient for MAC, and may play a role in pathogenesis (14).

Antibodies against MAC are produced in response to MAC infection in normal hosts, but not in AIDS patients

The increased risk of MAC disease when the CD4$^+$ T-lymphocyte counts fall below 100 suggests that the intracellular killing of these organisms is very sensitive to CD4-mediated immunity, and direct CD4$^+$ cell killing of MAC-sensitized macrophages has been reported (89). However, at this stage of HIV infection, CD8$^+$ cell function, natural killer cell function, and humoral antibody production are also severely impaired. A recent report has suggested that CD3$^+$ CD4$^-$ CD8$^-$ cells may be important in the immune response to MAC infection in patients with AIDS (75). Some other conditions that cause severe immunosuppression also predispose to disseminated MAC infection, notably hairy cell leukemia, but, in general, disseminated MAC is rare in such patients (4).

Most MAC disease appears to result from primary exposure to the pathogen, rather than reactivation of previously controlled infection. This conclusion is supported by the lack of antibody that would suggest previous exposure (41), a frequency of MAC disease that greatly exceeds the expected prevalence of skin test positivity to MAC antigens (114), and the temporal sequence of colonization leading to dissemination (9).

Pathology

The histopathology of MAC varies with the immune status of the host and the site of infection. MAC in the immunodeficient host is usually disseminated. There is often minimal host response. Clusters of large foamy macrophages form sheets or loose aggregates that resemble granulomas; true granulomas are rare (66, 117). When present, necrosis is inflammatory (neutrophilic) rather than caseating (36). The mycobacteria are negatively stained within the cytoplasm, giving the macrophages a striated appearance (66). Acid-fast, periodic acid-Schiff, and silver impregnation techniques reveal masses of intracytoplasmic bacilli. Infection in the immunocompetent host may be localized in lung, cervical nodes, or skin. Patients with immunosuppressive conditions other than AIDS are able to mount a granulomatous response, and mycobacteria are less numerous.

Gastrointestinal Disease

Endoscopic examination often reveals normal epithelium in early infection

Infection probably starts in the area of Peyer's patches in the small intestine (28). Endoscopic examination often reveals normal epithelium in early infection; acid-fast stains may be required to detect single, infected cells in the lamina propria. As infection progresses, the mucosa often appears granular, with yellow to white patches. In severe cases, the mucosa is thickened and flat. Mesenteric adenopathy may occur prior to dissemination of the infection. The resulting thickening of the bowel wall can lead to intussusception with consequent gastrointestinal hemorrhage, or can cause obstruction, but these are rare (5). Histologically, epithelial cells are usually intact and may show mild inflammatory changes, but ulceration is uncommon. Sheets of foamy macrophages are present in the lamina propria; these massively infected cells may expand the villi, giving an appearance and clinical syndrome similar to Whipple disease (26, 93, 103). True granulomas with Langhans giant cells, epithelioid macrophages, and caseous necrosis are not typically seen (8).

MAC infection may be seen in the colon as well as the small bowel. In acute cases the mucosa may be friable with multiple erosions and ulceration, findings which may explain the occasional occurrence of diarrhea. In tissue section, the organisms are located within foamy macrophages in the lamina propria. There is sparing of the glands, but surface epithelium may show congestion and focal acute inflammation with erosions or ulcerations (116).

Disseminated Disease

Lymph node, liver, spleen, and bone marrow are the most common sites involved (66). Lymph node changes vary from tiny foci of infection to marked lymphadenopathy with replacement of the normal architecture by sheets of foamy macrophages containing masses of mycobacteria. Granulomas, abscesses, and necrosis with neutrophilic inflammation are seen in many cases (8, 21). Because MAC is an infection of patients with severe immunodeficiency, the normal architecture of the node is altered and often shows follicular atrophy. Mycobacterial spindle-cell lesions similar to histioid leprosy have been reported; the spindled macrophages contain bacilli (112, 126).

In the liver, the portal triads show mild nonspecific inflammation with foci of infected macrophages. Within the midzonal areas, individual Kupffer cells may be infected or there may be poorly formed granulomas. These granulomas contain admixtures of foamy macrophages, lymphocytes, and occasionally a few epithelioid macrophages or polymorphonuclear leukocytes. Langhans giant cells and central caseous necrosis are extremely uncommon (8). Bone marrow biopsy reveals small aggregates of foamy macrophages; granulomas are less common (66, 123). Mycobacteria are difficult to identify in the marrow, especially in patients receiving anti-mycobacterial prophylaxis. The spleen is the organ most likely to mount a granulomatous response. Miliary involvement with splenomegaly is not uncommon (66, 94).

Pulmonary Disease

The lesions of pulmonary disease are usually localized and often solitary and appear grossly as well-circumscribed nodules. Granulomatous pleuritis, bronchitis or bronchiolitis, and vasculitis have been reported (60, 72). The histologic features vary from well-formed to poorly formed granulomas. Giant cells are frequently seen, and in rare cases there is central caseating necrosis and cavitation. Lymph node involvement is uncommon. A subset of MAC pulmonary infection in the immunocompetent host presents as diffuse nodules or interstitial pneumonia (8, 60, 72).

Lymph Nodes and Skin

Lesions of cervical nodes and skin also reveal granulomatous inflammation (34); ulceration and fistulation are frequent complications. Acid-fast bacilli are found within macrophages or giant cells, but are often single. Foamy macrophages stuffed with myriad bacilli are rare (113, 125).

Differential Diagnosis

MAC infection must be differentiated from tuberculosis, other nontuberculous mycobacterial infections, histoplasmosis, cryptococcosis, coccidioidomycosis, and blastomycosis. In AIDS, where granulomas may not be present, the differential diagnosis includes other disseminated infections such as bacterial sepsis and cytomegalovirus and herpes simplex virus infection. Clinically these may be quite similar, and differentiation on purely clinical grounds is rarely possible. Special stains for microorganisms and cultures for viruses or fungi may be necessary to establish a diagnosis and to rule out other concurrent infections. MAC enteric disease with histologic features of Whipple disease can be differentiated from this condition by acid-fast stains (93). The histologic pattern of tuberculosis has some overlap with MAC infection and reliable species identification requires culture or molecular probes, but MAC tends to present as myriad bacilli in intact, foamy histiocytes whereas the single or scattered bacilli of M. *tuberculosis* are usually associated with significant necrosis.

Special stains for microorganisms and cultures for viruses or fungi may be necessary to establish a diagnosis and to rule out other concurrent infections

Clinical Syndromes

Disseminated Disease

Disseminated MAC disease begins as a localized process that progresses rapidly to include numerous organ systems (9, 41). Localized infection may begin in either the gastrointestinal tract (with abdominal pain, anorexia, weight loss, and, less frequently, diarrhea) or respiratory tract (with pneumonia), following acquisition of the organism through either ingestion or inhalation. In most cases, presenting signs and symptoms are those of the disseminated process, including fevers, night sweats, anemia, weight loss, and, in advanced cases, hepatosplenomegaly. Survival of AIDS patients with disseminated MAC is markedly shortened; the median survival after a diagnosis of disseminated MAC in one study was 4 months, compared to 11 months for AIDS patients without MAC (47, 52, 58). However, survival is prolonged by antimycobacterial therapy (47, 50, 57, 64, 99).

Pulmonary Disease

Pulmonary disease caused by MAC is similar in presentation to tuberculosis. Patients may have localized infiltrates, cavitation, or solitary or multiple pulmonary nodules (1, 2, 18, 49, 55, 61, 91, 106); hilar adenopathy alone is uncommon. Patients are usually febrile, with sputum that contains mycobacteria by culture if not by smear. Weight loss is less common but may occur in cases where the disease has remained untreated for a prolonged period of time or been refractory to therapy. Among persons with MAC pulmonary disease, isolates of the M. avium group are similar in number to those of the M. intracellulare group (32). No clinical differences distinguish the two groups.

Lymphadenitis and Other Manifestations

Children with cervical lymphadenitis have one or more enlarged, tender lymph nodes, but are otherwise asymptomatic; less commonly, they may have systemic illness with fevers, weight loss, and night sweats (73, 95, 96, 125). Draining sinus tracts may be seen, particularly if incision and drainage has been attempted. MAC cervical lymphadenitis is usually unilateral, and chest X-rays are routinely normal. MAC can also present as localized disease such as appendicitis, arthritis and tenosynovitis, and skin infection, although these presentations are uncommon (13, 38, 69).

Treatment

Disseminated Disease

Once disseminated MAC is detected, combination antimycobacterial therapy is required; monotherapy leads to drug resistance and clinical failure

Once disseminated MAC is detected, combination antimycobacterial therapy is required; monotherapy leads to drug resistance and clinical failure. A regimen of clarithromycin at 500 mg twice daily and ethambutol at 15 mg/kg daily (with or without rifabutin at 300 mg daily) is recommended for treatment of disseminated MAC disease (43). Such a regimen has been shown to be effective in disseminated disease in adults with AIDS (99). Presumptive treatment is not recommended, as the clinical ability to predict MAC disease is limited (10) and other treatable processes may be overlooked.

Most patients will show improvement in fevers and night sweats after treatment, and patients with alkaline phosphatase elevations usually show improvement in this parameter. Weight loss is arrested in most cases, but only about half of treated patients will regain lost weight. Anemia responds less frequently and often requires transfusions, while diarrhea may or may not respond to antimycobacterial therapy; in many cases it is likely that the diarrhea in these patients is due to agents other than MAC (90).

Patients who fail or relapse on a macrolide-containing regimen should have susceptibility testing of their isolate performed. Other agents available for use in therapy of MAC disease include ciprofloxacin and amikacin. For treatment of failure/relapse, the addition of amikacin (15 mg/kg/day 5 days a week) plus rifabutin (if not previously used) or ciprofloxacin (750 mg by mouth twice a day) is recommended. Amikacin is usually given for only 4 to 8 weeks because of the high risk of ototoxicity if continued longer. Patients with AIDS and MAC are at high risk of relapse of MAC if antimycobacterial therapy is discontinued. This, combined with the difficulty of documenting eradication of MAC from the host, has resulted in most patients with AIDS and MAC being treated indefinitely.

Pulmonary Disease

Pulmonary MAC disease in patients without AIDS is treated with the same regimen as is used for disseminated disease in AIDS (2, 118). Some authors recommend addition of streptomycin to this regimen, but the efficacy of this strategy has not been studied. Treatment should be continued for 1 year after sputum smears convert to negative. If the patient fails to clear the sputum of mycobacteria, particularly in cases where a necrotic tissue focus remains in the lung, adjunctive surgery may be required.

Lymphadenitis

Surgical removal of infected nodes has traditionally been the treatment of choice for cervical lymphadenitis due to MAC, but a recent report has suggested that macrolide-containing antimycobacterial regimens may also be curative in this manifestation of MAC disease (29). In some patients with hereditary predisposition to MAC disease, immunotherapy with gamma interferon may be useful (40), but such cases are rare, and immunotherapy of MAC disease is not generally recommended.

Prevention

The United States Public Health Service recommends that persons with HIV infection and less than 50 CD4$^+$ cells/µl receive prophylactic antibiotics (azithromycin at 1,200 mg once weekly or clarithromycin at 500 mg twice a day) to prevent MAC disease (6). These regimens can prevent 59 to 69% of disseminated disease (43).

In Sweden, the number of cases of cervical lymphadenitis in children increased after discontinuation of BCG vaccination, suggesting a possible protective effect of BCG against this clinical manifestation of MAC (63, 92, 109). Lower rates of disseminated MAC disease in Sweden have also been attributed to BCG given in childhood (62). However, because of the risk of disseminated disease after immunization with a live vaccine, BCG is not recommended for adults with HIV infection. Prior tuberculosis appears to

The U.S. Public Health Service recommends that persons with HIV infection and less than 50 CD4$^+$ cells/µl receive prophylactic antibiotics to prevent MAC disease

protect against MAC disease, suggesting the generation of antimycobacterial immunity by an episode of tuberculosis disease (46). Lifetime soil exposure has also been noted to be associated with protection against MAC (114); such exposure presumably represents immunization by soil mycobacteria. At this time, due to the lack of availability of a suitable vaccine, immunization is not recommended as a strategy for prevention of MAC disease in any risk group.

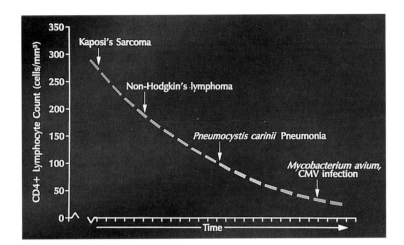

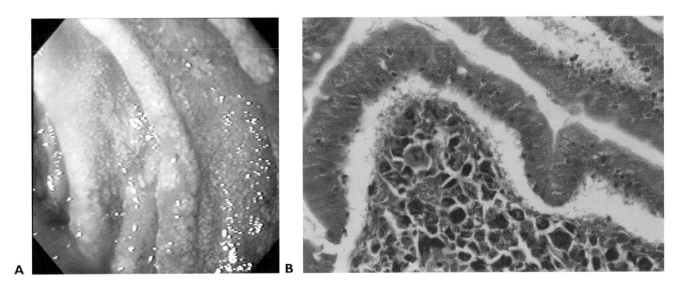

Figure 9.1   Occurrence of AIDS-indicating diagnoses in the natural history of HIV infection. Graph showing where conditions are likely to occur with declining CD4⁺ counts.

A   **B**

Figure 9.2   (A) Endoscopic appearance of duodenal mucosa of a patient with MAC disease. Note the thickened folds. (B) Histologic section of duodenal mucosa with expansion of lamina propria by macrophages stuffed with acid-fast bacilli. Ziehl-Neelsen stain; ×100.

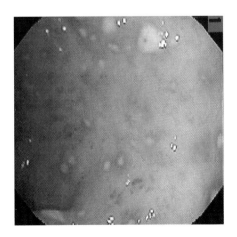

Figure 9.3   Endoscopic appearance of colonic mucosa of a patient with disseminated MAC disease. Note the yellow plaques and focal ulcerations. (Courtesy of Dr. Mark Sims.)

Figure 9.4 Mesenteric adenopathy secondary to disseminated MAC disease. (A) Computed tomographic scan shows thickening of the bowel wall, massive adenopathy, and splenomegaly. (B) Gross photograph of lymph nodes. On cut section the node has a homogeneous yellow surface due to the massive infiltration with MAC organisms. (C) Ziehl-Neelsen stain reveals myriad acid-fast bacilli in macrophages (×330).

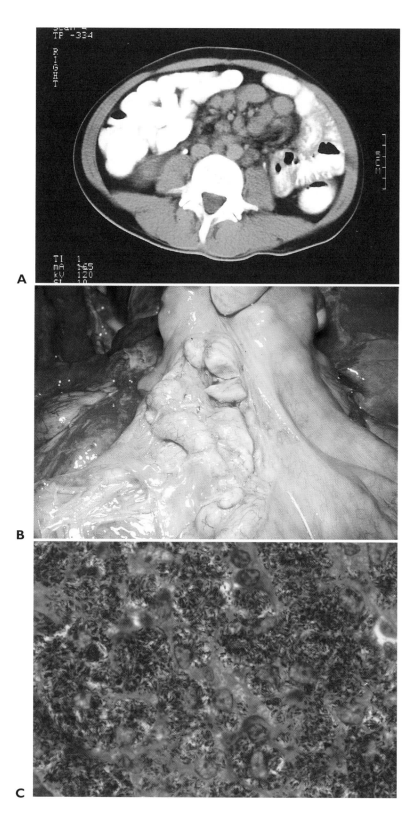

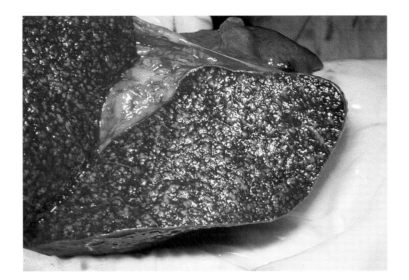

Figure 9.5   Spleen showing miliary lesions of MAC.

Figure 9.6   Lymph node with spindle cell lesion of MAC. Note the elongated macrophages stuffed with acid-fast bacilli. Ziehl-Neelsen stain; ×50.

References

1. **Ahn, C. H., S. S. Ahn, R. A. Anderson, D. T. Murphy, and A. Mammo.** 1986. A four-drug regimen for initial treatment of cavitary disease caused by *Mycobacterium avium* complex. *Am. Rev. Respir. Dis.* **134:**436–441.

2. **American Thoracic Society.** 1997. Diagnosis and treatment of disease caused by nontuberculous mycobacteria. American Thoracic Society Official Statement. *Am. J. Respir. Crit. Care Med.* **156:**S1–S25.

3. **Arbeit, R. D., A. Slutsky, T. W. Barber, J. N. Maslow, S. Niemczyk, J. O. Falkinham, G. T. O'Connor, and C. F. von Reyn.** 1993. Genetic diversity among strains of *Mycobacterium avium* causing monoclonal and polyclonal bacteremia in patients with AIDS. *J. Infect. Dis.* **167:**1384–1390.

4. **Bahmani, A., L. Elting, J. Tarrand, and K. Rolston.** 1997. *Mycobacterium avium* complex infection in cancer patients, p. 203, abstract 708. *In Program and Abstracts of the 35th Annual Meeting of the Infectious Diseases Society of America.* Alexandria, Va.

5. **Cappell, M. S., R. Hassan, S. Rosenthal, and M. Mascarenhas.** 1991. Gastrointestinal obstruction due to *Mycobacterium avium-intracellulare* associated with the acquired immunodeficiency syndrome. *Am. J. Gastroenterol.* **12:**1823–1827.

6. **Centers for Disease Control and Prevention.** 1997. USPHS/IDSA guidelines for the prevention of opportunistic infections in persons infected with human immunodeficiency virus. *Morbid. Mortal. Weekly Rep.* **46:**1–47.

7. **Chapman, J. S.** 1970. The atypical mycobacteria. *Hosp. Pract.* **5:**69–80.

8. **Chester, A. C., and W. C. Winn.** 1986. Unusual and newly recognized patterns of nontuberculous mycobacterial infection with emphasis on the immunocompromised host. *Pathol. Annu.* **1:**251–270.

9. **Chin, D. P., P. C. Hopewell, D. M. Yajko, E. Vittinghoff, C. R Horsburgh, Jr., W. K. Hadley, E. N. Stone, P. S. Nassos, S. M. Ostroff, M. A. Jacobson, C. C. Matkin, and A. L. Reingold.** 1994. *Mycobacterium avium* complex in the respiratory or gastrointestinal tract and the risk of developing *Mycobacterium avium* complex bacteremia in patients with the human immunodeficiency virus. *J. Infect. Dis.* **169:**289–295.

10. **Chin, D. P., A. L. Reingold, C. R. Horsburgh, D. M. Yajko, W. K. Hadley, E. P. Elkin, E. N. Stone, E. M. Simon, P. C. Gonzalez, S. M. Ostroff, M. A. Jacobson, and P. C. Hopewell.** 1994. Predicting *Mycobacterium avium* complex bacteremia in patients infected with human immunodeficiency virus: a prospectively validated model. *Clin. Infect. Dis.* **19:**668–674.

11. **Debrunner, M., M. Salfinger, O. Brandli, and A. von Graevenitz.** 1992. Epidemiology and clinical significance of nontuberculous mycobacteria in patients negative for human immunodeficiency virus in Switzerland. *Clin. Infect. Dis.* **15:**330–345.

12. **Del Beccaro, M. A., P. M. Mendelman, and C. Nolan.** 1989. Diagnostic usefulness of mycobacterial skin test antigens in childhood lymphadenitis. *Pediatr. Infect. Dis. J.* **8:**206–210.

13. **Disla, E., A. Reddy, G. Cuppari, and M. Mullen.** 1995. Primary *Mycobacterium avium* complex septic arthritis in a patient with AIDS. *Clin. Infect. Dis.* **20:**1432–1434.

14. **Douvas, G. S., M. H. May, J. R. Pearson, E. Lam, L. Miller, and N. Tsuchida.** 1994. Hypertriglyceridemic serum, very low density lipoprotein, and iron enhance *Mycobacterium avium* replication in human macrophages. *J. Infect. Dis.* **170:**1248–1255.

15. **du Moulin, G. C., K. D. Stottmeier, P. A. Pelletier, A. Y. Tsang, and J. Hed-
    ley-Whyte.** 1988. Concentration of *Mycobacterium avium* by hospital hot water
    systems. *JAMA* **260:**1599–1601.

16. **Eaton, T., J. O. Falkinham, III, and C. F. von Reyn.** 1995. Recovery of
    Mycobacterium avium from cigarettes. *J. Clin. Microbiol.* **33:**2757–2758.

17. **Eisenbach, K. D., M. D. Sifford, M. D. Cave, J. H. Bates, and J. T. Craw-
    ford.** 1991. Detection of *Mycobacterium tuberculosis* in sputum samples using a
    polymerase chain reaction. *Am. Rev. Respir. Dis.* **144:**1160–1163.

18. **Etzkorn, E. T., S. Aldarondo, C. K. McCallister, J. Matthews, and A. J.
    Ognibene.** 1986. Medical therapy of *Mycobacterium avium-intracellulare* pul-
    monary disease. *Am. Rev. Respir. Dis.* **134:**442–445.

19. **Fakih, M., S. Chapalamadugu, A. Ricart, N. Corriere, and D. Amsterdam.**
    1996. *Mycobacterium malmoense* bacteremia in two AIDS patients. *J. Clin.
    Microbiol.* **34:**731–733.

20. **Falkinham, J. O., III.** 1996. Epidemiology of nontuberculous mycobacteria.
    Clin. Microbiol. Rev. **9:**177–215.

21. **Farhi, D. C., U. G. Mason, and C. R. Horsburgh.** 1986. Pathologic findings in
    disseminated *Mycobacterium avium-intracellulare* infection: a report of 11 cases.
    Am. J. Clin. Pathol. **85:**67–72.

22. **Finkelstein, D. M., P. L. Williams, G. Molenberghs, J. Feinberg, W. G. Pow-
    derly, J. Kahn, R. Dolin, and D. Cotton.** 1996. Patterns of opportunistic infec-
    tions in patients with HIV infection. *J. Acquired Immune Defic. Syndr.*
    12:38–45.

23. **Frederick, T., B. Caldwell, and L. Mascola.** 1996. The pediatric spectrum of
    HIV disease project, abstract We.C3445, p. 134–135. *In Abstracts of the XI Inter-
    national Conference on AIDS,* Vancouver.

24. **Gamboa, F., J. M. Manterola, J. Lonca, L. Matas, B. Viñado, M. Giménez, P.
    J. Cardona, E. Padilla, and V. Ausina.** 1997. Detection and identification of
    mycobacteria by amplification of RNA and DNA in pretreated blood and bone
    marrow aspirates by a simple lysis method. *J. Clin. Microbiol.* **35:**2124–2128.

25. **Gilks, C. F., R. J. Brindle, C. Mwachari, B. Batchelor, J. Bwayo, J. Kimari,
    R. D. Arbeit, and C. F. von Reyn.** 1995. Disseminated mycobacterium infec-
    tion among HIV-infected patients in Kenya. *J. Acquired Immune Defic. Syndr.*
    8:195–198.

26. **Gillin, J. S., C. Urmacher, R. West, and M. Shike.** 1983. Disseminated
    Mycobacterium avium-intracellulare infection in acquired immunodeficiency syn-
    drome mimicking Whipple's disease. *Gastroenterology* **85:**1187–1191.

27. **Grange, J. M., M. D. Yates, and A. Pozniak.** 1995. Bacteriologically confirmed
    non-tuberculous mycobacterial lymphadenitis in southeast England: a recent
    increase in the number of cases. *Arch. Dis. Child.* **72:**516–517.

28. **Gray, J. R., and L. Rabeneck.** 1989. Atypical mycobacterial infection of the
    gastrointestinal tract in AIDS patients. *Am. J. Gastroenterol.* **84:**1521–1524.

29. **Green, P. A., C. F. von Reyn, and R. P. Smith, Jr.** 1993. *Mycobacterium avium*
    complex parotid lymphadenitis: successful therapy with clarithromycin and
    ethambutol. *Pediatr. Infect. Dis. J.* **12(7):**615–617.

30. **Greenberg, A. E., S. Lucas, O. Tossou, I. M. Coulibaly, D. Coulibaly, S. Kas-
    sim, A. Ackah, and K. M. De Cock.** 1995. Autopsy-proven causes of death in
    HIV-infected patients treated for tuberculosis in Abidjan, Côte d'Ivoire. *AIDS*
    9:1251–1254.

31. **Gruft, H., J. Katz, and D. C. Blanchard.** 1975. Postulated source of *Mycobacterium intracellulare* (Battey) infection. *Am. J. Epidemiol.* **102:**311–318.

32. **Guthertz, L. S., B. Damsker, E. J. Bottone, E. G. Ford, T. F. Midura, and J. M. Janda.** 1989. *Mycobacterium avium* and *Mycobacterium intracellulare* infections in patients with and without AIDS. *J. Infect. Dis.* **160:**1037–1041.

33. **Haas, W. H., W. R. Butler, C. L. Woodley, and J. T. Crawford.** 1993. Mixed-linker polymerase chain reaction: a new method for rapid fingerprinting of isolates of the *Mycobacterium tuberculosis* complex. *J. Clin. Microbiol.* **31:**1293–1298.

34. **Haas, W. H., P. Kirschner, S. Ziesing, H. J. Bremer, and E. C. Bottger.** 1993. Cervical lymphadenitis in a child caused by a previously unknown mycobacterium. *J. Infect. Dis.* **167:**237–240.

35. **Hampson, S. J., J. Thompson, M. T. Moss, F. Portaels, E. P. Green, J. Hermon-Taylor, and J. J. Mcfadden.** 1989. DNA probes demonstrate a highly conserved strain of *Mycobacterium avium* infecting AIDS patients. *Lancet* **i:**65–68.

36. **Harawi, S. J.** 1989. The microorganisms: mycobacteria, p. 68–73. *In* S. J. Harawi and C. J. O'Hara (ed.), *Pathology and Pathophysiology of AIDS and HIV-Related Diseases.* C.V. Mosby Company, St. Louis, Mo.

37. **Haug, C. J., P. Aukrust, E. Lien, F. Muller, T. Espevik, and S. S. Froland.** 1996. Disseminated *Mycobacterium avium* complex infection in AIDS: immunopathogenic significance of an activated tumor necrosis factor system and depressed serum levels of 1, 25 dihydroxyvitamin D. *J. Infect. Dis.* **173:**259–262.

38. **Hellinger, W. C., J. D. Smilack, J. L. Greider, Jr., S. Alverez, S. D. Trigg, N. S. Brewer, and R. S. Edson.** 1995. Localized soft-tissue infections with *Mycobacterium/Mycobacterium intracellulare* complex in immunocompetent patients: granulomatous tenosynovitis of the hand or wrist. *Clin. Infect. Dis.* **21:**65–69.

39. **Hide, M., T. Hondo, S. Yonehara, S. Motohiro, and S. Okano.** 1997. Infection with *Mycobacterium avium-intracellulare* with abscess, ulceration and fistula formation. *Br. J. Dermatol.* **136:**121–123.

40. **Holland, S. M., E. M. Eisenstein, D. B. Kuhns, M. L. Turner, T. A. Fleishner, W. Strober, and J. I. Gallin.** 1994. Treatment of disseminated nontuberculous mycobacterial infection with interferon gamma. A preliminary report. *N. Engl. J. Med.* **330:**1348–1355.

41. **Horsburgh, C. R.** 1991. *Mycobacterium avium* complex infection in the acquired immunodeficiency syndrome. *N. Engl. J. Med.* **324:**1332–1338.

42. **Horsburgh, C. R.** 1994. Epidemiology of human disease caused by *Mycobacterium avium* complex. *Can. J. Infect. Dis.* **5**(Suppl. B):5B–9B.

43. **Horsburgh, C. R.** 1996. Advances in the prevention and treatment of *Mycobacterium avium* disease. *N. Engl. J. Med.* **335:**428–430.

44. **Horsburgh, C. R., M. B. Caldwell, and R. J. Simonds.** 1993. Epidemiology of disseminated nontuberculous mycobacterial infection in children with AIDS. *Pediatr. Infect. Dis. J.* **12:**219–222.

45. **Horsburgh, C. R., D. P. Chin, D. M. Yajko, O. C. Hopewell, P. S. Nassos, E. P. Elkin, W. K. Hadley, E. N. Stone, E. M. Simon, P. Gonzalez, S. Ostroff, and A. L. Reingold.** 1994. Environmental risk factors for acquisition of *Mycobacterium avium* complex in persons with human immunodeficiency virus infection. *J. Infect. Dis.* **170:**362–367.

46. Horsburgh, C. R., D. L. Hanson, J. L. Jones, and S. E. Thompson. 1996. Protection from *Mycobacterium avium* complex disease in HIV-infected persons with a history of tuberculosis. *J. Infect. Dis.* **174**(6):1212–1217.

47. Horsburgh, C. R., Jr., J. A. Havlik, D. A. Ellis, E. Kennedy, S. A. Fann, R. E. Dubois, and S. E. Thompson. 1991. Survival of AIDS patients with disseminated *Mycobacterium avium* complex infection with and without antimycobacterial chemotherapy. *Am. Rev. Respir. Dis.* **144**:557–559.

48. Horsburgh, C. R., Jr., U. G. Mason, D. C. Farhi, and M. D. Iseman. 1985. Disseminated infection with *Mycobacterium avium-intracellulare*: a report of 13 cases and a review of the literature. *Medicine* **64**:36–48.

49. Horsburgh, C. R., U. G. Mason, III, L. Heifets, K. Southwick, J. LaBrecque, and M. D. Iseman. 1987. Response to therapy of pulmonary *Mycobacterium avium-intracellulare* infection correlates with the results of in vitro susceptibility testing. *Am. Rev. Respir. Dis.* **135**:418–421.

50. Horsburgh, C. R., B. Metchock, S. M. Gordon, J. A. Havlik, Jr., J. E. McGowan, Jr., and S. E. Thompson, III. 1994. Predictors of survival in patients with AIDS and disseminated *Mycobacterium avium* complex disease. *J. Infect. Dis.* **170**:573–577.

51. Horsburgh, C. R., Jr., J. R. Schoenfelder, F. M. Gordin, D. L. Cohn, P. M. Sullam, and B. A. Wynne. 1997. Geographic and seasonal variation in *Mycobacterium avium* bacteremia among North American patients with AIDS. *Am. J. Med. Sci.* **313**(6):341–345.

52. Horsburgh, C. R., and R. M. Selik. 1989. The epidemiology of disseminated nontuberculous mycobacterial infection in the acquired immunodeficiency syndrome (AIDS). *Am. Rev. Respir. Dis.* **139**:4–7.

53. Humphrey, D. M., and M. H. Weiner. 1987. Mycobacterial antigen detection by immunohistochemistry in pulmonary tuberculosis. *Hum. Pathol.* **18**:701–708.

54. Ichiki, Y., M. Hirose, C. Esaki, and Y. Kitajima. 1997. Skin infection caused by *Mycobacterium avium*. *Br. J. Dermatol.* **136**:260–263.

55. Iseman, M. D. 1996. Pulmonary disease due to *Mycobacterium avium* complex, p. 45–77. *In* J. A. Korvick and C. A. Benson (ed.), *Mycobacterium avium-Complex Infection*. Marcel Dekker, Inc., New York.

56. Iseman, M. D., D. L. Buschman, and L. M. Ackerson. 1991. Pectus excavatum and scoliosis. Thoracic abnormalities associated with pulmonary disease caused by *Mycobacterium avium* complex. *Am. Rev. Respir. Dis.* **144**:914–916.

57. Ives, D. V., R. B. Davis, and J. S. Currier. 1995. Impact of clarithromycin and azithromycin on patterns of treatment and survival among AIDS patients with disseminated *Mycobacterium avium* complex. *AIDS* **9**:261–266.

58. Jacobson, M. A., P. C. Hopewell, D. M. Yajko, W. K. Hadley, E. Lazarus, P. K. Mohanty, G. W. Modin, D. W. Feigal, P. S. Cusick, and M. A. Sande. 1991. Natural history of disseminated *Mycobacterium avium* complex infection in AIDS. *J. Infect. Dis.* **164**:994–998.

59. Jones, J. L., D. L. Hanson, S. Y. Chu, P. L. Fleming, D. J. Hu, J. W. Ward, and the Adult/Adolescent Spectrum of HIV Disease Project Group. 1994. Surveillance of AIDS-defining conditions in the United States. *AIDS* **8**:1489–1493.

60. Kahana, L. M., M. Kay, M. A. Yakrus, and S. Wasserman. 1997. *Mycobacterium avium* complex infection in an immunocompetent young adult related to hot tub exposure. *Chest* **111**:242–245.

61. **Kalayjian, R. C., Z. Toossi, J. F. Tomashefski, Jr., J. T. Carey, J. A. Ross, J. W. Tomford, and R. J. Blinkhorn, Jr.** 1995. Pulmonary disease due to infection by *Mycobacterium avium* complex in patients with AIDS. *Clin. Infect. Dis.* **20:**1186–1194.

62. **Kallenius, G., S. E. Hoffner, and S. B. Svenson.** 1989. Does vaccination with bacille Calmette-Guerin protect against AIDS? *Rev. Infect. Dis.* **11:**349–351.

63. **Katila, M. L., E. Brander, and A. Backman.** 1987. Neonatal BCG vaccination and mycobacterial cervical adenitis in childhood. *Tubercle* **68:**291–296.

64. **Kerlikowske, K. M., M. H. Katz, A. K. Chan, and J. Perez-Stable.** 1992. Antimycobacterial therapy for disseminated *Mycobacterium avium* complex infection in patients with acquired immunodeficiency syndrome. *Arch. Intern. Med.* **152:**813–817.

65. **Kilby, J. M., P. H. Gilligan, J. R. Yankaskas, W. E. Highsmith, Jr., L. J. Edwards, and M. R. Knowles.** 1992. Nontuberculous mycobacteria in adult patients with cystic fibrosis. *Chest* **102:**70–75.

66. **Klatt, E. C., D. F. Jensen, and P. R. Meyer.** 1987. Pathology of Mycobacterium avium-intracellulare infection in acquired immunodeficiency syndrome. *Hum. Pathol.* **709:**714.

67. **Kullavanijaya, P., S. Sirimachan, and S. Surarak.** 1997. Primary cutaneous infection with *Mycobacterium avium intracellulare* complex resembling lupus vulgaris. *Br. J. Dermatol.* **136:**264–266.

68. **Li, Z., G. H. Bai, C. F. von Reyn, P. Marino, M. J. Brennan, N. Gine, and S. L. Morris.** 1996. Rapid detection of *Mycobacterium avium* in stool samples from AIDS patients by immunomagnetic PCR. *J. Clin. Microbiol.* **34:**1903–1907.

69. **Livingston, R. A., G. K. Siberry, C. N. Paidas, and J. J. Eiden.** 1995. Appendicitis due to *Mycobacterium avium* complex in an adolescent infected with the human immunodeficiency virus. *Clin. Infect. Dis.* **20:**1579–1580.

70. **Llewelyn, D. M., and D. Dorman.** 1971. Mycobacterial lymphadenitis. *Aust. Pediatr. J.* **7:**97–102.

71. **Mapother, M. E., and J. C. Songer.** 1984. In vitro interaction of *Mycobacterium avium* with intestinal epithelial cells. *Infect. Immun.* **45:**67–73.

72. **Marchevsky, A., B. Damsker, A. Gribetz, S. Tepper, and S. A. Geller.** 1982. The spectrum of pathology of non-tuberculous mycobacterial infections in open-lung biopsy specimens. *Am. J. Clin. Pathol.* **78:**695–700.

73. **Margileth, A. M., R. Chandra, and P. Altman.** 1984. Chronic lymphadenopathy due to mycobacterial infection. Clinical features, diagnosis, histopathology, and management. *Am. J. Dis. Child.* **138:**917–922.

74. **Mattila, J. O., M.-L. Katila, and M. Vornanen.** 1996. Slowly growing mycobacteria and chronic skin disorders. *Clin. Infect. Dis.* **23:**1043–1048.

75. **Moreau, J.-F., J.-L. Taupin, M. Dupon, J.-C. Carron, J.-M. Ragnaud, C. Marimoutou, N. Bernard, J. Constans, J. Texier-Maugein, P. Barbeau, V. Journot, F. Dabis, M. Bonneville, and J.-L. Pellegrin.** 1996. Increases in CD3$^+$ CD4$^-$ CD8$^-$ T lymphocytes in AIDS patients with disseminated *Mycobacterium avium* complex infection. *J. Infect. Dis.* **174:**969–976.

76. **Morris, A., L. B. Reller, M. Salfinger, K. Jackson, A. Sievers, and B. Dwyer.** 1993. Mycobacteria in stool specimens: the non-value of smears for predicting culture results. *J. Clin. Microbiol.* **31:**1358–1387.

77. **Musial, C. E., and G. D. Roberts.** 1987. Tuberculosis and other mycobacteria, p. 539–580. *In* B. B. Wentworth (ed.), *Diagnostic Procedures for Bacterial Infections*, 7th ed. American Public Health Association, Washington, D.C.

78. **Nightingale, S. D., L. T. Byrd, P. M. Southern, J. D. Jockusch, S. X. Cal, and B. A. Wynne.** 1992. Incidence of *Mycobacterium avium-intracellulare* complex bacteremia in human immunodeficiency virus-positive patients. *J. Infect. Dis.* **165:**1082–1085.

79. **Nightingale, S. D., D. W. Cameron, F. M. Gordin, P. M. Sullam, D. L. Cohn, R. E. Chaisson, L. J. Eron, P. D. Sparti, B. Bihari, D. L. Kaufman, J. J. Stern, D. D. Pearce, D. O. Winkler, G. Weinberg, A. LaMarca, and F. P. Siegal.** 1993. Two controlled trials of rifabutin prophylaxis against *Mycobacterium avium* complex infection in AIDS. *N. Engl. J. Med.* **329:**828–833.

80. **O'Brien, R. J., L. J. Geiter, and D. E. Snider.** 1987. The epidemiology of nontuberculous mycobacterial diseases in the United States. Results from a national survey. *Am. Rev. Respir. Dis.* **135:**1007–1014.

81. **Okello, D. O., N. Sewankambo, R. Goodgame, T. O. Aisu, M. Kwezi, A. Morrissey, and J. J. Ellner.** 1990. Absence of bacteremia with *Mycobacterium avium-intracellulare* in Ugandan patients with AIDS. *J. Infect. Dis.* **162:**208–210.

82. **Orenstein, J. M., C. Fox, and S. M. Wahl.** 1997. Macrophages as a source of HIV during opportunistic infections. *Science* **276:**1857–1861.

83. **Parker, B. C., M. A. Ford, H. Gruft, and J. O. Falkinham.** 1983. Epidemiology of infection by nontuberculous mycobacteria. IV. Preferential aerosolization of *Mycobacterium intracellulare* from natural waters. *Am. Rev. Respir. Dis.* **128:**652–656.

84. **Pethel, M. L., and J. O. Falkinham, III.** 1989. Plasmid-influenced changes in *Mycobacterium avium* catalase activity. *Infect. Immun.* **57:**1714–1718.

85. **Pfaller, M. A.** 1994. Application of new technology to detection, identification, and antimicrobial susceptibility testing of mycobacteria. *Am. J. Clin. Pathol.* **101:**329–337.

86. **Pierce, M., S. Crampton, D. Henry, L. Heifets, A. LaMarca, M. Montecalvo, G. P. Wormser, H. Jablonowski, J. Jemsek, M. Cynamon, B. G. Yangco, G. Notario, and J. C. Craft.** 1996. A randomized trial of clarithromycin as prophylaxis against disseminated *Mycobacterium avium* complex infection in patients with advanced acquired immunodeficiency syndrome. *N. Engl. J. Med.* **335:**384–391.

87. **Pinto-Powell, R., K. N. Olivier, B. J. Marsh, S. Donaldson, H. W. Parker, W. Boyle, M. Knowles, M. Magnusson, and C. F. von Reyn.** 1996. Skin testing with *Mycobacterium avium* sensitin to identify infection with M. *avium* complex in patients with cystic fibrosis. *Clin. Infect. Dis.* **22:**560–562.

88. **Prince, D. S., D. D. Peterson, R. M. Steiner, J. E. Gottlieb, R. Scott, H. L. Israel, W. G. Figueroa, and J. E. Fish.** 1989. Infection with *Mycobacterium avium* complex in patients without predisposing conditions. *N. Engl. J. Med.* **321:**863–868.

89. **Ravn, P., and B. K. Pedersen.** 1996. *Mycobacterium avium* and purified protein derivative-specific cytotoxicity mediated by CD4[+] lymphocytes from healthy HIV-seropositive and -seronegative individuals. *J. Acquired Immune Defic. Syndr.* **2:**433–441.

90. **Ray, S. M., S. E. Thompson, and C. R. Horsburgh.** 1995. Role of *Mycobacterium avium* complex (MAC) in AIDS patients with diarrhea, abstract 473, p. 135. *In IDSA 33rd Annual Meeting Program, September 16–18*, San Francisco.

91. **Reich, J. M., and R. E. Johnson.** 1991. *Mycobacterium avium* complex pulmonary disease. Incidence, presentation, and response to therapy in a community setting. *Am. Rev. Respir. Dis.* **143:**1381–1385.

92. **Romanus, V., H. O. Hallander, P. Wahlen, A. M. Olinder-Nielsen, P. H. W. Magnusson, and I. Juhlin.** 1995. Atypical mycobacteria in extrapulmonary disease among children. Incidence in Sweden from 1969 to 1990, related to changing BCG-vaccination coverage. *Lancet* **76:**300–310.

93. **Roth, R. I., R. L. Owen, D. F. Keren, and P. A. Volberding.** 1985. Intestinal infection with *Mycobacterium avium* in acquired immune deficiency syndrome (AIDS). Histological and clinical comparison with Whipple's disease. *Dig. Dis. Sci.* **30:**497–504.

94. **Rotterdam, H.** 1997. *Mycobacterium avium* complex (MAC) infection, p. 657–669. *In* D. H. Connor, F. W. Chandler, D. A. Schwarz, H. J. Manz, and E. E. Lack (ed.), *Pathology of Infectious Diseases*, vol. 1. Appleton and Lange, Philadelphia.

95. **Saitz, E. W.** 1981. Cervical lymphadenitis caused by atypical mycobacteria. *Pediatr. Clin. North Am.* **28:**823–839.

96. **Schaad, U. B., T. P. Votteler, G. H. McCracken, and J. D. Nelson.** 1979. Management of atypical mycobacterial lymphadenitis in childhood: a review based on 380 cases. *J. Pediatr.* **95:**356–360.

97. **Schnittman, S., H. C. Lane, F. G. Witebsky, L. L. Gosey, M. D. Hoggan, and A. S. Fauci.** 1988. Host defense against *Mycobacterium-avium* complex. *J. Clin. Immunol.* **8(4):**234–243.

98. **Schulze-Robbecker, R., C. Feldmann, R. Fischeder, B. Janning, M. Exner, and G. Wahl.** 1995. Dental units: an environmental study of sources of potentially pathogenic mycobacteria. *Lancet* **76:**318–323.

99. **Shafran, S. D., J. Singer, D. P. Zarowny, P. Phillips, I. Salit, S. L. Walmsley, I. W. Fong, M. J. Gill, A. R. Rachlis, R. G. Lalonde, M. M. Fanning, and C. M. Tsoukas, for the Canadian HIV Trials Network Protocol 010 Study Group.** 1996. A comparison of two regimens for the treatment of *Mycobacterium avium* complex bacteremia in AIDS: rifabutin, ethambutol, and clarithromycin versus rifampin, ethambutol, clofazimine, and ciprofloxacin. *N. Engl. J. Med.* **335:**377–383.

100. **Shiratsuchi, H., J. L. Johnson, and J. J. Ellner.** 1991. Bidirectional effects of cytokines on growth of M. *avium* in human monocytes. *J. Immunol.* **146:**3165–3170.

101. **Shiratsuchi, H., J. L. Johnson, and J. J. Ellner.** 1994. Modulation of the effector function of human monocytes for *Mycobacterium avium* by human immunodeficiency virus envelope protein gp120. *J. Clin. Invest.* **93:**885–891.

102. **Shiratsuchi, H., Z. Toosi, M. A. Mettler, and J. J. Ellner.** 1993. Colonial morphotype as a determinate of cytokine expression by human monocytes infected with M. *avium. J. Immunol.* **150:**2945–2954.

103. **Strom, R. L., and R. P. Gruninger.** 1983. AIDS with *Mycobacterium avium-intracellulare* lesions resembling those of Whipple's disease. *N. Engl. J. Med.* **309:**1323–1324.

104. **Swenson, S. J., T. E. Hartman, and D. E. Williams.** 1994. Computer tomographic diagnosis of *Mycobacterium avium-intracellulare* complex in patients with bronchiectasis. *Chest* **105:**49–52.

105. **Tanaka, E., R. Amitani, A. Niimi, K. Suzuki, T. Murayama, and F. Kuze.** 1997. Yield of computed tomography and bronchoscopy for the diagnosis of *Mycobacterium avium* complex pulmonary disease. *Am. J. Respir. Crit. Care Med.* **155:**2041–2046.

106. **Tierstein, A. S., B. Damsker, P. A. Kirschner, D. J. Krellenstein, B. Robinson, and M. T. Chuang.** 1990. Pulmonary infection with *Mycobacterium avium-intracellulare*: diagnosis, clinical patterns, treatment. *Mt. Sinai J. Med.* **57:**209–215.

107. **Tisdall, P. A., D. R. DeYoung, G. D. Roberts, and J. P. Anhalt.** 1982. Identification of clinical isolates of mycobacteria with gas-liquid chromatography: a 10-month follow-up study. *J. Clin. Microbiol.* **16:**400–402.

108. **Tomashefski, J. F., Jr., R. C. Stern, C. A. Demko, and C. F. Doershuk.** 1996. Nontuberculous mycobacteria in cystic fibrosis. *Am. J. Respir. Crit. Care Med.* **154:**523–528.

109. **Trnka, L., D. Dankova, and E. Svandova.** 1994. Six years' experience with the discontinuation of BCG vaccination. 4. Protective effect of BCG vaccination against *Mycobacterium avium intracellulare* complex. *Lancet* **75:**348–352.

110. **Tsang, A. Y., J. C. Denner, P. J. Brennan, and J. K. McClatchy.** 1992. Clinical and epidemiological importance of typing of *Mycobacterium avium* complex isolates. *J. Clin. Microbiol.* **30:**479–484.

111. **Tsukamura, M., N. Kita, H. Shimoide, H. Arakawa, and A. Kuze.** 1988. Studies on the epidemiology of nontuberculous mycobacteriosis in Japan. *Am. Rev. Respir. Dis.* **137:**1280–1284.

112. **Umlas, J., M. Federman, C. Crawford, C. J. O'Hara, J. S. Fitzgibbon, and A. Modeste.** 1991. Spindle cell pseudotumor due to *Mycobacterium avium-intracellulare* in patients with acquired immunodeficiency syndrome (AIDS): positive staining of mycobacteria for cytoskeleton filaments. *Am. J. Surg. Pathol.* **15:**1181–1187.

113. **von Lichtenberg, F.** 1991. Mycobacterial diseases, p. 173–187. *In Pathology of Infectious Diseases.* Raven Press, New York.

114. **von Reyn, C. F., R. D. Arbeit, A. N. A. Tosteson, M. A. Ristola, T. W. Barber, R. Waddell, C. H. Sox, R. J. Brindle, C. F. Gilks, A. Ranki, C. Bartholomew, J. Edwards, J. O. Falkinham, III, G. T. O'Connor, and the International MAC Study Group.** 1996. The international epidemiology of disseminated *Mycobacterium avium* complex infection in AIDS. *AIDS* **10:**1025–1032.

115. **von Reyn, C. F., J. N. Maslow, T. W. Barber, J. O. Falkinham, III, and R. D. Arbeit.** 1994. Persistent colonisation of potable water as a source of *Mycobacterium avium* infection in AIDS. *Lancet* **343:**1137–1141.

116. **Waisman, J., H. Rotterdam, G. N. Niedt, K. Lewin, and P. Racz.** 1987. AIDS: an overview of the pathology. *Pathol. Res. Pract.* **182:**729–754.

117. **Wallace, J. M., and J. B. Hannah.** 1988. *Mycobacterium avium* complex infection in patients with the acquired immunodeficiency syndrome. *Chest* **93:**926–932.

118. **Wallace, R. J., Jr., B. A. Brown, D. E. Griffith, W. M. Girard, and D. T. Murphy.** 1996. Clarithromycin regimens for pulmonary *Mycobacterium avium* complex: the first 50 patients. *Am. J. Respir. Crit. Care Med.* **153:**1766–1772.

119. **Warren, J.** 1992. Mycobacterial infections, p. 190–207. *In* S. T. Shulman, J. P. Phair, and H. M. Sommers (ed.), *The Biological and Clinical Basis of Infectious Diseases,* 4th ed. Saunders, Philadelphia.

120. **Wayne, L. G., and H. P. Willet.** 1986. Mycobacteria, p. 1435–1457. *In* P. H. A. Sneath (ed.), *Bergeys Manual of Systemic Bacteriology*, vol. 2. The Williams and Wilkins Co., Baltimore.

121. **Whittier, S., R. L. Hopfer, M. R. Knowles, and P. H. Gilligan.** 1993. Improved recovery of mycobacteria from respiratory secretions of patients with cystic fibrosis. *J. Clin. Microbiol.* **31:**861–864.

122. **Wickman, K.** 1986. Clinical significance of nontuberculous mycobacteria. A bacteriological survey of Swedish strains isolated between 1973 and 1981. *Scand. J. Infect. Dis.* **18:**337–344.

123. **Wiley, E. L., A. Perry, S. D. Nightingale, and J. Lawrence.** 1993. Detection of *Mycobacterium avium intracellulare* complex in bone marrow specimens of patients with acquired immunodeficiency syndrome. *Am. J. Clin. Pathol.* **101:**446–451.

124. **Witty, L. A., V. F. Tapson, and C. A. Piantadosi.** 1994. Isolation of mycobacteria in patients with pulmonary alveolar proteinosis. *Medicine* **73:**103–109.

125. **Wolinsky, E.** 1995. Mycobacterial lymphadenitis in children: a prospective study of 105 nontuberculous cases with long-term follow-up. *Clin. Infect. Dis.* **20:**954–963.

126. **Wood, C., B. J. Nickeloff, and N. R. Todes-Taylor.** 1985. Pseudo-tumor resulting from atypical mycobacterial infection: a "histoid" variety of *Mycobacterium avium-intracellulare* complex infection. *Am. J. Clin. Pathol.* **83:**524–527.

127. **Yajko, D. M., D. P. Chin, P. C. Gonzalez, P. S. Nassos, P. C. Hopewell, A. L. Reingold, C. R. Horsburgh, Jr., M. A. Yakrus, S. M. Ostroff, and W. K. Hadley.** 1995. *Mycobacterium avium* complex in water, food, and soil samples collected from the environment of HIV-infected individuals. *J. Acquired Immune Defic. Syndr.* **9:**176–182.

chapter 10

Chancroid

George P. Schmid and Mary Klassen

Chancroid shares with donovanosis and lymphogranuloma venereum the dubious distinction of being one of the three "minor sexually transmitted diseases." Yet, chancroid is not a minor sexually transmitted disease (STD) for much of the world, as the worldwide incidence of chancroid may exceed that of syphilis (14). In the past decade, immigration, illegal drug use (principally crack cocaine), and the human immunodeficiency virus (HIV) epidemic have brought unprecedented interest in chancroid. Though chancroid was previously a disease of small numbers in industrialized countries, immigration from the developing world, where the disease is common, brought infected individuals into scattered locations; prostitution (particularly, in the United States, associated with crack cocaine) then created small epidemics. In both the industrialized and developing worlds, chancroid has been associated with enhanced transmission of HIV, and in the developing world chancroid plays an important role in the transmission of this virus.

George P. Schmid, Division of STD Prevention, National Center for HIV, STD, and TB Prevention, Centers for Disease Control and Prevention, Mailstop E-27, 1600 Clifton Road, N.E., Atlanta, GA 30333. **Mary Klassen,** Department of Infectious and Parasitic Disease Pathology, Armed Forces Institute of Pathology, Washington, DC 20306-6000.

Pathology of Emerging Infections 2
Edited by Ann Marie Nelson and C. Robert Horsburgh, Jr.
© 1998 American Society for Microbiology, Washington, D.C.

Microbiology

The etiologic agent of chancroid is *Haemophilus ducreyi*. In 1889, Auguste Ducrey at the University of Naples first described the bacillus following repeated inoculation of forearm skin with material from patients' own ulcers (1, 48). Many questions about the organism and host response to it remain unanswered.

The bacillus of Ducrey is in the genus *Haemophilus* because of its fastidious growth requirements and structural and antigenic properties (1, 2). On electron microscopy, the cell wall is trilaminar as in other gram-negative bacteria (2). Studies of respiratory quinones and DNA suggest that *H. ducreyi* is not closely related to the other species of its family, *Pasteurellaceae*, which includes the genera *Actinobacillus* and *Pasteurella*. There is limited DNA-DNA hybridization, with relative DNA homology of only 0.18 (2).

Extracellular tissue-degrading enzymes, such as proteases or elastases, have not been detected (1). Intradermal injection of purified *H. ducreyi* lipopolysaccharide leads to increased soluble interleukin-2 and tissue necrosis (1). Biochemical and molecular studies have identified macromolecular components that may be important in virulence (58). *H. ducreyi* has at least 11 plasmids conferring resistance to ampicillin, tetracycline, chloramphenicol, streptomycin, kanamycin, and sulfonamides (17, 48). Polymyxin resistance, which is accompanied by the loss of a 47,000-molecular-weight protein, correlates with virulence in *H. ducreyi* (39).

In 1900, Bezançon et al. cultured the organism on solid agar with fresh whole rabbit blood (1). In 1922, Teague and Diebert standardized the culture technology using heated human or rabbit blood (48). Following overnight incubation, the supernatant would be stained in search of gram-negative rods in "long parallel chains" or the "school of fish arrangement." During the Second World War, Beeson successfully cultivated *H. ducreyi* with humidity, CO_2, erythrocytes, and serum (48). During the 1978 outbreak of chancroid in Winnipeg, Canada, Hammond and colleagues developed a medium that has become the standard technique (18, 48).

Most laboratories use one or both of two types of media for primary isolation: gonococcal base or Mueller-Hinton agar (30, 38, 48). Both media are made selective by vancomycin and enriched with other ingredients such as bovine hemoglobin, fetal bovine serum, horse blood, or vitamins (48). High yields have been obtained by using gonococcal agar and Mueller-Hinton agar in a biplate fashion (25). Vancomycin (3 µg/ml) inhibits gram-positive organisms that may be present as contaminants or superinfecting bacteria (18, 55). Inoculation of media with and without vancomycin is recommended.

H. ducreyi does not grow well at 37°C (48). The optimal incubation temperature is probably 33 to 34°C (30, 48, 51). A high-humidity environment with 3 to 7% CO_2 improves growth (38, 48, 55). A candle extinction jar with moistened paper towel may be used if a CO_2 incubator is not available (30, 48).

Colonies are usually not visible until 48 h (30, 48). They vary in size and opacity, giving the impression of a mixed culture. Most are 0.5 to 1.0 mm in diameter, yellow-gray or tan, dome-shaped, nonmucoid, and extremely

---

The bacillus of Ducrey is in the genus Haemophilus because of its fastidious growth requirements and structural and antigenic properties

cohesive. They are difficult to pick up and produce a nonuniform suspension in saline (30). *H. ducreyi* produces alpha-hemolysis in stabs on rabbit blood agar (55).

H. ducreyi stains poorly with safranin and crystal violet. Gram staining of colonies shows small, faintly staining gram-negative coccobacilli (48). Sometimes they are in short chains, clumps, whorls, or "rail track" groupings (30, 48). Individual bacteria may show bipolar staining (30).

H. ducreyi is catalase negative (30, 48). It is oxidase positive but delayed to 15 to 20 s with the *N,N,N′,N′*-tetramethyl-*p*-phenylenediamine dihydrochloride reagent (30, 36, 37, 48, 55). The oxidase test is negative with the dimethyl-*p*-phenylenediamine oxalate reagent (36, 37). Hammond and colleagues demonstrated that *H. ducreyi* lacks hemin synthetase and is the only human pathogen in its genus with a requirement for exogenous hemin as demonstrated by a negative ALA-porphyrin test (18, 36, 37, 48). Clinical isolates may be beta-lactamase positive, although the reference strains may be beta-lactamase negative (30, 55). Nitrate reduction and alkaline phosphatase tests are positive, allowing identification by the RapID NH test kit system (19, 38, 48). *H. ducreyi* does not produce indole or H_2S (30, 48).

Epidemiology

A significant distinction between industrialized countries and developing countries is not only the relative different incidences of chancroid, but also the relative different incidences of diseases characterized by ulcers. In STD clinics in industrialized countries, patients with genital ulcers make up 1 to 5% of all clinic attendees, but in developing countries this percentage may be 20 to 70% (43). Markedly different, also, is the prevalence of chancroid among the two groups. The frequency, by percentage, of chancroid among individuals with genital ulcers in industrialized countries is low, from 0 to 5% unless an outbreak is occurring (44, 50). In the developing world, however, the frequency is often dramatically higher, 18 to 62%, and is not apparently related to outbreaks (44, 50).

In the industrialized world, even though chancroid is uncommon, it has increased in frequency in the past decade. This is best documented in the United States. Once a common disease in the United States, chancroid became rare following the introduction of antibiotics after World War II. Between 1970 and 1979, a mean of 878 cases was reported annually (52). In 1982, however, an outbreak occurred in California and was followed by multiple outbreaks elsewhere so that the annual number of cases in 1987–1991 was higher each year than any year since 1949 (52). Since reaching a peak of 4,986 cases in 1987, the number of cases reported each year has declined annually to 606 in 1995 (10). The reasons for this decline, unlike the reasons for the previous increase, are intriguingly uncertain.

In the United States and Canada, chancroid is localized to selected cities, and this is true of other industrialized countries, where recent years have seen outbreaks occurring in cities in Europe and Australia. It is often difficult to determine how common chancroid is because of lack of diagnostic

In the industrialized world, even though chancroid is uncommon, it has increased in frequency in the past decade

facilities, even in industrialized countries (53); relatively insensitive surveillance systems; and a relative lack of medical publication possibilities. Nevertheless, through a variety of sources, one can make reasonable guesses of relative frequencies of cases. These frequencies can be grouped into those countries in which there are scattered cases, more homogeneously spread numbers of cases but of low prevalence, and homogeneously spread numbers of cases but of high prevalence; for some areas, it is difficult to know whether chancroid is present. In general, the industrialized countries have scattered cases, the developing countries of Latin America, North Africa, and the Middle East have low prevalences, and the developing countries of sub-Saharan Africa and Asia have high prevalences.

The varying prevalences of chancroid throughout the world relate to four broad epidemiologic themes: immigration, poverty, commercial sex, and prevalence of circumcision. Immigration has been important in many of the outbreaks in industrialized countries, as disease has appeared in areas which previously had no cases of chancroid. In the United States, many of the early outbreaks involved immigrants from Hispanic countries (52), but other cases and small outbreaks were traced to individuals from the Caribbean and the Far East. In individuals seeking care for chancroid in the seaport of Rotterdam, The Netherlands, the probable country of acquisition of chancroid cases has been extremely varied, with patients acquiring their infection in at least 14 countries on five continents (35).

Poverty is historically linked to chancroid, more so than for other STDs, and is certainly a factor in many developing countries. Why poverty should be particularly associated with chancroid is not clear, unless it is simply a proxy for other risk factors such as commercial sex or lack of medical care. In the United States, cases in recent years have occurred almost invariably among individuals of low socioeconomic status. Years ago in the industrialized countries, however, wartime, with its disastrous effects on living conditions in the war-torn countries, provided opportunities for outbreaks; during the Korean War, chancroid was 14 times as common as syphilis among white American troops (3).

Commercial sex is a risk factor for chancroid universally. This is a feature well recognized by authors of older medical literature, who noted that traveling carnivals (and their women) often left cases of chancroid in their wake. In the United States, outbreaks of chancroid have fit one of two epidemiologic patterns. Both involve commercial sex, but of different forms.

The first pattern involves immigrant Hispanic males, in many instances illegal entrants to the United States (5, 16). Often, for economic and legal reasons, these men live closely together without integrating significantly into local society. Abrupt increases occur when infected professional commercial sex workers, working for money, sell their services to many men living closely together.

The second pattern, and more recently the predominant one, often involves black males and drugs, usually crack cocaine. This pattern lacks the abrupt onset of the first, but "informal" prostitution is directly or indirectly involved by the frequent exchange of sex for drugs or the money to buy

Poverty is historically linked to chancroid, more so than for other STDs

drugs. Multiple investigations of American chancroid outbreaks in multiple locations have documented the association of outbreaks with black race, commercial sex, and crack (13, 32, 52).

The first pattern may lead into the second, as occurred in Dallas, Texas, in 1986 (16). This outbreak originally began among Hispanic men, most of whom were undocumented workers living in boarding houses. Within the next 2 years, black Americans became the preponderant racial group affected and chancroid had spread widely throughout the city.

The distinction between prostitution, promiscuity, and nonpromiscuous high levels of sexual activity is, however, often a fine one and subject to cultural and situational interpretation. Sub-Saharan Africa has some of the highest rates of chancroid, and also has the fastest growing urban populations, in the world, with doubling times of every 10 to 14 years (29). Many residents come to cities seeking work; traditional family relationships in rural areas are disrupted, and prostitution out of situational "necessity" is common for males who are without spouses and for females who are unable to find other means of support. Also, in some African societies, high levels of sexual activity, perhaps with gifts being exchanged, are an accepted cultural norm. While commercial sex is an important epidemiologic marker of chancroid in every continent, the common feature is frequent sexual encounters with multiple individuals.

But it is commercial sex, particularly in the industrialized world, that yields the high male:female ratios of reported cases that are characteristic of chancroid. In the United States, for example, of nine outbreaks between 1981 and 1987, the male:female ratio was 3:1 to 25:1 and was highest in outbreaks highly associated with commercial sex workers (52). While one might argue that males outnumber females because males are symptomatic and females are not, that is unlikely to be the case or to contribute significantly to the reason for the large disparity in male-female differences (see below).

The lack of circumcision appears to predispose to the development of chancroid, although few formal studies have been performed to document this. Perhaps the best study has been by Cameron et al., who examined men in Kenya presenting with an STD following sex with a prostitute and determined the STD the men had and their circumcision status (6). Of men with a genital ulcer (89% of whom were diagnosed with chancroid), 38% had a foreskin, compared with only 15% of the men with another STD. A more recent case-control study from New York City found that 77% of the males with chancroid had a foreskin compared with 56% of the control men with gonorrhea (32).

It is commercial sex, particularly in the industrialized world, that yields the high male:female ratios of reported cases that are characteristic of chancroid

Clinical Features

Lesions arise in the areas of the male genital tract that are most easily traumatized: the prepuce of uncircumcised men and the coronal sulcus of circumcised men. In women, most lesions are found on the external genitalia and only occasionally on the vaginal walls or cervix; perianal lesions may occur, do not appear to necessarily result from sex, and have been confused as hemorrhoids (8). About one-half of patients will have a single ulcer, and more than four is unusual. The usual incubation period is 3 to 7 days.

At the site of inoculation, an inflamed macule or papule appears and rapidly erodes into an ulcer. Many patients simply recall a "sore" developing without a distinct macule or papule. Typically, an ulcer caused by *H. ducreyi*, compared to those of other ulcerative diseases, has a ragged, nonindurated margin with an erythematous edge and a beefy, deep, necrotic base. Superficial and atypical ulcers may occur, however. Ulcers may coalesce and form large, serpiginous ulcerations that partly encircle the penis. A diagnostic feature of chancroid is that the ulcers are exquisitely painful and tender, making examination difficult. Retraction of the prepuce may not be possible, due to phimosis. In women, ulcers of the cervix or vagina occasionally occur, with little or no symptomatology (20, 46).

As the disease progresses, as many as one-half of men develop unilateral or bilateral inguinal adenopathy. This adenopathy is characteristically painful even though the nodes may be small. Large, fluctuant nodes (buboes) may occur, a finding only occasionally seen in genital herpes and never in syphilis. In the absence of effective antimicrobial therapy or drainage, buboes frequently rupture. In women, lymphadenopathy in the inguinal area is unusual, presumably because of differences in lymphatic drainage.

Without treatment, tissue destruction may be significant, but *H. ducreyi* does not spread outside the genital tract. Patients' infections eventually heal after several unpleasant months, often with scarring, presumably due to the development of immunity.

Of all STDs, chancroid has been the one most associated with HIV infection and may augment HIV transmission as much as 300-fold (21). Chancroid has been associated with HIV infection both at the time of initial evaluation (with seropositivity resulting from previous risky sexual behavior) and later (with seropositivity resulting from HIV infection acquired at the time of *H. ducreyi* infection). The prevalence of HIV infection in individuals seeking medical attention can be striking, with prevalences of >45% (2) in Malawi, but also 18% in an American city (32). Seroconversion further increases these prevalences. In one study in Kenya, 43% of uncircumcised men who acquired chancroid following a single sexual encounter with a prostitute (who was HIV positive) developed HIV infection (6). Such seroconversion rates are <5% in the United States (57); here, fewer source patients are HIV positive. Because of the high risk of HIV seropositivity, an HIV test should be done at the time of a chancroid patient's initial visit and another 3 months later; a follow-up syphilis test should also be performed at both times (9).

There are several reasons for the firm association of chancroid with HIV transmission. First, the lesions of chancroid are deep, eroded, and often bloody. Second, the infiltrate in the base of the ulcer is highly cellular, very likely containing many cells bearing CD4 receptors which may contain virus

> *As the disease progresses, as many as one-half of men develop unilateral or bilateral inguinal adenopathy*

or be targets for viral attachment. HIV has been found in the exudates of 4 (11%) of 36 ulcers when tested by culture (28). Third, because chancroid enhances transmission of HIV, and does so in individuals who are often highly sexually active, populations characterized by chancroid are likely to be infected with HIV and act as efficient transmitters of the virus. Last, and unfortunately not uniquely to chancroid, patients continue to have sexual intercourse after onset of lesions—20% in one American study (13).

Pathophysiology

H. ducreyi penetrates the skin of the external genitalia, possibly through minor abrasions, colonizes subcutaneous tissues, and then produces tissue damage or induces the production of cytokines that result in ulcer formation. Contact between organisms and undamaged skin does not lead to any reaction or damage of mouse skin (1). Intradermal injection of either live or heat-killed organisms causes tissue necrosis, although ulcer formation requires viable organisms (1). *H. ducreyi* shows adherence to different cell lines in vitro that might be mediated by pili or hemagglutinins. Pili have been detected by electron microscopy (7). Binding to extracellular matrix proteins has also been reported (1). Virulent strains are resistant to the complement-mediated lethal action of normal serum and are relatively resistant to phagocytosis and killing by polymorphonuclear leukocytes (39). Nonvirulent strains, that do not produce cutaneous lesions, are susceptible to killing by polymorphonuclear cells. An excessive supply of iron results in a more prolonged localized inflammatory response (1). Outer membrane proteins change with antibody modulation during in vivo growth and may be important factors for maintenance of infection (1).

*V*irulent strains are resistant to the complement-mediated lethal action of normal serum

In a human model of infection, subjects were infected with *H. ducreyi* by delivery of bacterial suspensions into the epidermis and dermis through puncture wounds made by an allergy-testing device (56). Subjects developed papular lesions that evolved into pustules resembling natural disease. Some papular lesions resolved spontaneously, indicating that host responses may clear infection. Papular lesions intermittently shed bacteria, suggesting that chancroid may be transmissible before ulceration.

There is experimental evidence for a cell-mediated immune response. Different antigen preparations of *H. ducreyi* induce proliferation of lymphocytes from both unexposed and chancroid-sensitized individuals (1). In a sensitized person, measured cell responses are much stronger. The dose-dependent phenomenon is associated with interleukin-2 production. The histology of the inflammatory infiltrate (described below) also suggests that there is a significant role for cell-mediated immunity, perhaps delayed hypersensitivity type (27, 31). Recruitment of CD4 T lymphocytes and macrophages may be critical to the role of chancroid in HIV transmission (27, 31, 56).

Virulent strains, as defined by the rabbit intradermal test, are resistant to serum, phagocytosis, and killing by polymorphonuclear cells, suggesting that these factors mediate the pathogenicity of *H. ducreyi* (39). In human models, there is little evidence for humoral or peripheral blood mononuclear cell responses to bacterial antigens (56).

Pathology

Classic histological descriptions of chancroid describe three zones of inflammation

Classic histological descriptions of chancroid describe three zones of inflammation. There is a superficial dermal infiltrate containing neutrophils and short parallel chains of gram-negative bacilli overlying granulation tissue with a subjacent plasma cell-rich infiltrate. The epidermis may show acanthosis, spongiosis, and neutrophilic permeation. Recently, it has been found that T lymphocytes (predominantly CD4$^+$) and histiocytes (many Langerhans) often dominate the inflammatory infiltrate (27, 31, 56). The mononuclear infiltrate extends deep into the dermis and may be perivascular with areas of granulomatous inflammation and vasculitis (27). In one study, plasma cells were a minor component of the inflammatory cell population (31). These features are typical of a cell-mediated immune reaction.

Diagnosis

Health care workers often make the diagnosis of chancroid on the basis of its clinical features; however, the signs and symptoms overlap considerably with syphilis, herpes simplex, and lymphogranuloma venereum. Isolation and culture of *H. ducreyi* may sometimes be unacceptably insensitive. Inability to grow the organism may be due to strain differences in nutritional requirements, improper handling, delayed inoculation, use of less than optimal growth conditions, and vancomycin-sensitive organisms (25, 51). Recent advances in non-culture techniques have enhanced the diagnosis of chancroid.

For specimen collection, either cotton or calcium alginate swabs are suitable (48). One swab is used to remove superficial debris and another to collect the exudate. Because the organisms will survive for only 2 to 4 h on the swab, the specimen should be immediately inoculated onto agar or stored in the refrigerator. Ulcer exudate can yield large numbers of organisms, but inguinal lymph nodes are unlikely to yield positive cultures unless they have ruptured. Gram staining of smears of the specimen may show *H. ducreyi* as pale-staining, gram-negative coccobacilli. They may be arranged in groups having a "school of fish" appearance and may be within polymorphonuclear cells.

Dot-immunobinding assays have demonstrated that sera from patients with chancroid have higher levels of immunoglobulin M (IgM) and IgG reactivity with outer membrane from *H. ducreyi* than with outer membrane from *Haemophilus influenzae* or *Haemophilus parainfluenzae* (49). In contrast, sera from control patients and patients with disease caused by *H. influenzae* do not react with any of the outer membrane preparations.

Enzyme immunoassay may be useful for the serologic diagnosis and epidemiological study of *H. ducreyi* infection. Systems for the detection of IgG and IgM have been developed (12, 34). Patients with clinical chancroid have circulating antibodies, especially during the period of early convalescence from acute primary chancroid. Antibody production is not diminished in the presence of HIV infection (12).

An enzyme-linked immunosorbent assay (ELISA) antigen detection test uses polyclonal serum against *H. ducreyi* antigens (47). Adsorption on a mixture of *Haemophilus* spp., *Escherichia coli*, *Candida albicans*, and *Corynebacterium* spp. removed nonspecific antibodies. The adsorbed serum reacted with all *H. ducreyi* isolates tested, but not with other bacterial species. When this test was evaluated with clinical specimens from chancroid-positive African patients and chancroid-negative controls, it yielded a sensitivity and specificity of 100%.

Indirect immunofluorescence assays with monoclonal antibodies detect organisms in smears from genital ulcers (26, 49). An assay using an outer membrane-reactive monoclonal antibody stained organisms in smears from three of six chancroid ulcer patients and none from controls (49). Another assay is more sensitive than culture or Gram staining, detecting less than four organisms per sample (26). It detected *H. ducreyi* in 95% of animal lesions compared with 14% detected by culture. The assay identified over 90% of culture-positive cases of chancroid but also detected organisms in some culture-negative cases where clinical evidence for the diagnosis was strong.

Parsons et al. have produced radiolabeled DNA probes for *H. ducreyi* and used them to identify the organism and to detect it in specimens from experimental animals (42). They selected three DNA fragments for use as probes on the basis of their ability to encode *H. ducreyi*-specific proteins. With DNA-DNA hybridization, the three probes, labeled with ^{32}P, reacted strongly with 16 strains of *H. ducreyi* from various sources; 76% of 33 other bacterial isolates, including *Neisseria gonorrhoeae*, showed no hybridization. A further 24% of the isolates reacted weakly and belonged to other *Haemophilus* and *Pasteurella* species.

PCR (polymerase chain reaction) is useful for detection of *H. ducreyi* in areas where the organism is endemic, particularly where testing by culture is difficult or impossible (59). *Taq* polymerase inhibitors in specimens from genital ulcers and sodium phosphate in transport medium reduce the sensitivity of PCR (24). Addition of detergents in preparing nucleic acids and a dialysis step prior to amplification improves sensitivity (24). Two of the several assays that have been developed are described here.

Chui et al. used the published nucleotide sequences of the 16S rRNA gene of *H. ducreyi* to develop primer sets and probes (11). One set of broad-specificity primers yields a 303-bp PCR product from all bacteria tested. Two 16-base probes internal to this sequence are species specific for *H. ducreyi* when tested with 12 species of the families *Pasteurellaceae* and *Enterobacteriaceae*. The two probes in combination with the broad-specificity primers are 100% sensitive with 51 strains of *H. ducreyi* isolated from six continents over a 15-year period. The direct detection of *H. ducreyi* from 100 clinical specimens by PCR showed a sensitivity of 83 to 98% and a specificity of 51 to 67%, depending on the number of amplification cycles.

When the ELISA was evaluated with clinical specimens from chancroid-positive African patients and chancroid-negative controls, it yielded a sensitivity and specificity of 100%

A simplified method for detection of *H. ducreyi* in patient samples includes sample preparation by chloroform extraction, one-tube nested PCR to minimize contamination, and colorimetric detection (59). The primers were designed from published nucleotide sequences of the 16S rRNA gene of *H. ducreyi*. The outer primers are longer, for annealing at a higher temperature. The inner primers are shorter and labeled with biotin and digoxigenin for binding with avidin and colorimetric detection. The PCR technique has detected all 35 strains of *H. ducreyi* tested, from four different geographical regions, and is negative for related strains of bacteria and common contaminating bacteria.

Treatment

H. ducreyi has developed resistance to several antimicrobial agents, primarily through plasmids, and as a result, antimicrobials that were once effective are not any longer. Treatment with erythromycin (500 mg orally four times a day for 7 days), ceftriaxone (250 mg intramuscularly once), or azithromycin (1 g orally once) is recommended therapy for cases or sex partners in the United States (9). As a result of a meeting held in February 1997 to formulate new Centers for Disease Control and Prevention treatment guidelines, ciprofloxacin (500 mg orally twice a day for 3 days) will also become recommended therapy. Outside the United States, erythromycin (500 mg orally three times a day for 5 days) has been shown to be effective and is recommended by the World Health Organization (60). A single dose of ceftriaxone may not be effective in some locations outside the United States, and multiple doses of trimethoprim-sulfamethoxazole cannot now be relied on due to the development of antimicrobial resistance. Patients with HIV infection do not respond as well as patients without HIV infection, particularly to single-dose therapy, and more intensive regimens and follow-up may be needed in such individuals (4, 54).

In many clinical situations, it is impossible to diagnose the cause of a genital ulcer adequately. Multiple clinical studies have shown that the ability to clinically diagnose the etiology of genital ulcers is difficult, as low as 50%, depending upon the etiology and prevalences of varying causes of ulcers (33, 40). In addition, ulcers may have more than one pathogen, with coinfection of *H. ducreyi* and either *Treponema pallidum* or herpes simplex virus being found in >10% of cases (33, 41). The sensitive PCR assay has recently identified coinfection to occur more frequently than previously thought. In areas where chancroid and syphilis are common, treatment for both diseases is an acceptable therapeutic strategy (9, 50).

Fluctuant buboes should be drained. Needle aspiration through noninflamed skin has been traditional therapy. A recent study showed that incision and drainage appears to require less frequent reaspiration, however (0 of 11 patients receiving incision and drainage versus 6 of 12 receiving needle aspiration only), and may be preferable in some settings (15).

Individuals who have been sex partners of cases while the case was symptomatic or for 10 days prior to the onset of symptoms should be examined and treated.

> *H. ducreyi has developed resistance to several antimicrobial agents*

Prevention

There is little evidence that asymptomatic carriage of H. ducreyi is common. Although asymptomatic infection of males has been reported from England, there is doubt as to the identity of the isolates made. Occasional isolations of H. ducreyi have been made from asymptomatic women (20, 46), including one study using PCR that showed a prevalence of 2% among commercial sex workers in The Gambia (20); in this latter study, 8 of the 12 women who tested positive had ulcers upon examination, although they were asymptomatic. Epidemiologic investigations indicate that men and women who are important in transmission of H. ducreyi are largely symptomatic (45, 46). Thus, control efforts should focus on identifying persons at risk for chancroid and who are symptomatic rather than spending scarce resources screening asymptomatic individuals.

In communities where chancroid is first appearing, successful control depends on prompt recognition of the disease and immediate identification and treatment of partners. This is particularly important because H. ducreyi appears to be highly transmissible, with a transmission efficiency of 63% for male-to-female transmission found in one small study (45). If the individual introducing chancroid into the community has sex with a limited number of partners and these partners are not highly sexually active, control efforts may be successful in eliminating the disease from the community (8). Even large epidemics may be eliminated with prompt and aggressive control efforts (5, 22). Identifying and locating commercial sex workers is crucial in these efforts, but often difficult because of the anonymity of prostitution and evidence that exchange of illegal drugs for sex has been the form of payment in some outbreaks. If initial control efforts fail, elimination becomes very difficult, although experience indicates that outbreaks will subsequently diminish in severity for unknown reasons.

Control of chancroid is widely thought to be important in the control of HIV infection, at least in the developing world (23). Nevertheless, attributable risks of chancroid on HIV infection have not been well characterized. One study attributed 30% of HIV infections in an African cohort of women to genital ulcers, the majority of which were chancroid (23).

> *H. ducreyi appears to be highly transmissible*

Figure 10.1 Numbers of cases of chancroid reported in the United States, 1981–1995.

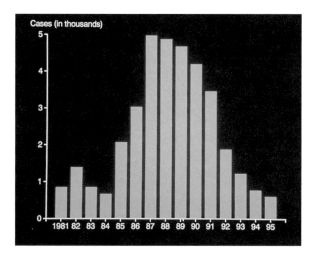

Figure 10.2 "Guesstimated" prevalence of chancroid worldwide.

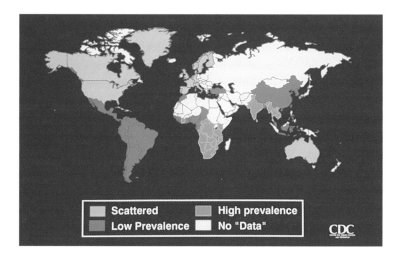

Figure 10.3 Characteristic ulcer caused by *H. ducreyi*, showing an undermined border with a deep, bleeding base.

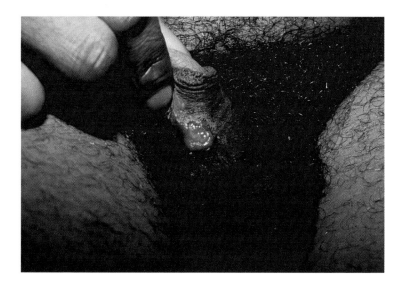

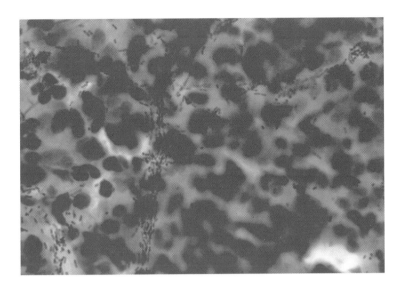

Figure 10.4   Gram stain of base of ulcer, showing dense cellular infiltrate and gram-negative coccobacilli.

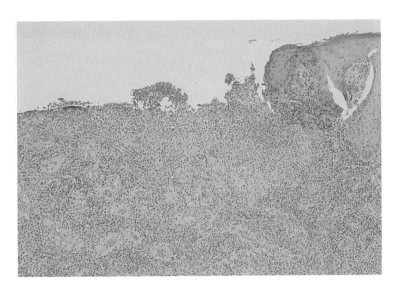

Figure 10.5   Penile ulcer. Sections show the three zones of inflammation: a superficial dermal infiltrate with acute inflammation; a mononuclear infiltrate of T lymphocytes (predominantly CD4$^+$) and histiocytes; and areas of granulomatous inflammation and vasculitis. Hematoxylin and eosin stain; ×25.

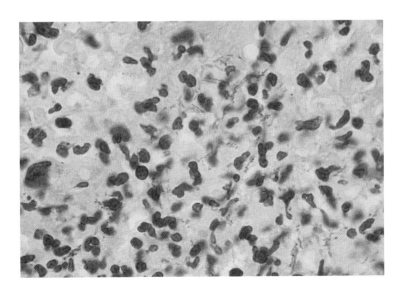

Figure 10.6   Penile ulcer. Tissue Gram stain reveals pale-staining gram-negative coccobacilli arranged in "school of fish" groups. Brown-Hopps stain; ×330.

References

1. **Abeck, D., and H. C. Korting.** 1992. Mechanisms of skin adherence, penetration and tissue necrosis production by *Haemophilus ducreyi*, the causative agent of chancroid. *Acta Dermatol. Venereol. Suppl.* **174:**1–20.

2. **Albritton, W. L.** 1989. Biology of *Haemophilus ducreyi*. *Microbiol. Rev.* **53:**377–389.

3. **Asin, J.** 1952. Chancroid: a report of 1402 cases. *Am. J. Syph.* **36:**483–487.

4. **Behets, F. M. T., G. Liomba, G. Lule, G. Dallabetta, I. F. Hoffman, H. A. Hamilton, S. Moeng, and M. S. Cohen.** 1995. Sexually transmitted diseases and human immunodeficiency virus control in Malawi: a field study of genital ulcer disease. *J. Infect. Dis.* **171:**451–456.

5. **Blackmore, C. A., K. Limpakarnjanarat, J. G. Rigau-Perez, W. L. Albritton, and J. R. Greenwood.** 1985. An outbreak of chancroid in Orange County, California. *J. Infect. Dis.* **151:**840–844.

6. **Cameron, D. W., J. N. Simonsen, L. J. D'Costa, A. R. Ronald, G. M. Maitha, M. N. Gakinya, M. Cheang, J. O. Ndinya-Achola, P. Piot, R. C. Brunham, and F. A. Plummer.** 1989. Female to male transmission of human immunodeficiency virus type 1: risk factors for seroconversion in men. *Lancet* **ii:**403–407.

7. **Castellazzo, A., M. Shero, M. A. Apicella, and S. M. Spinola.** 1992. Expression of pili by *Haemophilus ducreyi*. *J. Infect. Dis.* **165**(Suppl. 1):S198–S199.

8. **Centers for Disease Control and Prevention.** 1985. Chancroid—Massachusetts. *Morbid. Mortal. Weekly Rep.* **34:**711–718.

9. **Centers for Disease Control and Prevention.** 1993. Sexually transmitted diseases treatment guidelines. *Morbid. Mortal. Weekly Rep.* **42**(RR-14):20–22.

10. **Centers for Disease Control and Prevention.** 1996. *Sexually Transmitted Diseases Surveillance, 1995.* Division of STD Prevention, Centers for Disease Control and Prevention, Atlanta.

11. **Chui, L., W. Albritton, B. Paster, I. Maclean, and R. Marusyk.** 1993. Development of the polymerase chain reaction for diagnosis of chancroid. *J. Clin. Microbiol.* **31:**659–664.

12. **Desjardins, M., C. E. Thompson, L. G. Filion, J. O. Ndinya-Achola, F. A. Plummer, A. R. Ronald, P. Piot, and D. W. Cameron.** 1992. Standardization of an enzyme immunoassay for human antibody to *Haemophilus ducreyi*. *J. Clin. Microbiol.* **30:**2019–2024.

13. **DiCarlo, R. P., B. S. Armentor, and D. H. Martin.** 1995. Chancroid epidemiology in New Orleans men. *J. Infect. Dis.* **172:**446–452.

14. **Editorial.** 1982. Chancroid. *Lancet* **ii:**747–748.

15. **Ernst, A. A., E. Marvez-Valls, and D. H. Martin.** 1995. Incision and drainage versus aspiration of fluctuant buboes in the emergency department during an epidemic of chancroid. *Sex. Transm. Dis.* **22:**217–220.

16. **Farris, J. R., D. Hutcheson, G. Cartwright, and J. H. Glover.** 1991. Chancroid in Dallas: new lessons from an old disease. *Texas Med. J.* **87:**78–81.

17. **Fiumara, N. J., K. Rothman, and S. Tang.** 1986. The diagnosis and treatment of chancroid. *J. Am. Acad. Dermatol.* **15:**939–943.

18. **Hammond, G. W., C. J. Lian, J. C. Wilt, and A. R. Ronald.** 1978. Comparison of specimen collection and laboratory techniques for isolation of *Haemophilus ducreyi*. *J. Clin. Microbiol.* **7:**39–43.

19. **Hannah, P., and J. R. Greenwood.** 1982. Isolation and rapid identification of *Haemophilus ducreyi*. *J. Clin. Microbiol.* **16:**861–864.

20. **Hawkes, S., B. West, S. Wilson, H. Whittle, and D. Mabey.** 1995. Asymptomatic carriage of *Haemophilus ducreyi* confirmed by the polymerase chain reaction. *Genitourin. Med.* **71:**224–227.

21. **Hayes, R. J., K. F. Schulz, and F. A. Plummer.** 1995. The cofactor effect on genital ulcers on the per-exposure risk of HIV transmission in sub-Saharan Africa. *J. Trop. Med. Hyg.* **98:**1–8.

22. **Jessamine, P. G., and R. C. Brunham.** 1990. Rapid control of a chancroid outbreak: implications for Canada. *Can. Med. Assoc. J.* **142**(10)**:**1081–1085.

23. **Jessamine, P. G., F. A. Plummer, J. O. Ndinya-Achola, M. A. Wainberg, I. Wamola, L. J. D'Costa, D. W. Cameron, J. N. Simonson, P. Plourde, and A. R. Ronald.** 1990. Human immunodeficiency virus, genital ulcers and the male foreskin: synergism in HIV-1 transmission. *Scand. J. Infect. Dis.* **69**(Suppl.)**:**181–186.

24. **Johnson, S. R., D. H. Martin, C. Cammarata, and S. A. Morse.** 1995. Alterations in sample preparation increase sensitivity of PCR assay for diagnosis of chancroid. *J. Clin. Microbiol.* **33:**1036–1038.

25. **Jones, C. C., and T. Rosen.** 1991. Cultural diagnosis of chancroid. *Arch. Dermatol.* **127:**1823–1827.

26. **Karim, Q. N., G. Y. Finn, C. S. Easmon, Y. Dangor, D. A. Dance, Y. F. Ngeow, and R. C. Ballard.** 1989. Rapid detection of *Haemophilus ducreyi* in clinical and experimental infections using monoclonal antibody: a preliminary evaluation. *Genitourin. Med.* **65:**361–365.

27. **King, R., J. Gough, A. Ronald, J. Nasio, J. O. Ndinya-Achola, F. Plummer, and J. A. Wilkins.** 1996. An immunohistochemical analysis of naturally occurring chancroid. *J. Infect. Dis.* **174:**427–430.

28. **Kreiss, J. K., R. Coombs, F. Plummer, K. K. Holmes, B. Nikora, W. Cameron, E. Ngugi, J. O. Ndinya-Achola, and L. Corey.** 1989. Isolation of human immunodeficiency virus from genital ulcers in Nairobi prostitutes. *J. Infect. Dis.* **160:**380–384.

29. **Larson, A.** 1989. Social context of human immunodeficiency virus transmission in Africa: historical and cultural bases of East and Central African sexual relations. *Rev. Infect. Dis.* **11:**716–731.

30. **Lubwama, S. W., F. A. Plummer, J. Ndinya-Achola, H. Nsanze, W. Namaara, L. J. D'Costa, and A. R. Ronald.** 1986. Isolation and identification of *Haemophilus ducreyi* in a clinical laboratory. *J. Med. Microbiol.* **22:**175–178.

31. **Magro, C. M., A. N. Crowson, M. Alfa, A. Nath, A. Ronald, J. O. Ndinya-Achola, and J. Nasio.** 1996. A morphological study of penile chancroid lesions in human immunodeficiency virus (HIV)-positive and -negative African men with a hypothesis concerning the role of chancroid in HIV transmission. *Hum. Pathol.* **27:**1066–1070.

32. **McLaughlin, M., M. Wilkes, S. Blum, A. Hermoso, and G. Schmid.** 1989. Risks associated with acquiring chancroid genital ulcerative disease and HIV infection, abstr. A.615. *In* V International Conference on AIDS, Montreal, Canada, June 4–9.

33. **Morse, S. A., D. A. Trees, Y. Htun, F. Radebe, K. A. Orle, Y. Dangor, C. M. Beck-Sague, S. Schmid, G. Fehler, J. B. Weiss, and R. C. Ballard.** 1997. Comparison of clinical diagnosis and standard laboratory and molecular methods for the diagnosis of genital ulcer disease in Lesotho: association with human immunodeficiency virus infection. *J. Infect. Dis.* **175:**583–589.

34. **Museyi, K., E. Van Dyck, T. Vervoort, D. Taylor, C. Hoge, and P. Piot.** 1988. Use of an enzyme immunoassay to detect serum IgG antibodies to *Haemophilus ducreyi. J. Infect. Dis.* **157:**1039–1043.

35. **Nayyar, K. C., E. Stolz, and M. F. Michel.** 1979. Rising incidence of chancroid in Rotterdam: epidemiological, clinical, diagnostic and therapeutic aspects. *Br. J. Vener. Dis.* **55:**439–441.

36. **Nobre, G. N.** 1982. Identifying *Haemophilus ducreyi. Lancet* **ii:**1043. (Letter.)

37. **Nobre, G. N.** 1982. Identification of *Haemophilus ducreyi* in the clinical laboratory. *J. Med. Microbiol.* **15:**243–245.

38. **Oberhofer, T. R., and A. E. Back.** 1982. Isolation and cultivation of *Haemophilus ducreyi. J. Clin. Microbiol.* **15:**625–629.

39. **Odumeru, J. A., G. M. Wiseman, and A. R. Ronald.** 1984. Virulence factors of *Haemophilus ducreyi. Infect. Immun.* **43:**607–611.

40. **O'Farrell, N., A. A. Hoosen, K. D. Coetzee, and J. Van den Ende.** 1994. Genital ulcer disease: accuracy of clinical diagnosis and strategies to improve control in Durban, South Africa. *Genitourin. Med.* **70:**7–11.

41. **Orle, K. A., C. A. Gates, D. H. Martin, B. A. Body, and J. B Weiss.** 1996. Simultaneous PCR detection of *Haemophilus ducreyi, Treponema pallidum,* and herpes simplex virus types 1 and 2 from genital ulcers. *J. Clin. Microbiol.* **34:**49–54.

42. **Parsons, L. M., M. Shayegani, A. L. Waring, and L. H. Bopp.** 1989. DNA probes for the identification of *Haemophilus ducreyi. J. Clin. Microbiol.* **27:**1441–1445.

43. **Piot, P., and A. Meheus.** 1985. Genital ulcerations. *In* D. Taylor-Robinson (ed.), *Clinical Problems in Sexually Transmitted Diseases.* Martinus Nyhoff Publishers, Boston.

44. **Piot, P., and F. A. Plummer.** 1990. Genital ulcer adenopathy syndrome, p. 711–716. *In* K. Holmes, P.-A. Mardh, P. F. Sparling, P. Wiesner, W. Cates, Jr., S. M. Lemmon, and W. E. Stamm (ed.), *Sexually Transmitted Diseases,* 2nd ed. McGraw Hill Publishers, New York.

45. **Plummer, F. A., L. J. D'Costa, and H. Nsanze.** 1983. Epidemiology of chancroid and *Haemophilus ducreyi* in Nairobi, Kenya. *Lancet* **ii:**1293–1295.

46. **Plummer, F. A., L. J. D'Costa, H. Nsanze, P. Karasira, I. W. Maclean, P. Piot, and A. R. Ronald.** 1985. Clinical and microbiologic studies of genital ulcers in Kenyan women. *Sex. Transm. Dis.* **12:**193–197.

47. **Roggen, E. L., R. Pansaerts, E. Van Dyck, and P. Piot.** 1993. Antigen detection and immunological typing of *Haemophilus ducreyi* with a specific rabbit polyclonal serum. *J. Clin. Microbiol.* **31:**1820–1825.

48. **Ronald, A. R., and F. A. Plummer.** 1989. Chancroid and granuloma inguinale. *Clin. Lab. Med.* **9:**535–543.

49. **Schalla, W. O., L. L. Sanders, G. P. Schmid, M. R. Tam, and S. A. Morse.** 1986. Use of dot-immunobinding and immunofluorescence assays to investigate clinically suspected cases of chancroid. *J. Infect. Dis.* **153:**879–887.

50. **Schmid, G. P.** 1990. Approach to the patient with genital ulcer disease. *Med. Clin. North Am.* **74:**1559–1574.

51. **Schmid, G. P., Y. C. Faur, J. A. Valu, S. A. Sikandar, and M. M. McLaughlin.** 1995. Enhanced recovery of *Haemophilus ducreyi* from clinical specimens by incubation at 33 versus 35°C. *J. Clin. Microbiol.* **33:**3257–3259.

52. **Schmid, G. P., L. L. Sanders, Jr., J. H. Blount, and E. R. Alexander.** 1987. Chancroid in the United States. Reestablishment of an old disease. *JAMA* **258:**3265–3268.

53. **Schulte, J. M., F. A. Martich, and G. P. Schmid.** 1992. Chancroid in the United States, 1981–1990. *Morbid. Mortal. Weekly Rep.* **41**(SS-3)**:**57–61.

54. **Schulte, J. M., and G. P. Schmid.** 1995. The management of chancroid. *Clin. Infect. Dis.* **51**(Suppl.)**:**539–546.

55. **Sottnek, F. O., J. W. Biddle, S. J. Kraus, R. E. Weaver, and J. A. Stewart.** 1980. Isolation and identification of *Haemophilus ducreyi* in a clinical study. *J. Clin. Microbiol.* **12:**170–174.

56. **Spinola, S. M., A. Orazi, J. N. Arno, K. Fortney, P. Kotylo, C. Y. Chen, A. A. Campagnari, and A. F. Hood.** 1996. *Haemophilus ducreyi* elicits a cutaneous infiltrate of CD4 cells during experimental human infection. *J. Infect. Dis.* **173:**394–402.

57. **Telzak, E. E., M. A. Chaisson, P. J. Bevier, R. L. Stoneburner, K. G. Castro, and H. W. Jaffe.** 1993. HIV-1 seroconversion in patients with and without genital ulcer disease. *Ann. Intern. Med.* **119:**1181–1186.

58. **Trees, D. L., and S. A. Morse.** 1995. Chancroid and *Haemophilus ducreyi*: an update. *Clin. Microbiol. Rev.* **8:**357–375.

59. **West, B., S. M. Wilson, J. Changalucha, S. Patel, P. Mayaud, R. C. Ballard, and D. Mabey.** 1995. Simplified polymerase chain reaction for detection of *Haemophilus ducreyi* and diagnosis of chancroid. *J. Clin. Microbiol.* **33:**787–790.

60. **World Health Organization.** 1995. Chancroid, p. 27–28. *In WHO Model Prescribing Information: Drugs Used in Sexually Transmitted Diseases and HIV Infection.* World Health Organization, Geneva.

chapter 11

Meningococcal Disease

Jo Marie Lyons and Robert W. Pinner

*N*eisseria meningitidis causes the severe and dramatic syndromes of acute meningitis and a distinctive sepsis called meningococcemia. The severity of the disease and the potential for secondary spread focus the attention of clinicians and communities when sporadic cases occur. When meningococcal disease occurs in large epidemics, as it has a predilection to do in certain parts of the world, its impact multiplies, as it causes considerable illness and death and challenges national and international public health efforts.

Microbiology

The *Neisseria* species are non-sporeforming, nonmotile, oxidase-positive, aerobic, gram-negative diplococci that are nutritionally fastidious and require extra CO_2 for growth (62). Of the *Neisseria* species, *N. meningitidis*

Jo Marie Lyons, Department of Anatomical Pathology, Emory University School of Medicine, Grady Memorial Hospital, Box 268, 80 Butler Street, S.E., Atlanta, GA 30335. **Robert W. Pinner,** National Center for Infectious Diseases, Centers for Disease Control and Prevention, Building 1, Room 6029, Mailstop C-12, 1600 Clifton Road, N.E., Atlanta, GA 30333.

Pathology of Emerging Infections 2
Edited by Ann Marie Nelson and C. Robert Horsburgh, Jr.
© 1998 American Society for Microbiology, Washington, D.C.

(meningococcus) and *N. gonorrhoeae* (gonococcus) are the principal pathogens in humans, but illness caused by other species has been reported.

N. meningitidis can be classified into serogroups based on the structural and antigenic differences in the capsular polysaccharide expressed. Although 13 serogroups of *N. meningitidis* have been defined, five (A, B, C, Y, and W135) account for nearly all disease.

Epidemiology

Place and Person

Meningococcal disease occurs throughout the world, but its current pattern of occurrence demonstrates substantial geographic variation. In the United States, for example, the incidence of meningococcal disease is approximately 1 per 100,000 population (8, 9, 48). It occurs seasonally in the United States, with the highest attack rates in mid- to late winter and the lowest in late summer (8, 9, 37). In contrast, in the "meningitis belt" of sub-Saharan Africa, endemic rates may be as high as 10 to 25 per 100,000 (42). Moreover, this region is susceptible to seasonal epidemics, during which the attack rate may reach 1% in some locales (Fig. 11.1). Epidemics in the meningitis belt occur during the dry season and end in early spring when the rainy season begins (18). Meningitis belt epidemics tend to be periodic, occurring approximately every 8 to 12 years. This periodicity is not precise, however, and some have suggested that the interval between epidemics has shortened recently.

Humans are the only natural host of meningococci, transmission of which occurs through close contact with nasopharyngeal secretions. Only a tiny fraction of those who are exposed to meningococci develop clinical infections; a higher proportion of those exposed will carry the organism in the nasopharynx for periods of time and can transmit the infection.

Meningococcal disease primarily affects children. In the United States, the highest age-specific incidence occurs in children 3 to 5 months old, with approximately half the cases occurring in children 2 years or younger (Fig. 11.2) (9). Epidemics of meningococcal disease are characterized by a shift in age-specific attack rates, when a higher proportion of cases occur in older children and young adults. The case fatality rate of meningococcal disease is 5 to 25%, and among survivors, long-term sequelae including persistent neurological problems can occur. Prior to the use of antibiotics, the case fatality rate for meningococcal meningitis was 50 to 80% (4).

Several host characteristics influence susceptibility to meningococcal disease, including asplenia, properdin deficiency, and terminal complement deficiency. Individuals with human immunodeficiency virus may be at increased risk for meningococcal disease (53), although the issue is not settled.

Other factors, such as dust or smoke which may damage mucosal membranes; other respiratory infections which may damage mucosal membranes and cause transient immune suppression (28); crowding; and poor living

In the "meningitis belt" of sub-Saharan Africa, endemic rates may be as high as 10 to 25 per 100,000

conditions may all increase risk of meningococcal disease. However, the relative contributions of these potential risk factors have been difficult to quantify.

Strain Characteristics and Molecular Epidemiology

Strain characteristics of N. meningitidis play an important role in patterns of disease. Serogroup A is the group most commonly responsible for epidemics, especially in the meningitis belt. In the United States, serogroup A has been essentially absent since the end of World War II, and serogroups B and C account for the vast majority of cases (9, 37). In the past few years in the United States, serogroup Y has accounted for an increasing proportion of cases (from 0% to 32.5% between 1989 and 1995, in a Centers for Disease Control and Prevention [CDC]-coordinated laboratory-based active surveillance effort) (8).

In addition to serogrouping, subtyping schemes based on differences among strains in the outer membrane proteins or lipopolysaccharide (LPS), on electrophoretic patterns of expressed enzymes (multilocus enzyme electrophoresis), and on pulsed-field gel electrophoresis have also been devised, which have revealed important and interesting features about the epidemiology of meningococcal disease. Sporadic cases are caused by a variety of different strains. During epidemics, however, a single strain is generally responsible for nearly all disease, although a variety of different strains have been responsible for epidemics over the years.

Subtyping schemes have revealed important and interesting features about the epidemiology of meningococcal disease

For example, a clonal group of N. meningitidis (named ET III-1 clonal group) caused epidemics of group A meningococcal disease in Nepal in 1983 and 1984 and in Pakistan and New Delhi, India, in 1985 (2, 13) and may have caused earlier epidemics in China. In 1987, an outbreak of group A meningococcal disease caused by ET III-1 strains occurred in association with the annual Moslem pilgrimage (Haj) to Mecca (34). The epidemic started among persons from south Asian countries, including Nepal, in whom the highest attack rate also occurred. The pilgrims carried these strains home with them, with the result that strains of this ET III-1 complex were implicated in several subsequent epidemics in countries of sub-Saharan Africa outside the traditional meningitis belt (Kenya, 1989; Uganda, 1990; and Burundi, 1992) (30).

ET III-1 strains had not previously been implicated in disease in the traditional African meningitis belt until 1996, when they were responsible for the large epidemics that occurred in the region (36). Several countries recorded large increases in the number of cases of serogroup A meningococcal disease, which totaled the highest number ever of annual reported cases in the meningitis belt. The total number of cases was reported by the World Health Organization as 152,813, undoubtedly a substantial underestimate, with 15,783 (10%) deaths (Fig. 11.3).

Serogroup B meningococci are an important cause of sporadic disease in industrialized countries and have also been associated with epidemics (with attack rates in the range of 10 to 50/100,000 population, generally lower than in the major serogroup A epidemics). In the late 1970s, serogroup B strains belonging to a clonal group known as ET-5 caused epidemics in Europe (Norway, 1974–1975; Great Britain, 1974–1976; Iceland, 1976; and Denmark, 1981) (16). Intercontinental spread of clones was probably responsible for subsequent epidemics in Cuba (1980), Chile (1985), and Brazil (1987) (Fig. 11.4). In the United States, serogroup B ET-5 strains have been associated with an increased incidence of meningococcal disease in Oregon since 1989 and have also been identified in the state of Washington (11, 16) (Fig. 11.5).

Serogroup C may cause endemic disease, small clusters, and epidemics (though usually with lower attack rates than the large group A epidemics). Since the early 1990s, clusters of cases of group C meningococcal disease have been occurring with increasing frequency in the United States (Fig. 11.6) (20). These outbreaks have been caused by closely related strains of group C. The interesting recent observation of switching of capsular type from B to C among strains of *N. meningitidis* emphasizes the capacity of this organism for genetic exchange, and this switching may confound epidemiologic conclusions based only on traditional serogrouping (57).

Clinical Features

Clinical presentations of meningococcal disease include the syndromes of acute meningitis and septicemia as well as local infections

Clinical presentations of meningococcal disease include the syndromes of acute meningitis and septicemia as well as local infections. Headache, fever, and stiff neck are the most common symptoms in patients presenting with meningococcal meningitis. Alteration in mental status may also occur, and the patient may have a rash. In infants under 1 year of age, the presentation may be atypical with slow onset, absence of stiff neck, and presence of bulging fontanelle. Fever, rash, and prostration of acute onset are the principal manifestations of meningococcemia. Rarely, patients with meningococcal bacteremia may present with prolonged intermittent fevers, rash, arthralgias, and headaches, a syndrome known as *chronic meningococcemia*. Sensineural hearing impairment, seizures, and mental retardation can result from meningococcal meningitis. When limb necrosis complicates meningococcal sepsis, surgical debridement or amputation may be required. Table 11.1 summarizes the clinical features of meningococcal disease syndromes (39).

Pathophysiology

The central nervous system (CNS) is usually protected from bacterial invasion by an intact blood-brain barrier, requiring a bacterial species such as *N. meningitidis* to possess certain specific factors in order to enhance invasiveness and subsequent infection. All the major CNS pathogens including *N. meningitidis* are encapsulated. This outer capsule possesses certain properties which play an important role in the ability of the bacteria to invade and ultimately produce disease within the subarachnoid space (SAS). The situation is further complicated by the fact that once the bacteria enter the CNS, the host defense mechanisms are inadequate to control the infection (58). It is this interplay between the bacterial virulence factors and host defense

Table 11.1 Clinical features of syndromes of meningococcal disease[a]

Syndrome	Common clinical features
Meningococcal meningitis	Headache, fever, stiff neck, alteration of mental status, vomiting; physical findings of meningismus and other meningeal signs, including cranial nerve palsies; occasional petechial or maculopapular rash; neutrophilic leukocytosis in CSF, low CSF glucose, elevated CSF protein
Meningococcemia	Fever; petechial, purpuric, or maculopapular rash
Fulminant meningococcemia (purpura fulminans, Waterhouse-Friderichsen syndrome)	Fever, extensive petechial purpuric rash, hypotension, circulatory collapse, disseminated intravascular coagulation
Focal infection (may be primary infection or late complication of meningococcemia)	
Septic arthritis	Fever; pain, swelling, effusion in joint
Pneumonia	Productive cough, fever, purulent sputum containing gram-negative diplococci, rales, infiltrates on chest roentgenogram
Purulent pericarditis	Fever, chest pain, pericardial friction rub, pericardial effusion
Conjunctivitis	Pain, conjunctival erythema, purulent ocular discharge
Urethritis	Dysuria, purulent urethral discharge
Chronic meningococcemia	Persistent fever, petechial rash or rash resembling gonococcemia, joint aches, headache, illness of 6 to 8 weeks

[a]Source, reference 39.

mechanisms that ultimately determines the clinical expression that the infection will take and whether or not there will be any SAS involvement.

The first step in developing meningococcal meningitis begins with colonization of the nasopharyngeal mucosa by the bacteria. The adherence of the bacteria to the mucosa is enhanced by the presence of pili or fimbriae on the bacterial surface (19, 58). The meningococci tend to adhere preferentially to the nonciliated nasopharyngeal columnar epithelial cells and, once attached, are transported across the cells within phagocytic vacuoles, which leads to hematogenous dissemination (25, 52, 54). The bacteria have also been found to be able to produce a nonpilate, nonattaching phase, allowing them to desorb from initial attachment sites and move to another location. By this means the organisms may be able to be transferred from one host to another (19). Normally immunoglobulin A (IgA), which is primarily found within mucosal secretions, would be expected to help block the adherence of the bacteria to the mucosal cells. However, in *N. meningitidis* infections high concentrations of circulating IgA antibodies may actually allow for the development of invasive disease by preferentially binding to the organisms and blocking the additional beneficial effects of IgM and IgG (58). In addition, meningococci produce IgA1 proteases which act to cleave the antibody in the hinge region. In some cases this leads to inactivation of the antibody, thus helping to facilitate the bacterial adherence to the mucosal surface (6).

The bacteria produce a nonpilate, nonattaching phase, allowing them to desorb from initial attachment sites and move to another location

Once the bacteria have successfully crossed the epithelial cells and entered into the bloodstream, they must effectively evade host defense mechanisms in order to survive to invade the CNS. They are able to accomplish this successfully by virtue of the fact that they are encapsulated. The bacterial capsule enhances survival within the bloodstream and aids in the development of a high-grade bacteremia by effectively inhibiting phagocytosis and resisting complement pathway activation. Normal host mechanisms available to defend against the antiphagocytic activity of the bacterial capsule consist of the humoral response, which is responsible for the production of antibody-antigen complexes to the capsule, and the activation of the classical, as well as the alternative, complement pathways. It has been found that systemic infections with neisserial species more commonly occur in individuals with inherited deficiencies in one of the terminal complement components (i.e., C5, C6, C7, C8, and perhaps C9), the so-called membrane attack complex. While these individuals have a markedly greater frequency of developing invasive meningococcal disease, they actually have a lower mortality rate with treatment than do those individuals who develop meningococcal meningitis with a normal complement system (46). The reasons for this decreased mortality rate in complement-deficient individuals remain unclear. A qualitative relationship has been shown to exist between the concentration of circulating meningococcal endotoxin (i.e., outer capsular membrane proteins on lipopolysaccharides [LPS]), a fatal outcome, and the degree of complement activation (5). This suggests that the presence of excessive complement-activating products along with other inflammatory mediators in non-deficient persons may actually help contribute to the development of multisystem failure and death. All of this would indicate that the way the host handles the immune complexes may have a profound effect on the immunopathological response and hence on the entire clinical course and outcome of the infection.

The various sites and mechanisms by which bacteria invade the SAS are really not known, but may be related to the concentration of the organisms in the blood. What is known is that once the bacteria have entered the SAS they are now in an area of impaired host defense (58). This is due in part to the fact that the quantitated levels of most complement components within the cerebrospinal fluid (CSF) are either very low or negative (49). Since complement is necessary to help with the opsonization and subsequent phagocytosis of encapsulated organisms such as *N. meningitidis*, this host defense mechanism is severely compromised within the SAS. As a result the bacteria are able to easily survive and rapidly replicate. Once in the SAS the bacterial endotoxins (capsular LPS) may help in the induction and release of inflammatory mediators such as interleukin-1, tumor necrosis factor, and/or prostaglandins (58). The source of these inflammatory mediators within the CSF in bacterial meningitis is still unclear. However, it is the inflammatory response within the SAS that results in the development of neurological symptoms seen in meningitis. If this is left untreated, it can set into motion those pathological events that will ultimately culminate in death.

Once the bacteria have entered the SAS they are now in an area of impaired host defense

Pathology

As noted above, once *N. meningitidis* has successfully crossed the nasopharyngeal epithelial cells it invades the bloodstream to establish a bacteremia. The subsequent clinical manifestations and pathological findings are then determined by whether or not an actual septicemia and/or meningitis develops. It has been shown that the outer capsular membrane LPS of *N. meningitidis* is its major toxic factor (19). This molecular substance is particularly toxic for human endothelial and epithelial cells. As previously mentioned, the outer membrane LPS is an important activator of the complement system. In the process of complement activation, anaphylotoxins (C3a, C4a, C5a) are also formed. These are potent mediators of inflammation and help promote the activation of the clotting system (23). Thus, in a septicemia due to *N. meningitidis* there is direct bacterial damage to the endothelium, leading to an activation of the clotting system. This results in the production of fibrin split products, leukocyte and platelet thrombi, leading to disseminated intravascular coagulation. It is this combination of injury to the endothelial cells and activation of the clotting system that is believed to underlie the widespread hemorrhages seen in meningococcal disease. Nowhere are the pathological effects of this process more dramatically seen than in the skin and adrenal glands. The characteristic purpuric skin lesions associated with meningococcal septicemia histologically show extensive dermal vascular damage with prominent endothelial swelling and fibrin thromboses. There is a marked extravasation of erythrocytes, and neutrophils are found around the affected vessels (Fig. 11.7, 11.8, and 11.9). This is frequently associated with necrosis of the epidermis and subepidermal blistering. Often special stains may reveal the bacteria lying free within the vascular lumen and/or perivascular spaces. Studies have shown these changes are indeed mediated by an immune-complex reaction (51). In a particularly catastrophic clinical presentation of the illness known as purpura fulminans, these hemorrhagic skin lesions converge and progress to gangrene with resulting deforming autoamputation of the extremities (12).

Severe bilateral cortical hemorrhages can occasionally be found in the adrenal glands with meningococcemia, and when this occurs the glands grossly appear dark red (Fig. 11.10). They usually retain their shape unless the hemorrhage is extensive and disrupts the normal anatomy with extension of the hemorrhage out into the surrounding adipose tissue (23). Histologically, numerous hemorrhagic infarcts are found which are associated with extensive fibrin thrombi within the adrenal cortical capillaries (14). This hemorrhagic cortical necrosis leading to adrenal failure as a result of meningococcal septicemia has come to be known as the Waterhouse-Friderichsen syndrome. It too is thought to be secondary to the immunological reaction triggered by the infection. The role this syndrome plays in contributing to the circulatory collapse in individuals with meningococcal septicemia has been questioned in recent times, but it still appears to be of some importance (26).

Severe bilateral cortical hemorrhages can occasionally be found in the adrenal glands with meningococcemia

The effects of meningococcal septicemia may also be found in other organs of the body such as the kidneys, heart, liver, lung, and joints. In all these other locations the histological changes are similar to those seen in the skin, namely, injury to the endothelial cells of small vessels and evidence of fibrin thrombi (12).

Meningococcal meningitis may occur with or without sepsis, but it is one of the dreaded complications of bacteremia. A bacteremia is noted to be present in 30 to 90% of meningitis cases. The gross and histological findings in meningococcal meningitis are nonspecific and similar to those of any acute bacterial meningitis. Grossly a purulent exudate is seen in the leptomeninges, especially in the sulci over the lateral convexities and base of the brain (Fig. 11.11). This purulent exudate can and frequently does spread to involve the ventricular surfaces and choroid plexus. The exudate is initially composed primarily of neutrophils and bacteria that are found lying free within the CSF or within the neutrophils (Fig. 11.12 and 11.13). The precise role and overall beneficial effects of the neutrophils in controlling the infectious process are not known (58). Within the first 48 to 72 h of the infection, inflammatory changes are found in the walls of the small to medium-sized arachnoid arteries. This results in swelling of the endothelial cells with narrowing of the lumen, and there may be focal necrosis of the vessel wall with secondary thrombosis. This in turn can lead to secondary cerebral infarction. Also, as each arachnoid vessel penetrates into the underlying brain parenchyma, it is surrounded by a sleeve of arachnoid membranes which forms a perivascular extension of the arachnoid space. This is known as the Virchow-Robin space. The meningeal inflammation can extend down into the superficial brain parenchyma via these spaces and, by virtue of its close proximity to the brain tissue, trigger localized inflammatory changes resulting in focal to diffuse cerebritis. If the patient survives this acute inflammatory phase and the infection persists unchecked, then the composition of the exudate within the SAS will begin to change. An outer layer in the exudate just beneath the arachnoid membrane develops which is composed mainly of neutrophils and fibrin. Beneath this is another inner layer of exudate adjacent to the pia mater which is composed of lymphocytes, plasma cells, and macrophages (Fig. 11.14). As the exudate continues to accumulate and organize, the flow of CSF through the cerebral aqueduct and out of the fourth ventricle can become obstructed, leading to hydrocephalus.

The most life-threatening consequence of meningitis is related to the development of cerebral edema and the resultant increase in intracranial pressure that it can produce. There may be varying amounts of cerebral edema present depending on the duration of the inflammation and any secondary consequences it may have caused. Cerebral edema is a process that results in an increase in the overall volume of the brain due to increased water content. The cerebral edema seen in meningitis is usually due to a combination of vasogenic (increased vascular permeability), cytotoxic (increased accumulation of intracellular water and sodium with secondary cellular swelling), and interstitial edema (due to obstruction and

The most life-threatening consequence of meningitis is related to the development of cerebral edema

failure of CSF resorption) (58). The increase in intracranial pressure can be further worsened if the situation is complicated by other processes that also can trigger increased cerebral edema, such as the development of cerebritis or cerebral infarction. In the end all of these factors contribute to an ever-increasing brain size and volume which cannot be sustained within the fixed, confined space of the intracranial bony vault. This results in a downward migration or herniation of the brain through the dural tentorium and foramen magnum with devastating effects on the cardiorespiratory centers located within the brain stem, leading to irreversible brain injury and death.

All the above pathological brain findings and course of events are not specific for *N. meningitidis* and can be seen in meningitis caused by any of the other major bacterial pathogens mentioned above. It is important to note that in meningococcal meningitis, the pathological changes are dependent on both the severity and duration of the illness. In acute fulminating meningococcemia, death may occur before a purulent exudate can accumulate in the SAS. In these cases autopsy findings show petechial hemorrhages throughout the brain gray and white matter and in the ventricular subependymal regions. It is this hemorrhagic ependymitis that is typically present in cases of severe lethal meningococcal infection. These findings may be more related to the changes caused by the activation of the clotting system (i.e., disseminated intravascular coagulation) than to any direct inflammatory process actually involving the arachnoid membranes.

Diagnosis

All acute bacterial infections of the meninges are life-threatening if not promptly treated. This is especially true in infections due to meningococci, which are known for their propensity to follow a fulminating clinical course that can rapidly lead to death. The diagnosis of meningitis has always depended on a high index of clinical suspicion supported by the isolation of the pathogen from the CSF or, in some cases, the blood. In cases of *N. meningitidis* infection the blood cultures are positive in only about one-third of the patients with meningitis and positive only 50 to 75% of the time in those patients with clinical meningococcemia or meningococcemia-meningitis (23). CSF cultures are positive in about 90% of patients with meningococcal meningitis. The CSF findings normally present in bacterial meningitis are neutrophilic pleocytosis, mild increase in protein, and decrease (often dramatic) in glucose. This is not always the case in meningococcal meningitis, where the initial results from examination of the CSF may be normal due to the rapid onset of the disease (50). Diagnosis in these cases rests first and foremost on a strong index of clinical suspicion even in the absence of classical skin lesions or CSF abnormalities (63). The CSF should be examined for the presence of gram-negative diplococci on smears and cultures obtained. However, it may take 12 to 24 h for the cultures to show growth and, as noted above, up to 10% of cultures may be

In cases of N. meningitidis infection the blood cultures are positive in only about one-third of the patients with meningitis

negative. This has resulted in the need to develop tests that can more rapidly confirm the diagnosis.

Tests now available for the rapid detection of bacterial antigens in the CSF or blood are latex agglutination, coagglutination, and counterimmuno-electrophoresis. The latex agglutination test is especially useful in cases of *N. meningitidis* because it can identify the responsible serogroup (31). Determining the concentration of C-reactive protein (CRP), which is an acute-phase reactant, can be valuable in differentiating bacterial from viral meningitis, since in the former it is usually elevated but in the latter it remains low. This is useful to know especially if the CSF findings are not helpful in making the determination between bacterial versus viral meningitis. The CRP, however, is not specific for bacterial meningitis. It can be elevated in other noninfectious CNS conditions or even be low in those cases of bacterial meningitis where a CSF pleocytosis in response to the infection has not yet occurred (17, 24). In spite of this, CRP level determinations performed on CSF can still be used as a rapid clinical test to exclude the presence of bacterial meningitis in a patient (1).

The most recent diagnostic tool to become available for the rapid and early detection of *N. meningitidis* is the molecular diagnostic technique of PCR (polymerase chain reaction). This technique has proven to be a very helpful test to confirm the diagnosis of meningococcal meningitis, especially in cases where the CSF Gram stains, bacterial antigen, and cultures are all negative or in those patients already begun on antibiotic therapy (7, 22, 33). While this technique was initially only applied to CSF, it has now been shown to be effective in confirming the diagnosis of meningococcal disease from peripheral blood samples (32).

All of these diagnostic tests will now make it easier to more readily confirm the diagnosis of *N. meningitidis* infection. It is important to emphasize that whenever bacterial meningitis is suspected, after the appropriate diagnostic material has been collected, antibiotic therapy should be initiated as soon as possible and not withheld waiting for the results of any of the diagnostic procedures. Rather, once these results are known, then a reassessment of the clinical situation can be performed, and at that time adjustments or changes to the antibiotic therapy can be made if needed. Hopefully this will eventually led to faster medical control of the infectious process, resulting in a decrease in the still-significant morbidity and mortality associated with meningococcal disease.

Whenever bacterial meningitis is suspected, after the appropriate diagnostic material has been collected, antibiotic therapy should be initiated as soon as possible

Treatment

In the United States, high-dose intravenous penicillin (20×10^6 to 24×10^6 U/day for adults) continues to be the preferred antibiotic to treat infections known to be caused by *N. meningitidis* (although initial coverage is usually broader if the causative organism is not known). Other antibiotics are also effective, including ampicillin; some of the newer cephalosporins, such as ceftriaxone, cefotaxime, and cefuroxime (but not other cephalosporins); and chloramphenicol (Table 11.2). The emergence of sulfa-resistant

Table 11.2 Antibiotic treatment, chemoprophylaxis, and vaccination for epidemic meningococcal meningitis[a]

Treatment options
For penicillin-susceptible *N. meningitidis*
  Penicillin G, 3×10^6–4×10^6 U every 4 h in adults; 250,000–300,000 U/kg every 24 h in children
Alternatives
  Ceftriaxone, 1–2 g intravenously every 12 h (100 mg/kg per day)
  Chloramphenicol, 100 mg/kg per day in doses every 6 h

Treatment in an outbreak setting in developing countries
Long-acting chloramphenicol in oil suspension (Tifomycin), single dose
  Adults, 3.0 g (6 ml)
  Children 1–15 yrs, 100 mg/kg
  Children <1 yr, 50 mg/kg

Chemoprophylaxis (use recommended for close contacts of cases)
Rifampin
  Adults, 600 mg twice daily for 2 days
  Children ≥1 month, 10 mg/kg twice daily for 2 days
  Children <1 month, 5 mg/kg twice daily for 2 days
Ciprofloxacin
  Adults, 500 mg, 1 dose
Ceftriaxone
  Adults, 250 mg intramuscularly, 1 dose
  Children <15 yrs, 125 mg intramuscularly, 1 dose

Vaccination (use generally limited to epidemics or smaller outbreaks in certain circumstances)
A, C, Y, W135 vaccine (Memomune; Squibb-Connaught) or AC vaccine:
  Single 0.5-ml subcutaneous injection
  (Decreased efficacy <2 yrs of age; vaccine efficacy wanes after 3–5 yrs)

[a]Source, references 9, 45, and 64.

meningococcal strains in the 1960s has made this class of drugs no longer suitable unless there is specific information that the strain being treated is susceptible. Recently, meningococcal isolates with intermediate resistance to penicillin have been identified in Europe, South Africa, and the United States, though it appears that most patients with meningitis due to these intermediately resistant strains can be treated successfully with penicillin. While the clinical significance of these isolates is unclear, trends in antibiotic susceptibility of *N. meningitidis* require monitoring (21, 40, 47, 55, 56). There is some evidence to suggest that glucocorticoids may be a helpful adjunctive therapy in bacterial meningitis in children, but their role in adults is unclear (40).

During meningococcal disease epidemics in developing countries, management of large numbers of patients with multiple injections of crystalline penicillin (or even ceftriaxone) is generally impractical. A single intramuscular dose of an oily suspension of chloramphenicol has been demonstrated to be an effective treatment, making it a valuable first-line therapy during epidemics in developing countries (Table 11.2) (35, 61).

Prevention

Chemoprophylaxis

Cases of meningococcal disease are most often a consequence of contact with asymptomatic carriers rather than with persons with meningitis (who are relatively few in number). However, close contacts of patients have a 500- to 800-fold-increased risk of developing disease (27). For this reason, antimicrobial chemoprophylaxis of close contacts (such as household members or persons with exposure to the patient's oral secretions) of patients with meningococcal disease is recommended to prevent secondary cases. Rifampin, which effectively eradicates nasopharyngeal carriage of *N. meningitidis*, is the most commonly recommended agent for prophylaxis of meningococcal disease. Other drugs are also effective (Table 11.2). Multiple sources of exposure, prolonged duration of risk, difficult logistics, and high cost make mass chemoprophylaxis inapplicable in the setting of large epidemics (16).

Vaccination

Meningococcal A, C, Y, and W135 vaccines are composed of purified capsular polysaccharides. In adults and children >2 years old, protection is achieved within 7 to 10 days after vaccination. These vaccines have high efficacy in adults (38, 41, 44), but antibody levels decline over 2 to 3 years (65). Their limited duration of efficacy and lower immunogenicity in young children have prevented these vaccines from being used in routine immunization practice.

Decisions about the use of vaccination to control epidemic meningococcal disease in developing countries, particularly in the meningitis belt, are complicated. Vaccination campaigns are expensive and logistically difficult. Vaccinating based on only a few cases of meningococcal disease may result in wasted efforts if the epidemic fails to materialize, while vaccinating too late in the natural course of an epidemic would prevent few cases. The World Health Organization has published guidelines for detecting and responding to meningococcal disease epidemics, including recommendations about surveillance, case management, formation of epidemic response teams, and the use of threshold incidence rates to predict epidemics and trigger early decisions to implement campaigns (29, 64). Use of polysaccharide vaccines can prevent substantial numbers of cases during epidemics, as demonstrated in Nairobi, Kenya (1989), in which vaccination campaigns reduced the number of cases by an estimated 20% (38, 60).

Protein-conjugated serogroup A and C vaccines are currently being developed using methods similar to those used for *Haemophilus influenzae* type b vaccines, in which capsular polysaccharides are covalently linked to carrier proteins to convert the T-cell-independent polysaccharide to a T-cell-dependent antigen (2, 3, 59). Although the effectiveness of such meningococcal conjugate vaccines has not yet been demonstrated, recent experience with *H. influenzae* type b vaccines may be a cause for optimism that improved tools to prevent epidemic meningococcal disease may be available soon.

Protein-conjugated serogroup A and C vaccines are currently being developed

The serogroup B polysaccharide capsule of *N. meningitidis* does not produce a good immune response in humans, which has prevented development of effective group B polysaccharide vaccines and forced vaccine development to focus on outer membrane protein vaccines. Recent results on immunogenicity and efficacy of vaccines against several serogroup B outer membrane proteins have been encouraging, but their effectiveness in young children is uncertain. No vaccine to prevent serogroup B meningococcal diseases is currently licensed in the United States (15, 16).

Recent increases in clusters of group C disease in the United States have focused attention on defining an appropriate use of vaccine to prevent serogroup C disease in suspected outbreaks (9). Recent CDC recommendations outline a public health approach when an outbreak of serogroup C meningococcal disease is suspected. This approach includes clearly establishing the diagnosis with reliable serogroup information about isolates, enhancing surveillance, defining the population at risk, and consideration of targeted vaccination.

Figure 11.1 African "meningitis belt."

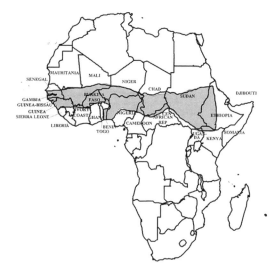

Figure 11.2 Incidence of meningococcal disease by age group, United States, 1989–1991. (Source, reference 9.)

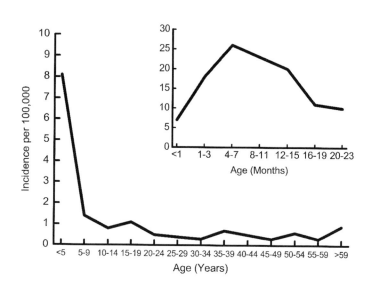

Figure 11.3 Comparison of group A *N. meningitidis* strains by multilocus enzyme electrophoretic typing (38). Each leg of the dendrogram represents a different enzyme type. Degree of relatedness between any two strains is estimated by the value of the relatedness index at the first node connecting them: the lower the relatedness index, the more closely related the two strains are. During 1996, ET III-1 strains were responsible for epidemics in the traditional African meningitis belt.

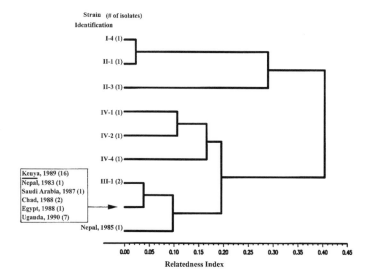

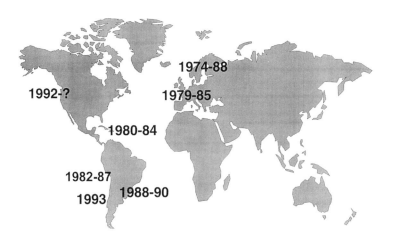

Figure 11.4   Global distribution of *N. meningitidis* ET-5 complex, 1974–1995 (16).

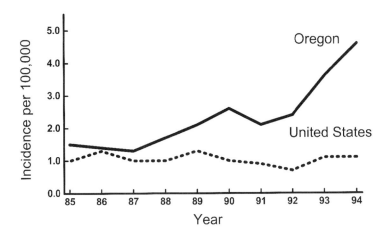

Figure 11.5   Incidence of meningococcal disease by year, Oregon versus the United States, 1985–1994 (16). Serogroup B ET-5 strains have been mainly responsible for the increased incidence of meningococcal disease in Oregon.

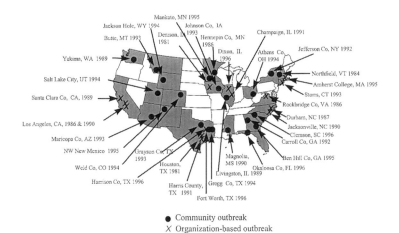

Figure 11.6   Serogroup C meningococcal disease outbreaks, 1981–1996 (20).

Figure 11.7 Typical diffuse purpuric skin lesions of meningococcal meningitis.

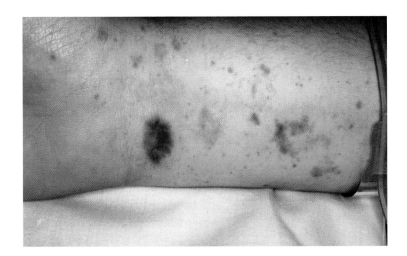

Figure 11.8 Skin with acute inflammatory infiltrate present within the superficial and deep dermis in a perivascular distribution. Hematoxylin and eosin (H&E) stain; ×100.

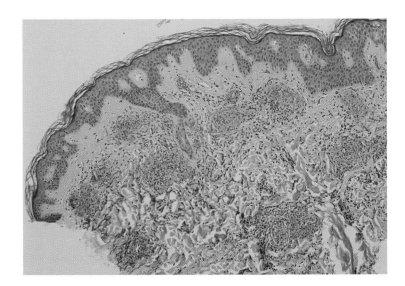

Figure 11.9 Same sample as Fig. 11.8. At higher power, infiltration of the vessel walls by neutrophils with early fibrinoid necrosis and extravasation of red blood cells into the surrounding stroma can be seen. H&E stain; ×400.

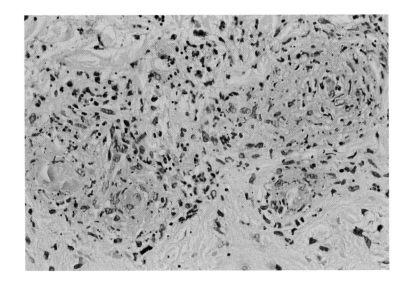

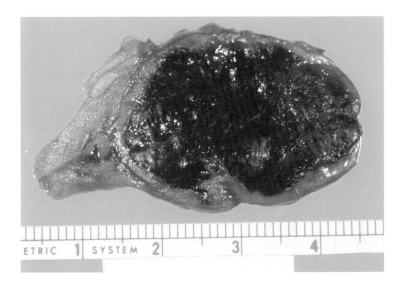

Figure 11.10   Adrenal gland with acute cortical hemorrhage resulting in marked expansion and enlargement of the entire gland.

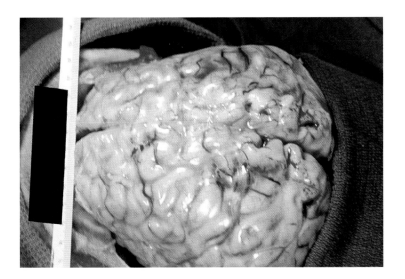

Figure 11.11   Gross brain lying within the cranial vault with prominent green-gray purulent exudate present within the leptomeninges over the superior and lateral surfaces.

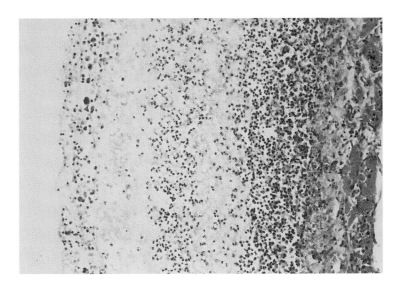

Figure 11.12   Acutely inflamed leptomeninges which are expanded by a proteinaceous exudate filled with a dense cellular infiltrate composed at this time primarily of neutrophils. H&E stain; ×200.

Figure 11.13 CSF containing numerous neutrophils and rare gram-negative diplococci lying
free within the fluid (center of photograph). Even
in fulminant cases of meningococcal meningitis it
may be difficult to identify the organisms within
the CSF. Gram stain; ×1,000.

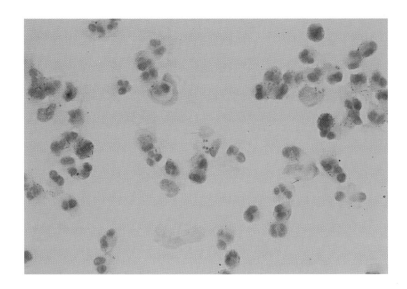

Figure 11.14 Chronically inflamed
leptomeninges being expanded by a more organizing fibrinous exudate. Beneath this exudate and
adjacent to the brain a dense cellular infiltrate
now composed of both acute and chronic inflammatory cells can be found. H&E stain; ×100.

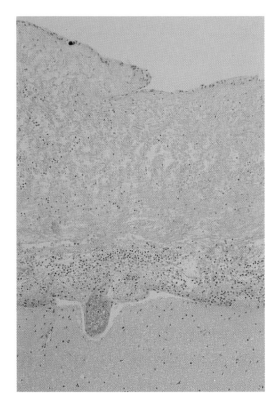

References

1. **Abramson, J. S., K. D. Hampton, S. Babu, B. L. Wasilauskas, and M. J. Marcon.** 1985. The use of C-reactive protein from cerebrospinal fluid for differentiating meningitis from other central nervous system diseases. *J. Infect. Dis.* **151:**854–858.

2. **Achtman, M.** 1990. Molecular epidemiology of epidemic bacterial meningitis. *Rev. Med. Microbiol.* **1:**29–38.

3. **Anderson, E. L., T. Bowers, and C. M. Mink.** 1994. Safety and immunogenicity of meningococcal A and C polysaccharide conjugate vaccines in adults. *Infect. Immun.* **62:**3391–3395.

4. **Apicella, M. A.** 1995. *Neisseria meningitidis,* p. 1896–1909. *In* G. L. Mandell, J. E. Bennett, and R. Dolin (ed.), *Principles and Practice of Infectious Diseases,* 4th ed. Churchill Livingstone, New York.

5. **Brandtzaeg, P., T. E. Mollnes, and P. Kierulf.** 1989. Complement activation and endotoxin levels in systemic meningococcal disease. *J. Infect. Dis.* **160:**58–65.

6. **Brooks, G. F., C. J. Lammel, M. S. Blake, B. Kusecek, and M. Achtman.** 1992. Antibodies against IgA1 protease are stimulated both by clinical disease and asymptomatic carriage of serogroup A *Neisseria meningitidis. J. Infect. Dis.* **166:**1316–1321.

7. **Caugant, D. A., E. A. Hoiby, L. O. Froholm, and P. Brandtzaeg.** 1996. Polymerase chain reaction for case ascertainment of meningococcal meningitis: application to the cerebrospinal fluids collected in the course of the Norwegian meningococcal serogroup B protection trial. *Scand. J. Infect. Dis.* **28:**149–153.

8. **Centers for Disease Control and Prevention.** 1993. Surveillance for diabetes mellitus—United States, 1980–1989, and laboratory-based surveillance for meningococcal disease in selected areas—United States, 1989–1991. *Morbid. Mortal. Weekly Rep.* **42:**21–30.

9. **Centers for Disease Control and Prevention.** 1995. Control and prevention of meningococcal disease and control and prevention of serogroup C meningococcal disease: evaluation and management of suspected outbreaks. *Morbid. Mortal. Weekly Rep.* **46:**1–21.

10. **Centers for Disease Control and Prevention.** 1995. Serogroup B meningococcal disease—Oregon, 1994. *Morbid. Mortal. Weekly Rep.* **44:**121–124.

11. **Centers for Disease Control and Prevention.** 1996. Serogroup Y meningococcal disease—Illinois, Connecticut, and selected areas, United States, 1989–1996. *Morbid. Mortal. Weekly Rep.* **45:**1010–1013.

12. **Chu, D. Z. J., and F. W. Blaisdell.** 1982. Purpura fulminans. *Am. J. Surg.* **143:**356–362.

13. **Cochi, S. L., L. Markowitz, D. D. Joshi, R. C. Owens, D. H. Stenhouse, D. N. Regmi, R. P. B. Shrestha, I. L. Acharya, M. Kanandhar, V. L. Gurubacharya, D. Owens, and A. L. Reingold.** 1987. Control of epidemic group A meningococcal meningitis in Nepal. *Int. J. Epidemiol.* **16:**91–97.

14. **Dalldorf, F. G., and J. C. Jennette.** 1977. Fatal meningococcal septicemia. *Arch. Pathol. Lab Med.* **101:**6–9.

15. **de Moraes, J. C., B. A. Perkins, M. C. Camargo, N. T. Hidalgo, H. A. Barbosa, C. T. Sacchi, I. M. Landgraf, V. L. Gattas, H. de G. Vasconcelos, B. D. Plikaytis, J. D. Wenger, and C. V. Broome.** 1992. Protective efficacy of a serogroup B meningococcal vaccine in Sao Paulo, Brazil. *Lancet* **340:**1074–1078.

16. **Fischer, M., and B. A. Perkins.** 1997. *Neisseria meningitidis* serogroup B: emergence of the ET-5 complex. *Semin. Pediatr. Infect. Dis.* **8:**50–56.

17. **Gray, B. M., D. R. Simmons, H. Mason, S. Barnum, and J. E. Volanakis.** 1986. Quantitative levels of C-reactive protein in cerebrospinal fluid in patients with bacterial meningitis and other conditions. *J. Pediatr.* **108:**665–670.

18. **Greenwood, B. M.** 1987. The epidemiology of acute bacterial meningitis in tropical Africa, p. 61–91. *In* J. D. Williams and J. Burnie (ed.), *Bacterial Meningitis.* Academic Press, London.

19. **Hart, C. A., and T. R. F. Rogers.** 1993. Meiningococcal disease. *J. Med. Microbiol.* **39:**3–25.

20. **Jackson, L. A., A. Schuchat, M. W. Reeves, and J. D. Wenger.** 1995. Serogroup C meningococcal outbreaks in the United States: an emerging threat. *JAMA* **273:**383–389.

21. **Jackson, L. A., F. C. Tenover, C. Baker, B. D. Plikaytis, M. W. Reeves, S. A. Stocker, R. E. Weaver, and J. D. Wenger.** 1994. Prevalence of *Neisseria meningitidis* relatively resistant to penicillin in the United States, 1991. Meningococcal Disease Study Group. *J. Infect. Dis.* **169:**438–441.

22. **Kristiansen, B., E. Ask, A. Jenkins, C. Fermer, P. Radstrom, and O. Skold.** 1991. Rapid diagnosis of meningococcal meningitis by polymerase chain reaction. *Lancet* **337:**1568–1569.

23. **Ladich, E. R., and E. E. Lack.** 1997. Meningococcal infections, p. 690–699. *In* D. E. Connor, F. W. Chandler, D. A. Schwartz, H. J. Manz, and E. E. Lack (ed.), *Pathology of Infectious Dieases,* vol. 1. Appleton and Lange, Stamford, Conn.

24. **Marzouk, O., K. Bestwick, A. P. J. Thomson, J. A. Sills, and C. A. Hart.** 1993. Variation in serum C-reactive protein across the clinical spectrum of meningococcal disease. *Acta Paediatr.* **82:**729–733.

25. **McGee, Z. A., D. S. Stephens, L. H. Hoffman, W. F. Schlech III, and R. G. Horn.** 1983. Mechanisms of mucosal invasion by pathogenic *Neisseria. Rev. Infect. Dis.* **5**(Suppl. 4):708–714.

26. **McWhinney, P. H. M., A. Patel, and E. Walker.** 1990. Adrenal failure in fulminant meningococcal septicemia: a clinical reality. *Scand. J. Infect. Dis.* **22:**755–756.

27. **Meningococcal Disease Surveillance Group.** 1976. Analysis of endemic meningococcal disease by serogroup and evaluation of chemoprophylaxis. *J. Infect. Dis.* **134:**201–204.

28. **Moore, P. S., J. Hierholzer, W. DeWitt, K. Gouan, D. Djore, T. Lippeveld, B. Plikaytis, and C. V. Broome.** 1990. Respiratory viruses and mycoplasma as cofactors for epidemic group A meningococcal meningitis. *JAMA* **264:**1271–1275.

29. **Moore, P. S., B. D. Plikaytis, G. A. Bolan, M. J. Oxtoby, A. Yada, A. Zoubga, A. L. Reingold, and C. V. Broome.** 1992. Detection of meningitis epidemics in Africa: a population-based analysis. *Int. J. Epidemiol.* **21:**155–162.

30. **Moore, P. S., M. W. Reeves, B. Schwartz, B. G. Gellin, and C. V. Broome.** 1989. Intercontinental spread of an epidemic group A *Neisseria meningitidis* strain. *Lancet* **ii:**260–263.

31. **Nato, F., J. C. Mazie, J. M. Fournier, B. Slizewicz, N. Sagot, M. Guibourdenche, D. Postic, and J. Y. Riou.** 1991. Production of polyclonal and monoclonal antibodies against group A, B, and C capsular polysaccharides of *Neisseria meningitidis* and preparation of latex reagents. *J. Clin. Microbiol.* **29:**1447–1452.

32. Newcombe, J., K. Cartwright, W. H. Palmer, and J. McFadden. 1996. PCR of peripheral blood for diagnosis of meningococcal disease. *J. Clin. Microbiol.* **34:**1637–1640.

33. Ni, H., A. I. Knight, K. Cartwright, W. H. Palmer, and J. McFadden. 1992. Polymerase chain reaction for diagnosis of meningococcal meningitis. *Lancet* **340:**1432–1434.

34. Novelli, V. M., R. G. Lewis, and S. T. Dawood. 1987. Epidemic group A meningococcal disease in Haj pilgrims. *Lancet* **ii:**863.

35. Pecoul, B., F. Varaine, M. Keita, G. Soga, A. Djibo, G. Soula, A. Abdou, J. Etinne, and M. Rey. 1991. Long-acting chloramphenicol versus intravenous ampicillin for treatment of bacterial meningitis. *Lancet* **338:**862–866.

36. Perkins, B. A. (Centers for Disease Control and Prevention). 1997. Personal communication.

37. Pinner, R. W., B. G. Gellin, W. F. Bibb, C. N. Baker, R. Weaver, S. B. Hunter, S. H. Waterman, L. F. Mooca, C. E. Frasch, and C. V. Broome. 1991. Meningococcal disease in the United States, 1986. *J. Infect. Dis.* **164:**368–374.

38. Pinner, R. W., F. Onyango, B. A. Perkins, N. B. Mirza, D. M. Ngacha, M. Reeves, W. DeWitt, E. Njeru, N. N. Agata, and C. V. Broome. 1992. Epidemic meningococcal disease in Nairobi, Kenya, 1989. *J. Infect. Dis.* **166:**359–364.

39. Pinner, R. W., and D. S. Stephens. 1992. Infections caused by meningococci, p. 384–387. *In* J. W. Hurst (ed.), *Medicine for the Practicing Physician,* 3rd ed. Butterworth-Heinemann, Boston.

40. Quagliarello, V. J., and W. M. Scheld. 1997. Treatment of bacterial meningitis. *N. Engl. J. Med.* **10:**708–716.

41. Reingold, A. L., C. V. Broome, A. W. Hightower, G. W. Ajello, G. A. Bolan, C. Adamsbaum, E. E. Jones, C. Phillips, H. Tiendrebeogo, and A. Yada. 1985. Age-specific differences in duration of clinical protection after vaccination with meningococcal polysaccharide A vaccine. *Lancet* **ii:**114–118.

42. Riedo, F. X., B. D. Plikaytis, and C. V. Broome. 1995. Epidemiology and prevention of meningococcal disease. *Pediatr. Infect. Dis. J.* **14:**643–657.

43. Roos, K. L., A. R. Tunkel, and W. M. Scheld. 1997. Acute bacterial meningitis in children and adults, p. 336–401. *In* W. M. Scheld, R. J. Whitley, and D. T. Durack (ed.), *Infections of the Central Nervous System,* 2nd ed. Lippincott-Raven, Philadelphia.

44. Rosenstein, N., O. Levine, J. Taylor, M. Weldon, B. Ray, B. Plikaytis, J. Wenger, and B. A. Perkins. 1996. Persistent serogroup C meningococcal disease outbreak in a vaccinated population, Gregg County, Texas, abstr. G84, p. 185. *In Abstracts of the 36th Interscience Conference on Antimicrobial Agents and Chemotherapy 1996.* American Society for Microbiology, Washington, D.C.

45. Rosenstein, N., R. W. Pinner, and D. S. Stephens. Epidemic bacterial meningitis. *In* D. Armstrong and J. Cohen (ed.), *Infectious Diseases.* Mosby, London, in press.

46. Ross, S. C., and P. Densen. 1984. Complement deficiency states and infection: epidemiology, pathogenesis and consequences of neisserial and other infections in an immune deficiency. *Medicine* **63:**243–273.

47. Sáez-Nieto, J. A., R. Lujan, S. Berrón, J. Campos, M. Viñas, C. Fusté, J. A. Vazquez, Q. Zhang, L. D. Bowler, J. V. Martinez-Suarez, and B. G. Scott. 1992. Epidemiology and molecular basis of penicillin-resistant *Neisseria meningitidis* in Spain: a 5-year history (1985–1989). *Clin. Infect. Dis.* **14:**394–402.

48. Schuchat, A., K. Robinson, J. D. Wenger, L. H. Harrison, M. Farley, A. L. Reingold, L. Lefkowitz, and B. A. Perkins. 1997. Bacterial meningitis in the United States in 1995. *N. Engl. J. Med.* **337:**970–976.

49. Simberkoff, M. S., N. H. Moldover, and J. J. Rahal, Jr. 1980. Absence of detectable bactericidal and opsonic activities in normal and infected human cerebrospinal fluids. A regional host defense deficiency. *J. Lab. Clin. Med.* **95:**362–372.

50. Sivakmaran, M., S. A. Nachman, E. Spitzer, and J. Aronson. 1997. Meningococcal meningitis revisited: normocellular CSF. *Clin. Pediatr.* **36:**351–355.

51. Sotto, M. N., B. Langer, S. Hoshino-Shimizu, and T. de Brito. 1976. Pathogenesis of cutaneous lesions in acute meningococcemia in humans: light, immunofluorescent, and electron microscopic studies of skin biopsy specimens. *J. Infect. Dis.* **133:**506–514.

52. Stephens, D. S., and M. M. Farley. 1991. Pathogenic events during infection of the human nasopharynx with *Neisseria meningitidis* and *Haemophilus influenzae*. *Rev. Infect. Dis.* **13:**22–33.

53. Stephens, D. S., R. A. Hajjeh, W. S. Baughman, R. C. Harvey, J. D. Wenger, and M. M. Farley. 1995. Sporadic meningococcal disease in adults: results of a 5-year population-based study. *Ann. Intern. Med.* **123:**937–939.

54. Stephens, D. S., L. H. Hoffman, and Z. A. McGee. 1993. Interaction of *Neisseria meningitidis* with human nasopharyngeal mucosa: attachment and entry into columnar epithelial cells. *J. Infect. Dis.* **148:**369–376.

55. Stocker, S. A., J. D. Wenger, and F. C. Tenover. 1996. Antimicrobial susceptibility testing of recent isolates of *Neisseria meningitidis* from the United States, abstr. D21, p. 64. *In Abstracts of the 36th Interscience Conference on Antimicrobial Agents and Chemotherapy 1996.* American Society for Microbiology, Washington, D.C.

56. Sutcliffe, E. M., D. M. Jones, S. El-Sheikh, and A. Percival. 1988. Penicillin-insensitive meningococci in the U.K. *Lancet* **i:**567–568.

57. Swartley, J. S., A. A. Marfin, S. Edupuganti, L. J. Liu, P. Cieslak, B. Perkins, J. D. Wenger, and D. S. Stephens. 1997. Capsule switching of *Neisseria meningitidis*. *Proc. Natl. Acad. Sci. USA* **94:**271–276.

58. Tunkel, A. R., and W. M. Scheld. 1993. Pathogenesis and pathophysiology of bacterial meningitis. *Clin. Microbiol. Rev.* **6:**118–136.

59. Twumasi, P. A., S. Kumah, and A. Leach. 1995. A trial of a group A plus group C meningococcal polysaccharide-protein conjugate vaccine in African infants. *J. Infect. Dis.* **171:**632–638.

60. Varaine, F., D. A. Caugant, J. Y. Riou, M. K. Konde, G. Soga, D. Nshimirimana, G. Muhirwa, D. Ott, E. A. Hoiby, F. Fermon, and A. Moren. 1997. Meningitis outbreaks and vaccination strategy. *Trans. R. Soc. Trop. Med. Hyg.* **91:**3–7.

61. Wali, S. S., J. T. Macfarlane, W. R. Weir, P.G. Cleland, P. A. J. Ball, M. Hassan-King, H. C. Whittle, and B. M. Greenwood. 1979. Single injection treatment of meningococcal meningitis. 2. Long-acting chloramphenicol. *Trans. R. Soc. Trop. Med. Hyg.* **73:**698–702.

62. Winn, W. C., Jr., and J. M. Kissane. 1996. Bacterial diseases, p. 780–781. *In* I. Damjanov and J. Linder (ed.), *Anderson's Pathology*, 10th ed., vol. 1. Mosby-Yearbook, Inc., St. Louis.

63. Wong, V. K., W. Hitchcock, and W. H. Mason. 1989. Meningococcal infections in children: a review of 100 cases. *Pediatr. Infect. Dis. J.* **8:**224–227.

64. **World Health Organization Working Group.** 1995. *Control of Epidemic Meningococcal Diseases. WHO Practical Guidelines.* Edition Fondation Marcel Merieux, Lyon, France.

65. **Zangwill, K. M., R. W. Stout, G. M. Carlone, L. Pais, H. Harekeh, S. Mitchell, W. H. Wolfe, V. Blackwood, B. D. Plikaytis, and J. D. Wenger.** 1994. Duration of antibody response after meningococcal polysaccharide vaccination in US Air Force personnel. *J. Infect. Dis.* **169:**847–852.

chapter 12

Escherichia coli O157:H7

Laurence Slutsker, Jeannette Guarner, and Patricia Griffin

*E*scherichia coli O157:H7 was first recognized as a human pathogen in 1982, when it was identified as the cause of two outbreaks of hemorrhagic colitis (77). Infection with this pathogen has subsequently been recognized as an important cause of bloody diarrhea and post-diarrheal hemolytic uremic syndrome (HUS) in the United States and Canada and has emerged as a major public health concern in these and many other countries. In 1993, *E. coli* O157:H7 was brought to prominent national attention when an outbreak in the western United States affected over 700 persons and caused the death of four children (9, 36). Since then, concern about this pathogen has played a major role in focusing national attention on food-borne illness.

Laurence Slutsker, Foodborne and Diarrheal Diseases Branch, Division of Bacterial and Mycotic Diseases, National Center for Infectious Diseases, Centers for Disease Control and Prevention, Mailstop A-38, 1600 Clifton Road, N.E., Atlanta, GA 30333. **Jeannette Guarner,** Infectious Disease Pathology Activity, National Center for Infectious Diseases, Centers for Disease Control and Prevention, Mailstop D-17, 1600 Clifton Road, N.E., Atlanta, GA 30333. **Patricia Griffin,** Foodborne and Diarrheal Diseases Branch, Division of Bacterial and Mycotic Diseases, National Center for Infectious Diseases, Centers for Disease Control and Prevention, Mailstop A-38, 1600 Clifton Road, N.E., Atlanta, GA 30333.

Pathology of Emerging Infections 2
Edited by Ann Marie Nelson and C. Robert Horsburgh, Jr.
© 1998 American Society for Microbiology, Washington, D.C.

E. coli serotype O157:H7 is designated by its somatic (O) and flagellar (H) antigens and produces either or both of two phage-encoded toxins. These toxins have been referred to as Shiga-like toxins because of their homology to the cytotoxin produced by *Shigella dysenteriae* type 1 (44, 86), or as verocytotoxins because of their toxicity to Vero tissue culture cells (44). In this chapter, we will use current nomenclature, which refers to the toxins simply as Shiga toxins (17). *E. coli* strains, such as serotype O157:H7, that produce one or more Shiga toxins are referred to as Shiga toxin-producing *E. coli* (STEC). The term enterohemorrhagic *E. coli* (EHEC) refers here to STEC that cause diarrhea or HUS.

Epidemiology

Transmission

E. coli O157:H7 is most often transmitted through consumption of contaminated food and water, but also may be spread directly from person to person and occasionally through occupational exposure. Outbreak investigations have provided most of the information about modes of transmission of *E. coli* O157:H7. In the United States, more outbreaks have been caused by ground beef than by any other vehicle. In the largest United States outbreak, 732 cases including deaths in four children were reported from four western states; the outbreak was traced to undercooked hamburgers from a fast-food restaurant chain (9, 36). Several large outbreaks of *E. coli* O157:H7 infections and 11 deaths occurred in Japan during the summer of 1996; the largest outbreak affected more than 6,000 schoolchildren (63, 98).

E. coli O157:H7 has been found in the intestines of ruminant food animals but does not cause illness in those animals. Healthy cattle constitute the major reservoir for this pathogen; approximately 1% may have the organism in their intestines (39). Beef may be contaminated during slaughter, and the process of grinding beef may transfer pathogens from the surface of the meat to the interior. If cooking is incomplete, the bacteria can survive and be ingested. Because ground beef may include meat from many carcasses, a small number of infected animals can contaminate a large supply of ground beef. *E. coli* O157:H7 has also been found in deer feces, and it caused an outbreak among persons who consumed venison jerky (46). Recently, the organism has been isolated from the feces of sheep (51) and from lamb products (27).

Foods other than ground beef that have been linked to outbreaks include roast beef, raw milk, salami, unpasteurized apple cider and juice, sandwiches, and ranch dressing. Any food that can be contaminated by beef, by cow manure, by contaminated water, or by an infected food handler can transmit this pathogen. Recently, fruits and vegetables have accounted for an increasing number of outbreaks. Radish sprouts were implicated in several outbreaks in Japan, including the massive Sakai City outbreak in 1996 (63). In the United States, recent outbreaks of *E. coli* O157:H7 infections have been caused by lettuce and alfalfa sprouts (3, 24). Produce-associated *E. coli*

> *E. coli* O157:H7 is most often transmitted through consumption of contaminated food and water

O157:H7 outbreaks probably are caused by either cross-contamination from meat products or direct contamination of produce in the field with feces of wild or domestic animals (23). Alfalfa sprouts may be especially problematic, because the sprouting process can dramatically amplify the number of pathogenic bacteria present, and alfalfa sprouts are not typically cooked before consumption (24).

Unchlorinated municipal water and swimming water have also caused outbreaks (4, 45). Person-to-person spread is common and is especially important in child care centers and chronic-care facilities (11, 19, 70). The occurrence of waterborne transmission and the ease with which *E. coli* O157:H7 is spread from person to person suggest that the infectious dose is low. Although studies of human ingestion of the organism to determine the infectious dose have not been performed, in one outbreak that was traced to salami the mean infectious dose was estimated to be fewer than 50 organisms (94).

Unchlorinated municipal water and swimming water have also caused outbreaks

Incubation Period and Fecal Excretion

The usual incubation period for illness is 3 to 4 days but may range from 1 to 8 days. It is likely that incubation periods longer than 8 days represent secondary spread (80). Fecal excretion of *E. coli* O157:H7 may occur for several weeks following resolution of symptoms. Young children tend to have longer periods of shedding than do older children or adults (11, 66, 82, 88). In one study of sporadic cases, 53% of children less than 5 years of age had the organism isolated from their stool 3 weeks after the onset of illness, compared with only 8% of older children and adults (66). In another study, the median duration of fecal excretion among children in an outbreak at a day care center was 29 days; 92% shed the organism in their stools for ≥3 weeks (82). Factors other than age that affect duration of shedding are unknown. Although asymptomatic infection and prolonged carriage occasionally occur, *E. coli* O157:H7 is not part of the normal human intestinal flora (35).

Geographic and Seasonal Factors

Human infection with *E. coli* O157:H7 has been reported from at least 30 countries on six continents, but in many of these locations, its frequency of isolation in comparison with other bacterial enteric pathogens is unknown. *E. coli* O157:H7 has most commonly been reported from Canada, the United States, and the United Kingdom (35). In the United States, sporadic cases and outbreaks are more frequently reported from northern than southern states. In the multicenter United States study (85), the isolation rate of *E. coli* O157:H7 from fecal specimens was fourfold higher in northern compared with southern sites. Whether this indicates the true distribution of the organism is unknown.

Infections with *E. coli* O157:H7 are most common in warmer months, with a peak incidence from June through September (65, 85, 99). The reason for this seasonal variation is unknown; it may reflect factors related to similar seasonal changes in prevalence in its reservoir in cattle and other animals, to seasonal changes in farming practices, or to variations in ground beef consumption or cooking practices.

> *Because most laboratories in the United States do not routinely culture stool specimens for E. coli O157:H7, the actual incidence of infection with the organism is unknown*

Incidence

Because most laboratories in the United States do not routinely culture stool specimens for *E. coli* O157:H7, the actual incidence of infection with the organism is unknown. Following publicity from the large American outbreak in 1993, reports of *E. coli* O157:H7 outbreaks in the United States increased markedly (9, 36), from 4 outbreaks in 1992 to 30 in 1994. Much of this increase was due to increased screening for *E. coli* O157:H7 by laboratories and increased reporting of infections. In a survey of a random sample of American clinical laboratories, the percentage screening at least all bloody stool specimens for *E. coli* O157:H7 increased from 15% to 54% during 1992–1994 (13). The number of states requiring reporting of these infections increased from 10 in 1992 to 44 by the end of 1997.

A prospective, population-based study conducted in the Seattle area during 1985–1986 reported an incidence of 8 infections per 100,000 persons per year (56). Based on this figure, *E. coli* O157:H7 causes an estimated 21,000 infections in the United States annually. It can be argued that this figure is an overestimate because, as mentioned previously, infections with this pathogen are more common in northern states (85). Conversely, it can also be argued that this figure is an underestimate, because the only cases detected were those in persons sufficiently ill to visit a physician and from whom stool cultures were obtained (56). In United States and Canadian studies comparing the isolation rate of *E. coli* O157:H7 from stool specimens with those of other bacterial enteric pathogens, *E. coli* O157:H7 was isolated more frequently than *Shigella* sp. (12, 16, 34, 56, 58, 66). The isolation rate of *E. coli* O157:H7 is particularly high if the diarrhea is bloody. In Canada, studies of bloody stool specimens have demonstrated isolation rates of 15% to 39% (15, 57, 67, 73). In a United States multicenter study (85), the isolation rate of *E. coli* O157:H7 from stool specimens with visible blood was higher than that for any other bacterial pathogen (Fig. 12.1).

Infection occurs in all age groups. In the same United States multicenter study, stool specimens from children 5 to 9 years old and adults 50 to 59 years old had the highest proportion that yielded *E. coli* O157:H7 (Fig. 12.2).

Pathogenesis

Although multiple factors may play a role in the pathogenesis of disease caused by *E. coli* O157:H7, there are two well-recognized virulence attributes: the production of one or more Shiga toxins and attaching and effacing (A/E) lesions.

Shiga Toxin (Stx)

A major virulence factor, and a defining characteristic of *E. coli* O157:H7 and other STEC, is the production of one or more Shiga toxins (Stx). The genes for Stx are encoded on bacteriophages. Two major groups of Stx have been described immunologically. Stx 1 is highly conserved and is identical to the Stx of *S. dysenteriae* type 1. Stx 2 has several variants, and the amino acid sequences of the A and B subunits of Stx 2 are 55% and 57% identical to Stx 1 (81). Different strains of *E. coli* O157:H7 can express Stx 1, Stx 2, or both Stx 1 and Stx 2 (62). The toxin consists of a single A subunit associated with a pentamer of B subunits. A portion of the A subunit, A_1, has enzymatic activity, while the B pentamer binds specifically to a glycolipid receptor, globotriaosylceramide (Gb_3) (62). After binding to the Gb_3 receptor, the whole toxin is endocytosed through coated pits and is then transported to the Golgi apparatus and later to the endoplasmic reticulum. The A subunit is translocated to the cytoplasm, where it acts on the 60S ribosomal subunit. In the cytoplasm, an A_1 peptide removes an adenine residue from the 28S rRNA, causing disruption of protein synthesis and eventually cell death.

Data from animal models suggest that Stx may be essential for the development of hemorrhagic colitis and bloody diarrhea. In an in vivo model, oral inoculation of rabbits with an enteropathogenic *E. coli* (EPEC) strain that does not produce Stx caused nonbloody diarrhea, while the same EPEC strain with an added Stx-producing bacteriophage caused severe colitis with vascular changes, edema, and more inflammation (76). However, in piglets, the presence or absence of Stx in *E. coli* O157:H7 strains did not alter the type of diarrhea (96).

In humans, Stx produced in the intestine is assumed to translocate to the bloodstream across epithelial cells, probably through transcellular pathways, although it has not been detected in the blood of patients with HUS (2). Human renal endothelial cells have a high concentration of Gb_3 receptors, suggesting that binding of Stx to this tissue is important in causing renal injury and the subsequent development of HUS (62). Stx is believed to damage the glomerular endothelial cells, leading to narrowing of capillary lumina and occlusion of the glomerular microvasculature with platelets and fibrin (55). Renal failure in postdiarrheal HUS is a consequence of the pathology in the blood vessels, most likely mediated primarily by Stx (62). Epidemiologically, Stx 2 seems to be more important than Stx 1 in development of HUS (35). Stx induces macrophages to express tumor necrosis factor alpha and interleukin-6 (IL-6) in vitro; these cytokines also may have a role in the pathogenesis of renal damage (93).

Attachment and Effacement (A/E)

A/E lesions have been well described in infections caused by EPEC and can be observed in intestinal biopsy specimens from patients or animals infected with EPEC. The A/E lesion is characterized by effacement of microvilli and intimate adherence between the bacterium and the epithelial cell membrane. With EHEC infection, the classic A/E histopathology has been observed in animal models (e.g., gnotobiotic piglets [60, 95] and infant rabbits [68]). However, A/E lesions have not been reported from clinical specimens from patients with EHEC infection (48). This may be because colonic biopsy specimens are usually collected late in disease, while A/E lesions may be present only early in the course.

The steps involved leading to the A/E histopathology in EHEC infection have not been studied as completely as for EPEC infection, for which a

The A/E lesion is characterized by effacement of microvilli and intimate adherence between the bacterium and the epithelial cell membrane

three-stage model has been proposed consisting of (i) localized adherence, (ii) signal transduction, and (iii) intimate adherence (31, 32).

In EPEC infection, localized adherence is dependent on the presence of a 60-MDa plasmid designated the EPEC adherence factor (EAF). The factor mediating localized adherence has been further characterized as the "bundle-forming pilus" (BFP) (62). A cluster of 13 genes on the EAF plasmid are required for the expression and assembly of the BFP. The determinants of localized adherence have not been as well characterized for EHEC. Similarly, most STEC strains isolated from humans have a 60-MDa plasmid termed the EHEC plasmid, which encodes an enterohemolysin and a fimbrial antigen possibly involved in adherence (62).

The second step, signal transduction, is mediated in EPEC by genes encoded on a 35-kb pathogenicity island called the locus of enterocyte effacement (LEE) (62). The LEE contains genes encoding the protein intimin (61) and other secreted proteins. These secreted proteins have a variety of effects, including an intracellular increase in calcium that may produce cytoskeletal changes that break down actin. EHEC also have an LEE which contains genes encoding intimin and secreted proteins. During this signal transduction stage, cytokines (e.g., IL-8, which is a neutrophil chemoattractant) are up-regulated (43).

The third step, intimate adherence, is mediated by the chromosomal *eae* gene, which codes for the protein intimin. The *eae* gene is present in all EHEC capable of producing A/E histopathology and is absent in bacteria that do not produce this lesion (62). During this stage, microvilli are flattened in the area where the bacteria attach and a pedestal of polymerized filamentous actin is developed (49). The A/E lesion eventually ruptures the cell membrane and causes apoptosis. The A/E lesions appear to be the most important factor for the production of colonic disease in both the piglet (96) and infant rabbit (53) animal models.

Other Virulence Factors

Other potential virulence factors have been studied. An enterohemolysin encoded by a gene in the EHEC 60-MDa plasmid has been found in nearly all *E. coli* O157:H7 strains (62). By lysing erythrocytes present in bloody stools, it may provide a source of iron in the form of heme and hemoglobin, which are known to stimulate growth of *E. coli* O157:H7 (52, 62). Another potential pathogenic factor is bacterial lipopolysaccharide (LPS), either from *E. coli* O157:H7 or from other intestinal bacteria (62). It enhances the cytotoxic activity of Stx on human vascular endothelial cells in vitro, but its effects in vivo are unknown.

An enterohemolysin encoded by a gene in the EHEC 60-MDa plasmid has been found in nearly all E. coli O157:H7 strains

Pathology

Colitis

Reports describing the gastrointestinal pathologic changes caused by *E. coli* O157:H7 are uncommon, perhaps because colonic sampling may not usually be performed in the setting of hemorrhagic colitis or thrombocytopenia secondary to HUS. In addition, available pathology on *E. coli* O157:H7-associated colitis may not be representative of the histologic spectrum of this disease because intestinal biopsies in patients with hemorrhagic colitis tend to be performed on those who have the most severe symptoms. Moreover, colonic biopsies are usually obtained late in the course of disease and thus may not reflect the initial damage caused by the infection.

Available data suggest that the histopathologic features of *E. coli* O157:H7-associated colitis are nonspecific and similar to those caused by *Clostridium difficile*. Kelly et al. (48) described the histopathology of rectosigmoid biopsies in 20 patients with hemorrhagic diarrhea caused by STEC. Nine patients had acute colitis (neutrophilic infiltrate in the lamina propria and crypts); four of these had increased numbers of apoptotic cells in the surface epithelium. The remaining 11 cases did not have a neutrophilic or leukocytic infiltrate and either were normal or had a mild nonspecific mononuclear cell infiltrate in the lamina propria. More recent reports (37, 40) have demonstrated that it may be necessary to perform a complete colonoscopy to find pathologic changes. In a series of 11 patients with hemorrhagic colitis, all specimens showed hemorrhage (Fig. 12.3) and edema (Fig. 12.4) in the lamina propria (37). The most severe endoscopic findings were seen in the cecum and ascending colon, with the severity of the findings in the transverse and descending colon intermediate between the right colon and sigmoid colon. Biopsy specimens from five patients showed an ischemic pattern only (coagulative necrosis and acute inflammation involving the luminal portion of the mucosa with preservation of deep colonic crypts) (Fig. 12.5); four showed a combination of ischemic and infectious findings (infiltration of neutrophils into the lamina propria, focal cryptitis, and crypt abscess formation) (Fig. 12.6 and 12.7); and one showed an infectious but not ischemic pattern of injury (37). One patient, from whom the only biopsy obtained was from the rectosigmoid colon, had neither pattern. Specimens from four patients with the ischemic pattern of injury had poorly formed inflammatory pseudomembranes (Fig. 12.8).

In patients with colitis associated with HUS or thrombotic thrombocytopenic purpura (TTP), the full length of the colon may be damaged with widespread microangiopathy, and the necrosis can extend to the submucosa and muscle layers. These patients may have prominent acute inflammation with pseudomembrane formation and necrosis of the lymphoid follicles in the Peyer's patches (75).

The differential diagnosis of colitis due to *E. coli* O157:H7 includes diseases in which either ischemia or infectious histopathology is present (47). Clinical factors that may suggest a diagnosis of ischemic colitis include a history of atherosclerosis or diabetes and a patchy distribution of intestinal disease that is more frequent and more prominent in the splenic flexure. Histologically, a feature present in cases with long-standing ischemic disease is crypt atrophy and distortion, which is not seen in *E. coli* O157:H7-associated colitis. Ulcerative colitis and Crohn's disease also need to be considered in the differential diagnosis of *E. coli* O157:H7-associated colitis. Histologic features that suggest the diagnosis of ulcerative colitis include crypt distortion (branching, nonparallel architecture and shortened crypts), homogeneous

In patients with colitis associated with HUS or TTP, the full length of the colon may be damaged

mucus depletion, and fibrosis of the lamina propria. In Crohn's disease, the differentiating histopathologic characteristics include patchy inflammation composed primarily of lymphocytes and plasma cells, presence of granulomas and fissures, and uneven depletion of mucus in the cell surface. It is difficult to distinguish the histopathology of infectious colitis due to *E. coli* O157:H7 from other infectious etiologies; other methods such as stool culture are needed. The clinical history may be helpful. For example, *C. difficile*-associated colitis usually occurs after treatment with antibiotics. Histologically, infectious colitis secondary to *C. difficile* tends to have more prominent cryptitis without abscess formation and frequent pseudomembrane formation.

The last entity that needs to be considered in the histopathologic differential diagnosis is colitis caused by nonsteroidal anti-inflammatory drugs; in this condition there is usually focal or solitary ulceration, strictures, and diffuse lymphocytic inflammation, surrounded by entirely normal colonic tissue.

Hemolytic Uremic Syndrome (HUS)

The renal pathology in postdiarrheal HUS has been described as a glomerular thrombotic microangiopathy

The renal pathology in postdiarrheal HUS has been described as a glomerular thrombotic microangiopathy (41, 74). Initially numerous thrombi in the glomerular capillaries lead to focal necrosis (Fig. 12.9). As the lesions progress, the vessels show endothelial cell swelling and are obstructed by fibrin thrombi, particularly in the afferent arterioles (Fig. 12.10), which can show myointimal proliferation when the thrombi resolve. The glomerular capillary walls thicken and present a prominent double contour on silver staining. Immunofluorescence studies demonstrate fibrinogen or fibrin-related antigens within the capillary walls and mesangium. By electron microscopy, the endothelium becomes detached from the basement membrane of the glomerulus, and granular material accumulates. As the acute lesions subside, evidence of glomerulosclerosis can be detected because of ischemic damage, and the progression to chronic renal failure may be related to the extent of the renal lesions. During the acute phase, the renal medulla may show acute tubular necrosis when there has been hypovolemic shock.

Clinical Manifestations

Following infection with *E. coli* O157:H7, a variety of clinical manifestations can ensue. *E. coli* O157:H7 can cause nonbloody diarrhea, bloody diarrhea (hemorrhagic colitis), HUS, TTP, and death (38). In United States outbreaks reported during 1982–1996, of approximately 3,000 ill persons, 22% were hospitalized, 6% developed HUS or TTP, and 0.6% died (25).

Diarrhea

Following an average incubation period of 3 days, illness caused by *E. coli* O157:H7 infection typically begins with severe abdominal cramps and nonbloody diarrhea; the diarrhea often becomes bloody by the second or third day of illness. About one-third of patients have vomiting, and two-thirds have abdominal tenderness. However, unlike most bacterial diarrheal illnesses, fever is usually low-grade or absent (38, 85). The lack of fever, along with impressive abdominal pain and tenderness, can lead clinicians to suspect other diagnoses such as Crohn's disease, ulcerative colitis, diverticulosis, and ischemic colitis. In children, misdiagnoses of intussusception and appendicitis may prompt exploratory laparotomy (38, 64).

The amount of blood in bowel movements may vary from a few small streaks to stools that are almost entirely blood (77). In the United States multicenter study, 63% of patients with *E. coli* O157:H7 infection had visible blood in their stool specimens (85). In reported outbreaks, the proportion of patients with *E. coli* O157:H7 infection who gave a history of bloody diarrhea has varied widely, from 35% (89) to 90% (9). Thus, although bloody stools are common with *E. coli* O157:H7 infection, the diagnosis must also be considered for patients with nonbloody diarrhea. Symptoms from infection with *E. coli* O157:H7 usually subside in approximately 1 week with no obvious sequelae.

HUS, TTP, and Death

Based on data from outbreaks, approximately 6% of patients with *E. coli* O157:H7 infection develop HUS (25). HUS is usually diagnosed 2 to 14 days (median, 6 days) after onset of diarrhea (44). HUS is characterized by microangiopathic hemolytic anemia, thrombocytopenia, renal failure, and central nervous system manifestations and probably is the most common cause of acute renal failure in children (71). Factors reported to increase the risk for developing postdiarrheal HUS include extremes of age (especially children less than 5 years of age), bloody diarrhea, vomiting, elevated leukocyte count, and treatment with antimotility agents (10, 19, 29, 30, 39, 70). Of patients who develop HUS, approximately one-half require dialysis, and three-quarters receive blood transfusions. It is estimated that ≥85% of cases of postdiarrheal HUS in North America are caused by infection with *E. coli* O157:H7 (35). Most of the remaining cases are caused by other *E. coli* strains that produce Shiga toxins.

Patients with *E. coli* O157:H7 infection are sometimes diagnosed with TTP. TTP is a syndrome usually diagnosed in adults that includes all the clinical features of HUS, although renal injury is typically less severe and neurologic involvement frequently is more prominent (79). Few cases of TTP are preceded by diarrhea (39); however, when diarrhea is present, the most likely cause is *E. coli* O157:H7 or another STEC (6, 39, 79).

The mortality rate for children who develop HUS is 3 to 5% (59, 78, 84); the proportion of fatal cases in adults is not known. Approximately 5% of patients with HUS who survive suffer severe sequelae, such as end-stage renal disease or permanent neurologic injury (47). Not all deaths of patients with *E. coli* O157:H7 infection are caused by HUS or TTP. In a review of published United States outbreaks in which at least one death was reported, 7 of 19 deaths occurred among patients who did not have HUS or TTP; those 7 persons who died were elderly (14).

Approximately 6% of patients with E. coli O157:H7 infection develop HUS

Diagnosis

Stool specimens from all patients with a history of bloody diarrhea should be cultured for *E. coli* O157:H7 (20, 85). In some age groups and in some geographic areas, *E. coli* O157:H7 may be isolated more frequently than *Shigella* spp. (85); in these situations, it may be reasonable to screen all stool specimens for *E. coli* O157:H7.

Culturing stools early in the course of diarrheal illness is important; the rate of recovery of *E. coli* O157:H7 declines rapidly after the first 6 days of illness (92, 100). In one study, the rate of recovery of *E. coli* O157:H7 was ≥90% from stool samples obtained within 2 days of onset of disease; this declined to 33% after 6 days (92). Early reports suggested that fecal leukocytes were found infrequently in patients with diarrhea due to *E. coli* O157:H7 (38). However, more recent data suggest that, similar to patients with enteritis due to other common enteric bacterial pathogens, fecal leukocytes are a common finding in patients with *E. coli* O157:H7 infection (85). Thus, the absence of fecal leukocytes in stool specimens is not an appropriate criterion for screening to determine which stool specimen should be cultured for *E. coli* O157:H7 (85).

E. coli O157:H7 will not be detected by standard methods for other common bacterial enteric pathogens in routine stool cultures because it is indistinguishable from the *E. coli* strains that are part of the normal fecal flora. Unlike 80 to 90% of other *E. coli* strains, *E. coli* O157:H7 does not ferment sorbitol rapidly (57). Sorbitol-MacConkey (SMAC) agar, in which lactose is replaced by sorbitol, is the medium of choice for screening. Modifying SMAC medium by adding cefixime, rhamnose, and tellurite can improve detection (28, 101).

Tests for the rapid detection of *E. coli* O157:H7 in stool using immunofluorescent (69) or enzyme immunoassay (87) methods have been developed. In addition, commercial test kits using either an enzyme immunoassay or latex agglutination methodology have been developed to detect Stx in bacterial colonies or directly from stool samples (1, 87). Use of one of these commercially available assays to detect Stx may make it feasible for laboratories that do not have access to reference methods to screen fecal samples for both *E. coli* O157:H7 and non-O157 STEC. However, the relatively high cost of these tests may limit their routine use in laboratories that process large numbers of stool specimens.

A limitation of assays that do not use culture methods is that the organism itself is not immediately available for study. Obtaining an isolate for further serologic and molecular subtyping is crucial for public health reasons, to enable rapid identification of outbreaks and implementation of appropriate control strategies. Therefore, a positive reaction in any of these assays should be followed by appropriate methods to isolate the organism (87). Sorbitol-negative (colorless) colonies should be selected for subsequent testing with commercially available *E. coli* O157 antiserum (26) or latex reagents (87). Presumptive identification of *E. coli* O157:H7 can be reported for an organism that is sorbitol negative on SMAC agar and agglutinates in O157 antiserum (87). Presumptive O157 isolates should be confirmed biochemically as *E. coli* because this antiserum cross-reacts with a variety of organisms that also cause diarrhea, including *Salmonella* group N, *Vibrio cholerae, Yersinia enterocolitica* serotype O9, and others (35). Confirmation of *E. coli* O157:H7 requires identification of the H7 flagellar antigen. However, determination of the H7 antigen is not necessary for the presumptive identification of O157 STEC; reporting of such strains to clinicians should not be delayed by H7 antigen identification.

Antibodies against O157 LPS have been detected in the serum of patients infected with *E. coli* O157:H7. Assays for this are not yet commercially available. Enzyme-linked immunosorbent assays (ELISAs) for immunoglobulin M (IgM), IgA, or IgG, immunoblotting, and indirect hemagglutination have been used by different groups. A study in the United States found that 92% of 26 persons with a positive *E. coli* O157:H7 stool culture had a positive IgG titer against O157 LPS, compared with 3% of controls (8). The response peaked 2 to 3 weeks after onset of illness. In outbreak situations, up to 33% of culture-negative ill persons can have positive titers. The response may be related to the severity of illness, because culture-positive patients with HUS developed higher titers than those without HUS (8).

Experimental assays to detect serum antibodies to Stx have been assessed. Antibody titers to Stx 1 were detected in 23% of 47 patients in an outbreak caused by a strain of *E. coli* O157:H7 that produced Stx 1 and Stx 2; specific antibodies to Stx 2 were not detected (8).

Treatment

No specific therapy has been proven effective in patients with *E. coli* O157:H7 infection; therefore, supportive measures are important. During the first week after onset of diarrhea, patients with documented infection should be monitored for signs and symptoms of HUS, such as pallor or oliguria. In high-risk patients, it may be prudent to monitor peripheral blood smears, blood counts, and urinalysis findings (90). Antimotility agents have been associated with an increased risk for developing HUS and are thus contraindicated in patients with diarrhea due to *E. coli* O157:H7 infection (10, 29). Management of HUS requires careful attention to fluid and electrolyte balance and other complications of renal failure such as azotemia and hypertension (83).

Although most *E. coli* O157:H7 strains are susceptible to antimicrobial agents used for enteric infections, antimicrobial treatment has not been demonstrated to improve the course of illness or to prevent complications. Two small retrospective studies have reported that patients who developed HUS were more likely to have received antimicrobial treatment; however, patients who received antimicrobial agents were more severely ill than those not treated (19, 70). A large retrospective study (10) and another case series (29, 30) did not confirm the association between HUS and antibiotic treatment. Only one prospective, randomized study of antimicrobial treatment with trimethoprim-sulfamethoxazole among patients with *E. coli* O157:H7

Antimicrobial treatment has not been demonstrated to improve the course of illness or to prevent complications infection has been reported (72). In that study, compared with no antimicrobial therapy, treatment with trimethoprim-sulfamethoxazole did not affect the duration or severity of illness nor subsequent fecal shedding of the organism. However, patients did not receive treatment until 7 days after onset of diarrhea. In vitro, subinhibitory concentrations of some antimicrobial agents increase Shiga toxin production by *E. coli* O157:H7 (97). Whether this phenomenon occurs in vivo or is clinically relevant is unknown.

Conclusions about the studies of the relations between antimicrobial therapy for persons infected with *E. coli* O157:H7 and subsequent development of HUS are limited by the lack of standardization of the type, timing, and duration of antimicrobial treatment, as well as the possibility that administration of antimicrobial agents could be a marker for a more severe illness (35). Large randomized, placebo-controlled, prospective treatment trials are needed to address this question. Other possible treatments for *E. coli* O157:H7 infection include orally administered Shiga toxin-binding resins and toxin-neutralizing antibodies (5, 54).

Other STEC

Many non-O157 STEC serotypes can cause bloody and nonbloody diarrhea and HUS

In humans, *E. coli* O157:H7 is the most frequently isolated and studied STEC. However, many other non-O157 STEC serotypes have also been isolated from humans and can cause bloody and nonbloody diarrhea and HUS (35). Outbreaks of non-O157 STEC infections have been reported from Australia, Italy (18), Japan (42), and the United States. In the United States, an outbreak linked to milk was caused by *E. coli* O104:H21, a previously unrecognized cause of illness (21). The only other reported United States outbreak was a family cluster of *E. coli* O111 infections (7). In Australia, an outbreak of *E. coli* O111 infections was linked to a commercially produced sausage; 23 children developed HUS, and 1 died (22, 33).

In North America, available data suggest that infections caused by the non-O157 STEC are less common than those caused by *E. coli* O157:H7. In a study in Canada, non-O157 STEC were identified in stools much less commonly than was *E. coli* O157:H7, but with similar frequency to *Shigella* spp. (66). In a small study in Seattle, non-O157 STEC were isolated about half as frequently as *E. coli* O157:H7 (12). However, non-O157 STEC infections probably occur much more frequently than is recognized because techniques to identify them are not routinely used by clinical laboratories (91).

Prevention

Prevention of *E. coli* O157:H7 infections requires close cooperation and good communication among clinicians, public health authorities, and clinical microbiologists. As with many food-borne diseases, efforts to decrease contamination of foods during production, distribution, processing, and preparation are needed to reduce the risk of infection. No human vaccine is available, although candidate vaccines are currently under investigation (50).

One critical component in the detection of outbreaks is the astute clinician who notices a cluster of patients with similar clinical features and alerts the health department. Notification of health departments by clinicians led to the first recognized outbreak of *E. coli* O157:H7 infections, as well as recognition of the large outbreak of *E. coli* O157:H7 infections in the western United States in 1993 and recognition of *E. coli* O104:H21 as a pathogen. Notification by clinicians can lead to public health investigations and actions that can prevent additional cases. For example, during the 1993 outbreak, an estimated 800 additional cases were prevented by the prompt recall of frozen hamburger patties after they were epidemiologically implicated as the source (9).

Rapid notification of the health department about *E. coli* O157:H7 cases in nursing home residents or attendees of child care centers is especially important to enable increased surveillance for diarrheal illness at the facility. Children with *E. coli* O157:H7 infection should be excluded from child care centers until two consecutive stool cultures performed at least 48 h after completion of antimicrobial therapy are negative. In addition, parents must be persuaded not to take children to another center, which could result in the spread of infection to other child care facilities.

Another important component in the detection of outbreaks is the comparison of strains from apparently sporadic cases using standardized molecular subtyping methodologies. One such method, pulsed-field gel electrophoresis (PFGE), is being implemented at state public health laboratories in the United States in 1997 as part of an electronic network. Use of PFGE can link together cases that do not appear to be associated and thus improve detection of dispersed outbreaks and facilitate prompt removal of contaminated foods from the marketplace.

We recommend that clinicians urge their clinical laboratories to culture diarrheal stool specimens for *E. coli* O157:H7 using SMAC medium, at a minimum from all stools with visible blood. Clinicians should consider *E. coli* O157:H7 when evaluating patients with diarrhea, especially when there is a history of bloody diarrhea, and should be aware that patients with *E. coli* O157:H7 infection are often mistakenly diagnosed with a noninfectious illness. Diagnosed cases should be reported to the health department, and the isolate should be referred to the state laboratory for subtyping. Clinicians also should consider that non-O157 STEC can cause both nonbloody and bloody diarrhea and should alert health authorities if they recognize a cluster of unexplained illnesses. Patients with diarrhea and parents of children with diarrhea should be advised that washing hands with soap after bowel movements is the most important measure in preventing the spread of infection.

One critical component in the detection of outbreaks is the astute clinician who notices a cluster of patients with similar clinical features and alerts the health department

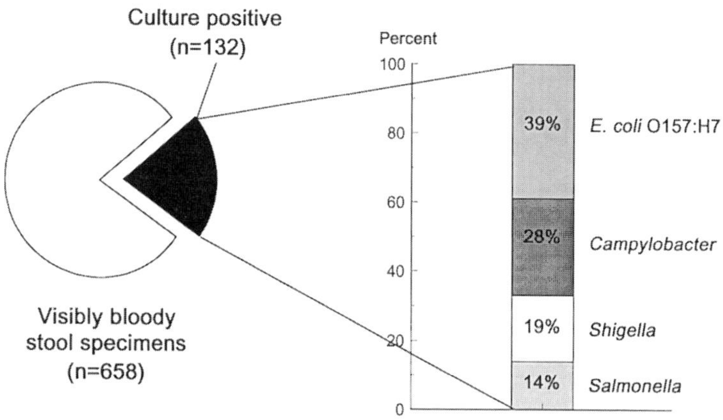

Figure 12.1 Percentage of bacterial pathogens isolated from visibly bloody stools, United States multicenter study, 1990–92. *E. coli* O157:H7 was the pathogen most commonly isolated from visibly bloody stools.

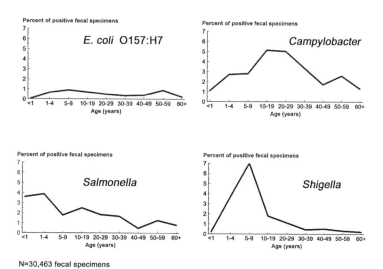

Figure 12.2 Age-specific isolation proportions from fecal specimens from patients with *E. coli* O157:H7 or other major bacterial enteric pathogens, United States multicenter study, 1990–1992. *E. coli* O157:H7 age-specific isolation proportions were highest in children aged 5 to 9 years (0.90%) and adults aged 50 to 59 years (0.89%), and it was isolated more frequently than *Shigella* spp. in adults over the age of 50 years.

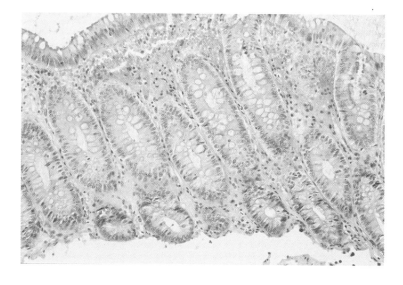

Figure 12.3 Ischemic pattern of *Escherichia coli* O157:H7 colitis: colonic mucosa showing hemorrhage in the luminal portion of the lamina propria with minimal inflammatory infiltrate. The mucosa demonstrates some cells with mucus depletion. (Hematoxylin and eosin [H&E] stain; original magnification ×20.)

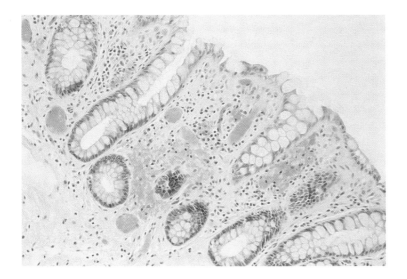

Figure 12.4   Ischemic pattern of *E. coli* O157:H7 colitis: colonic mucosa showing hemorrhage and edema of the entire lamina propria. The edema extends to the submucosa, and the blood vessels are congested and show fibrin thrombi. (H&E; original magnification ×20.)

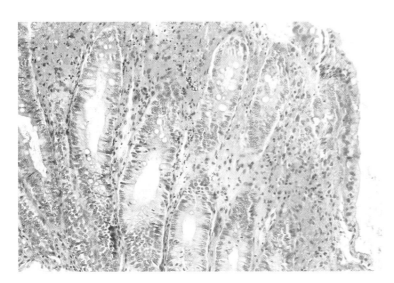

Figure 12.5   Ischemic pattern of *E. coli* O157:H7 colitis: colonic mucosa showing hemorrhage of the lamina propria, with partial coagulative necrosis of the surface epithelium and preservation of the deep colonic crypts. (H&E; original magnification ×20.)

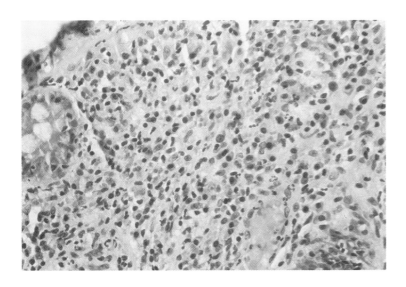

Figure 12.6   Infectious pattern of *E. coli* O157:H7 colitis: the lamina propria is expanded with acute (neutrophils) and chronic (lymphocytes) inflammatory cells. (H&E; original magnification ×40.)

Figure 12.7 Infectious pattern of *E. coli* O157:H7 colitis: lymphocytes and neutrophils invading the colonic crypts. (H&E; original magnification ×40.)

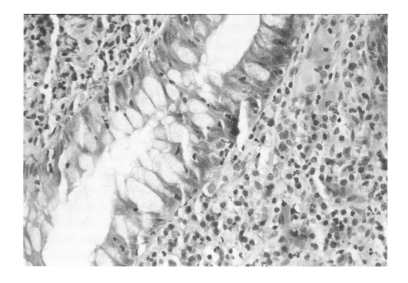

Figure 12.8 Pseudomembrane formation in *E. coli* O157:H7 colitis: in the luminal side a pseudomembrane composed of fibrin and both acute and chronic inflammatory infiltrate can be seen. (H&E; original magnification ×40.)

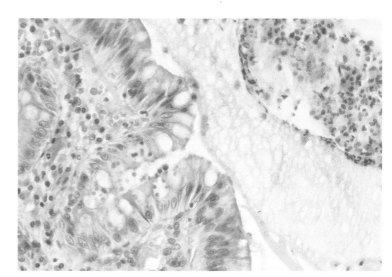

Figure 12.9 HUS following *E. coli* O157:H7 infection: glomerulus showing necrotic capillaries with fibrin deposition; in the peripheral tufts the capillary walls appear thickened and stiff. (H&E; original magnification ×40.)

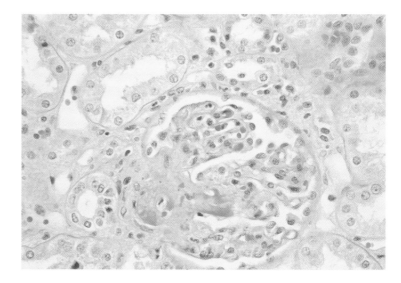

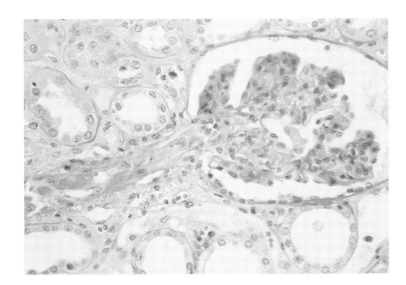

Figure 12.10 HUS following *E. coli* O157:H7 infection: glomerulus showing fibrin thrombus in the afferent arteriole and necrotic glomerular tufts. (H&E; original magnification ×40.)

References

1. **Acheson, D. W. K., S. DeBreuker, A. Donohue-Rolfe, K. Kozak, A. Yi, and G. T. Keusch.** 1994. Development of a clinically useful diagnostic enzyme immunoassay for enterohemorrhagic *Escherichia coli* infection, p. 109–112. *In* M. A. Karmali and A. G. Goglio (ed.), *Recent Advances in Verocytotoxin-Producing Escherichia coli Infections.* Elsevier Science Publishers, Amsterdam.

2. **Acheson, D. W. K., R. Moore, S. DeBreucker, L. L. Lincicome, M. Jacewicz, E. Skutelsky, and G. T. Keusch.** 1992. Translocation of Shiga toxin across polarized intestinal cells in tissue culture. *Infect. Immun.* **64:**3294–3300.

3. **Ackers, M., B. Mahon, E. Leahy, T. Damrow, L. Hutwagner, T. Barrett, W. Bibb, P. Hayes, P. Griffin, and L. Slutsker.** 1996. An outbreak of *Escherichia coli* O157:H7 infections associated with leaf lettuce consumption, Western Montana, abstr. K43, p. 257. *In Abstracts of the 36th Interscience Conference on Antimicrobial Agents and Chemotherapy, New Orleans, La.*

4. **Akashi, S., K. Joh, A. Tsuji, H. Ito, H. Hoshi, T. Hayakawa, J. Ihara, T. Abe, M. Hatori, and T. Mori.** 1994. A severe outbreak of haemorrhagic colitis and haemolytic uraemic syndrome associated with *Escherichia coli* O157:H7 in Japan. *Eur. J. Pediatr.* **153:**650–655.

5. **Armstrong, G. D., P. C. Rowe, P. Goodyer, E. Orrbine, T. P. Klassen, G. Wells, A. MacKenzie, H. Lior, C. Blanchard, F. Auclair, B. Thompson, D. J. Rafter, and P. N. McLaine.** 1995. A phase I study of chemically synthesized verotoxin (Shiga-like toxin) Pk-trisaccharide receptors attached to chromosorb for preventing hemolytic uremic syndrome. *J. Infect. Dis.* **171:**1042–1045.

6. **Ashkenazi, S.** 1993. Role of bacterial cytotoxins in hemolytic uremic syndrome and thrombotic thrombocytopenic purpura. *Annu. Rev. Med.* **44:**11–18.

7. **Banatvala, N., M. M. DeBeukelaer, P. M. Griffin, T. J. Barrett, K. D. Greene, J. H. Green, and J. G. Wells.** 1996. Shiga-like toxin-producing *Escherichia coli* O111 and associated hemolytic-uremic syndrome: a family outbreak. *Pediatr. Infect. Dis. J.* **15:**1008–1011.

8. **Barrett, T. J., J. H. Green, P. M. Griffin, A. T. Pavia, S. M. Ostroff, and I. K. Wachsmuth.** 1991. Enzyme-linked immunosorbent assays for detecting antibodies to Shiga-like toxin I, Shiga-like toxin II, and *Escherichia coli* O157:H7 lipopolysaccharide in human serum. *Curr. Microbiol.* **23:**189–195.

9. **Bell, B. P., M. Goldoft, P. M. Griffin, M. A. Davis, D. C. Gordon, P. I. Tarr, C. A. Bartleson, J. H. Lewis, T. J. Barrett, J. G. Wells, R. Baron, and J. Kobayashi.** 1994. A multistate outbreak of *Escherichia coli* O157:H7-associated bloody diarrhea and hemolytic uremic syndrome from hamburgers: the Washington experience. *JAMA* **272:**1349–1353.

10. **Bell, B. P., P. M. Griffin, P. Lozano, D. L. Christie, J. M. Kobayashi, and P. I. Tarr.** 1997. Predictors of hemolytic uremic syndrome in children during a large outbreak of *Escherichia coli* O157:H7 infections. *Pediatrics* **100:**e12.

11. **Belongia, E. A., M. T. Osterholm, J. T. Soler, D. A. Ammend, J. E. Braun, and K. L. MacDonald.** 1993. Transmission of *Escherichia coli* O157:H7 infection in Minnesota child day-care facilities. *JAMA* **269:**883–888.

12. **Bokete, T. N., C. M. O'Callahan, C. R. Clausen, N. M. Tang, N. Tran, S. L. Moseley, T. R. Fritsche, and P. I. Tarr.** 1993. Shiga-like toxin-producing *Escherichia coli* in Seattle children: a prospective study. *Gastroenterology* **105:**1724–1731.

13. **Boyce, T. G., A. G. Pemberton, J. G. Wells, and P. M. Griffin.** 1995. Screening for *Escherichia coli* O157:H7: a nationwide survey of clinical laboratories. *J. Clin. Microbiol.* **33:**3275–3277.

14. **Boyce, T. G., D. L. Swerdlow, and P. M. Griffin.** 1995. *Escherichia coli* O157:H7 and the hemolytic uremic syndrome. *N. Engl. J. Med.* **333:**364–368.

15. **Bryant, H. E., M. A. Athar, and C. H. Pai.** 1989. Risk factors for *Escherichia coli* O157:H7 infection in an urban community. *J. Infect. Dis.* **160:**858–864.

16. **Cahoon, F. E., and J. S. Thompson.** 1987. Frequency of *Escherichia coli* O157:H7 isolation from stool specimens. *J. Infect. Dis.* **33:**914–915.

17. **Calderwood, S. B., D. W. K. Acheson, G. T. Keusch, T. J. Barrett, P. M. Griffin, N. A. Strockbine, B. Swaminathan, J. B. Kaper, M. M. Levine, B. S. Kaplan, H. Karch, A. D. O'Brien, T. G. Obrig, P. I. Tarr, and I. K. Wachsmuth.** 1996. Proposed new nomenclature for Shiga-like toxin (verotoxin) family. *ASM News* **62:**118–119.

18. **Caprioli, A., I. Luzzi, F. Rosmini, C. Resti, A. Edefonti, F. Perfumo, C. Farina, A. Goglio, A. Gianviti, and G. Rizzoni.** 1994. Community-wide outbreak of hemolytic-uremic syndrome associated with non-O157 verocytotoxin-producing *Escherichia coli. J. Infect. Dis.* **169:**208–211.

19. **Carter, A. O., A. A. Borczyk, J. A. K. Carlson, B. Harvey, J. C. Hockin, M. A. Karmali, C. Krishnan, D. A. Korn, and H. Lior.** 1987. A severe outbreak of *Escherichia coli* O157:H7-associated hemorrhagic colitis in a nursing home. *N. Engl. J. Med.* **317:**1496–1500.

20. **Centers for Disease Control and Prevention.** 1993. Multistate outbreak of *Escherichia coli* O157:H7 infections from hamburgers—Western United States. *Morbid. Mortal. Weekly Rep.* **42:**258–263.

21. **Centers for Disease Control and Prevention.** 1995. Outbreak of acute gastroenteritis attributable to *Escherichia coli* serotype O104:H21—Helena, Montana, 1994. *Morbid. Mortal. Weekly Rep.* **44:**501–503.

22. **Centers for Disease Control and Prevention.** 1995. Community outbreak of hemolytic uremic syndrome attributable to *Escherichia coli* O111:NM—South Australia, 1995. *Morbid. Mortal. Weekly Rep.* **44:**550–558.

23. **Centers for Disease Control and Prevention.** 1997. Outbreaks of *Escherichia coli* O157:H7 infection and cryptosporidiosis associated with drinking unpasteurized apple cider—Connecticut and New York, October 1996. *Morbid. Mortal. Weekly Rep.* **46:**4–8.

24. **Centers for Disease Control and Prevention.** 1997. Outbreaks of *Escherichia coli* O157:H7 infections associated with eating alfalfa sprouts—Michigan and Virginia, June–July, 1997. *Morbid. Mortal. Weekly Rep.* **46:**741–744.

25. **Centers for Disease Control and Prevention.** 1998. Unpublished data.

26. **Chapman, P. A.** 1989. Evaluation of commercial latex slide test for identifying *Escherichia coli* O157. *J. Clin. Pathol.* **42:**1109–1110.

27. **Chapman, P. A., C. A. Siddons, A. T. C. Malo, and M. A. Harkin.** 1996. Lamb products as a potential source of *E. coli* O157. *Vet. Rec.* **139:**427–428. (Letter.)

28. **Chapman, P. A., C. A. Siddons, P. M. Zadik, and L. Jewes.** 1991. An improved selective medium for the isolation of *E. coli* O157. *J. Med. Microbiol.* **35:**107–110.

29. **Cimolai, N., S. Basalyga, D. G. Mah, B. J. Morrison, and J. E. Carter.** 1994. A continuing assessment of risk factors for the development of *Escherichia coli* O157:H7-associated hemolytic uremic syndrome. *Clin. Nephrol.* **42:**85–89.

30. **Cimolai, N., J. E. Carter, B. J. Morrison, and J. D. Anderson.** 1990. Risk factors for the progression of *Escherichia coli* O157:H7 enteritis to hemolytic-uremic syndrome. *J. Pediatr.* **116:**589–592.

31. **Donnenberg, M. S., and J. B. Kaper.** 1992. Enteropathogenic *Escherichia coli.* *Infect. Immun.* **60:**3953–3961.

32. **Donnenberg, M. S., S. Tzipori, M. L. McKee, A. D. O'Brien, J. Alroy, and J. B. Kaper.** 1993. The role of the *eae* gene of enterohemorrhagic *Escherichia coli* in intimate attachment in vitro and in a porcine model. *J. Clin. Invest.* **92:**1418–1424.

33. **Goldwater, P. N., and K. A. Bettelheim.** 1996. An outbreak of hemolytic uremic syndrome due to *Escherichia coli* O157:H–: or was it? *Emerg. Infect. Dis.* **2:**153–154.

34. **Gransden, W. R., M. A. Damm, J. D. Anderson, J. E. Carter, and H. Lior.** 1986. Further evidence associating hemolytic uremic syndrome with infection by verotoxin-producing *Escherichia coli* O157:H7. *J. Infect. Dis.* **154:**522–524.

35. **Griffin, P. M.** 1995. *Escherichia coli* O157:H7 and other enterohemorrhagic *Escherichia coli,* p. 739–761. *In* M. J. Blaser, P. D. Smith, J. I. Ravdin, H. B. Greenberg, and R. L. Guerrant (ed.), *Infections of the Gastrointestinal Tract.* Raven Press, Ltd., New York.

36. **Griffin, P. M., B. P. Bell, P. R. Cieslak, J. Tuttle, T. J. Barrett, M. P. Doyle, A. M. McNamara, A. M. Shefer, and J. G. Wells.** 1994. Large outbreak of *Escherichia coli* O157:H7 infections in the western United States: the big picture, p. 7–12. *In* M. A. Karmali and A. G. Goglio (ed.), *Recent Advances in Verocytotoxin-Producing Escherichia coli Infections.* Elsevier, New York.

37. **Griffin, P. M., L. C. Olmstead, and R. E. Petras.** 1990. *Escherichia coli* O157:H7-associated colitis, a clinical and histological study of 11 cases. *Gastroenterology* **99:**142–149.

38. **Griffin, P. M., S. M. Ostroff, R. V. Tauxe, K. D. Greene, J. G. Wells, J. H. Lewis, and P. A. Blake.** 1988. Illnesses associated with *Escherichia coli* O157:H7 infections: a broad clinical spectrum. *Ann. Intern. Med.* **109:**705–712.

39. **Griffin, P. M., and R. V. Tauxe.** 1991. The epidemiology of infections caused by *Escherichia coli* O157:H7, other enterohemorrhagic *E. coli,* and the associated hemolytic uremic syndrome. *Epidemiol. Rev.* **13:**60–98.

40. **Hunt, C. M., J. A. Harvey, E. R. Youngs, S. T. Irwin, and T. M. Reid.** 1989. Clinical and pathological variability of infection by enterohaemorrhagic (Vero cytotoxin producing) *Escherichia coli. J. Clin. Pathol.* **42:**847–852.

41. **Inward, C. D., A. J. Howie, M. M. Fitzpatrick, F. Rafaat, D. V. Milford, and C. M. Taylor.** 1997. Renal histopathology in fatal cases of diarrhoea-associated hemolytic uraemic syndrome. *Pediatr. Nephrol.* **11:**556–559.

42. **Itoh, T., A. Kai, K. Saito, Y. Yanagawa, M. Inaba, M. Takahashi, Y. Kudoh, S. Yamada, S. Matsushita, T. Terayama, and M. Ohashi.** 1988. Gastroenteritis associated with verocytotoxin producing *Escherichia coli* O145:NM, p. 21–28. *In* S. Kuwahara and N. F. Pierce (ed.), *Advances in Research on Cholera and Related Diarrheas.* KTK Scientific Publishers, Tokyo.

43. **Jung, H. C., L. Eckmann, S. Yang, A. Panja, J. Fierer, E. Morzycka-Wroblewska, and M. F. Kagnoff.** 1995. A distinct array of proinflammatory cytokines is expressed in human colon epithelial cells in response to bacterial invasion. *J. Clin. Invest.* **95:**55–65.

44. **Karmali, M. A., M. Petric, C. Lim, P. C. Fleming, G. S. Arbus, and H. Lior.** 1985. The association between idiopathic hemolytic uremic syndrome and infection by verotoxin-producing *Escherichia coli. J. Infect. Dis.* **151:**775–782.

45. **Keene, W. E., J. M. McAnulty, F. C. Hoesly, L. P. Williams, K. Hedberg, G. L. Oxman, T. J. Barrett, M. A. Pfaller, and D. W. Fleming.** 1994. A swimming-associated outbreak of hemorrhagic colitis caused by *Escherichia coli* O157:H7 and *Shigella sonnei*. *N. Engl. J. Med.* **331:**579–584.

46. **Keene, W. E., E. Sazie, J. Kok, D. H. Rice, D. D. Hancock, V. K. Balan, T. Zhao, and M. P. Doyle.** 1997. An outbreak of *Escherichia coli* O157:H7 infections traced to jerky made from deer meat. *JAMA* **277:**1229–1231.

47. **Kelly, J. K., and D. A. Owen.** 1997. *Escherichia coli* diarrhea, p. 555–564. *In* D. H. Connor, F. W. Chandler, D. A. Schwartz, H. J. Manz, and E. E. Lack (ed.), *Pathology of Infectious Diseases.* Appleton and Lange, Stamford, Conn.

48. **Kelly, J. K., C. H. Pai, I. H. Jadusingh, M. L. Macinnis, E. A. Shaffer, and N. B. Hershfield.** 1987. The histopathology of rectosigmoid biopsies from adults with bloody diarrhea due to verotoxin-producing *Escherichia coli*. *Am. J. Clin. Pathol.* **88:**78–82.

49. **Knutton, S., T. M. Baldwin, P. H. Williams, and A. S. McNeish.** 1989. Actin accumulation at sites of bacterial adhesion to tissue culture cells: basis of a new diagnostic test for enteropathogenic and enterohemorrhagic *Escherichia coli*. *Infect. Immun.* **57:**1290–1298.

50. **Konadu, E. Y., J. C. Parke, H. T. Tran, D. A. Bryla, J. B. Robbins, and S. C. Szu.** 1998. Investigational vaccine for *Escherichia coli* O157: phase 1 study of O157 O-specific polysaccharide-*Pseudomonas aeruginosa* recombinant exoprotein A conjugates in adults. *J. Infect. Dis.* **177:**383–387.

51. **Kudva, I. T., P. G. Hatfield, and C. J. Hovde.** 1996. *Escherichia coli* O157:H7 in microbial flora of sheep. *J. Clin. Microbiol.* **34:**431–433.

52. **Law, D., and J. Kelly.** 1995. Use of heme and hemoglobin by *Escherichia coli* O157 and other Shiga-like-toxin-producing *E. coli* serogroups. *Infect. Immun.* **63:**700–702.

53. **Li, Z., C. Bell, A. Buret, R. Robins-Browne, D. Stiel, and E. O'Loughlin.** 1993. The effect of enterohemorrhagic *Escherichia coli* O157:H7 on intestinal structure and solute transport in rabbits. *Gastroenterology* **104:**467–474.

54. **Lissner, R., H. Schmidt, and H. Karch.** 1996. A standard immunoglobulin preparation produced from bovine colostra shows antibody reactivity and neutralization activity against Shiga-like toxins and EHEC-hemolysin of *Escherichia coli* O157:H7. *Infection* **24:**378–383.

55. **Louise, C. B., and T. G. Obrig.** 1995. Specific interaction of *Escherichia coli* O157:H7-derived Shiga-like toxin II with human renal endothelial cells. *J. Infect. Dis.* **172:**1397–1401.

56. **MacDonald, K. L., M. J. O'Leary, M. L. Cohen, P. Norris, J. G. Wells, E. Noll, J. M. Kobayashi, and P. A. Blake.** 1988. *Escherichia coli* O157:H7, an emerging gastrointestinal pathogen: results of a one-year, prospective, population-based study. *JAMA* **259:**3567–3570.

57. **March, S. B., and S. Ratnam.** 1986. Sorbitol-MacConkey medium for detection of *Escherichia coli* O157:H7 associated with hemorrhagic colitis. *J. Clin. Microbiol.* **23:**869–872.

58. **Marshall, W. F., C. A. McLimans, R. E. Van Scoy, and J. P. Anhalt.** 1990. Results of a 6-month survey of stool cultures for *Escherichia coli* O157:H7. *Mayo Clin. Proc.* **65:**787–792.

59. **Martin, D. L., K. L. MacDonald, K. E. White, J. T. Soler, and M. T. Osterholm.** 1990. The epidemiology and clinical aspects of the hemolytic uremic syndrome in Minnesota. *N. Engl. J. Med.* **323:**1161–1167.

60. **McKee, M. L., A. R. Melton-Celsa, R. A. Moxley, D. H. Francis, and A. D. O'Brien.** 1995. Enterohemorrhagic *Escherichia coli* O157:H7 requires intimin to colonize the gnotobiotic pig intestine and to adhere to Hep-2 cells. *Infect. Immun.* **63:**3739–3744.

61. **McKee, M. L., and A. D. O'Brien.** 1996. Truncated enterohemorrhagic *Escherichia coli* (EHEC) O157:H7 intimin (EaeA) fusion proteins promote adherence of EHEC strains to Hep-2 cells. *Infect. Immun.* **64:**2223–2225.

62. **Nataro, J. P., and J. B. Kaper.** 1998. Diarrheagenic *Escherichia coli. Clin. Microbiol. Rev.* **11:**142–201.

63. **National Institute of Health and Infectious Disease.** 1997. Verocytotoxin-producing *Escherichia coli* (enterohemorrhagic *E. coli*) infections, Japan, 1996-June 1997. *Infect. Agents Surveill. Rep.* **18:**153–154.

64. **Ostroff, S. M., P. M. Griffin, R. V. Tauxe, L. D. Shipman, K. D. Greene, J. G. Wells, J. H. Lewis, P. A. Blake, and J. M. Kobayashi.** 1990. A statewide outbreak of *Escherichia coli* O157:H7 infections in Washington State. *Am. J. Epidemiol.* **132:**239–247.

65. **Ostroff, S. M., J. M. Kobayashi, and J. H. Lewis.** 1989. Infections with *Escherichia coli* O157:H7 in Washington State: the first year of statewide disease surveillance. *JAMA* **262:**355–359.

66. **Pai, C. H., N. Ahmed, H. Lior, W. M. Johnson, H. V. Sims, and D. E. Woods.** 1988. Epidemiology of sporadic diarrhea due to verocytotoxin-producing *Escherichia coli*: a two-year prospective study. *J. Infect. Dis.* **157:**1054–1057.

67. **Pai, C. H., R. Gordon, H. V. Sims, and L. E. Bryan.** 1984. Sporadic cases of hemorrhagic colitis associated with *Escherichia coli* O157:H7: clinical, epidemiologic, and bacteriologic features. *Ann. Intern. Med.* **101:**738–742.

68. **Pai, C. H., J. K. Kelly, and G. L. Meyers.** 1986. Experimental infection of infant rabbits with verotoxin-producing *Escherichia coli. Infect. Immun.* **51:**16–23.

69. **Park, C. H., D. L. Hixon, W. L. Morrison, and C. B. Cook.** 1994. Rapid diagnosis of enterohemorrhagic *Escherichia coli* O157:H7 directly from fecal specimens using immunofluorescence stain. *Am. J. Clin. Pathol.* **101:**91–94.

70. **Pavia, A. T., C. R. Nichols, D. P. Green, R. V. Tauxe, S. Mottice, K. D. Greene, J. G. Wells, R. L. Siegler, E. D. Brewer, D. Hannon, and P. A. Blake.** 1990. Hemolytic-uremic syndrome during an outbreak of *Escherichia coli* O157:H7 infections in institutions for mentally retarded persons: clinical and epidemiologic observations. *J. Pediatr.* **116:**544–551.

71. **Pickering, L. K., T. G. Obrig, and F. B. Stapleton.** 1994. Hemolytic-uremic syndrome and enterohemorrhagic *Escherichia coli. Pediatr. Infect. Dis. J.* **13:**459–476.

72. **Proulx, F., J. P. Turgeon, G. Delage, L. Lafleur, and L. Chicoine.** 1992. Randomized, controlled trial of antibiotic therapy for *Escherichia coli* O157:H7 enteritis. *J. Pediatr.* **121:**299–303.

73. **Ratnam, S., and S. B. March.** 1986. Sporadic occurrence of hemorrhagic colitis associated with *Escherichia coli* O157:H7 in Newfoundland. *Can. Med. Assoc. J.* **134:**43–46.

74. **Remuzzi, G., and P. Ruggenenti.** 1995. The hemolytic uremic syndrome. *Kidney Int.* **47:**2–19.

75. **Richardson, S. E., M. A. Karmali, L. E. Becker, and C. R. Smith.** 1988. The histopathology of the hemolytic uremic syndrome associated with verocytotoxin-producing *Escherichia coli* infections. *Hum. Pathol.* **19:**1102–1108.

76. **Richardson, S. E., T. A. Rotman, V. Jay, C. R. Smith, L. E. Becker, M. Petric, N. F. Olivieri, and M. A. Karmali.** 1992. Experimental verocytotoxemia in rabbits. *Infect. Immun.* **60:**4154–4167.

77. **Riley, L. W., R. S. Remis, S. D. Helgerson, H. B. McGee, J. G. Wells, B. R. Davis, R. J. Hebert, E. S. Olcott, L. M. Johnson, N. T. Hargrett, P. A. Blake, and M. L. Cohen.** 1983. Hemorrhagic colitis associated with a rare *Escherichia coli* serotype. *N. Engl. J. Med.* **308:**681–685.

78. **Rowe, P. C., E. Orrbine, M. Ogborn, G. A. Wells, W. Winther, H. Lior, D. Manuel, and P. N. McLaine.** 1994. Epidemic *Escherichia coli* O157:H7 gastroenteritis and hemolytic-uremic syndrome in a Canadian Inuit community: intestinal illness in family members as a risk factor. *J. Pediatr.* **124:**21–26.

79. **Ruggenenti, P., and G. Remuzzi.** 1990. Thrombotic thrombocytopenic purpura and related disorders. *Hematol. Oncol. Clin. North Am.* **4:**219–224.

80. **Ryan, C. A., R. V. Tauxe, G. W. Hosek, J. W. Wells, P. A. Stoesz, H. W. McFadden, P. W. Smith, G. F. Wright, and P. A. Blake.** 1986. *Escherichia coli* O157:H7 diarrhea in a nursing home: clinical, epidemiological, and and pathological findings. *J. Infect. Dis.* **154:**631–638.

81. **Sears, C. L., and J. B. Kaper.** 1996. Enteric bacterial toxins: mechanisms of action and linkage to intestinal secretion. *Microbiol. Rev.* **60:**167–215.

82. **Shah, S., R. Hoffman, P. Shillam, and B. Wilson.** 1996. Prolonged fecal shedding of *Escherichia coli* O157:H7 during an outbreak at a day care center. *Clin. Infect. Dis.* **23:**835–836.

83. **Siegler, R. L.** 1995. The hemolytic uremic syndrome. *Pediatr. Clin. North Am.* **42:**1505–1529.

84. **Siegler, R. L., A. T. Pavia, R. D. Christofferson, and M. K. Milligan.** 1994. A 20-year population-based study of postdiarrheal hemolytic uremic syndrome in Utah. *Pediatrics* **94:**35–40.

85. **Slutsker, L., A. A. Ries, K. D. Greene, J. G. Wells, L. Hutwagner, P. M. Griffin, and *Escherichia coli* O157:H7 Study Group.** 1997. *Escherichia coli* O157:H7 diarrhea in the United States: clinical and epidemiologic features. *Ann. Intern. Med.* **126:**505–513.

86. **Strockbine, N. A., L. R. M. Marques, J. W. Newland, H. W. Smith, R. K. Holmes, and A. D. O'Brien.** 1986. Two toxin-converting phages from *Escherichia coli* O157:H7 strain 933 encode antigenically distinct toxins with similar biologic activities. *Infect. Immun.* **53:**135–140.

87. **Strockbine, N. A., J. G. Wells, C. A. Bopp, and T. J. Barrett.** 1998. Detection and diagnosis of STEC infections: overview of detection and subtyping methods, p. 331–356. *In* J. B. Kaper and A. D. O'Brien (ed.), *Escherichia coli O157:H7 and Other Shiga Toxin-Producing E. coli Strains.* ASM Press, Washington, D.C.

88. **Swerdlow, D. L., and P. M. Griffin.** 1997. Duration of faecal shedding of *Escherichia coli* O157:H7 among children in day care centers. *Lancet* **349:**745–746.

89. **Swerdlow, D. L., B. A. Woodruff, R. C. Brady, P. M. Griffin, S. Tippen, H. D. Donnell, E. Geldreich, B. J. Payne, A. Meyer, J. G. Wells, K. D. Greene, M. Bright, N. H. Bean, and P. A. Blake.** 1992. A waterborne outbreak in Missouri of *Escherichia coli* O157:H7 associated with bloody diarrhea and death. *Ann. Intern. Med.* **117:**812–819.

90. **Tarr, P. I.** 1995. *Escherichia coli* O157:H7: clinical, diagnostic, and epidemiological aspects of human infection. *Clin. Infect. Dis.* **20:**1–10.

91. **Tarr, P. I., and M. A. Neill.** 1996. Perspective: the problem of non-O157 Shiga toxin (verocytotoxin)-producing *Escherichia coli*. *J. Infect. Dis.* **174**:1136–1139.

92. **Tarr, P. I., M. A. Neill, C. R. Clausen, S. L. Watkins, D. L. Christie, and R. O. Hickman.** 1990. *Escherichia coli* O157:H7 and the hemolytic uremic syndrome: importance of early cultures in establishing the etiology. *J. Infect. Dis.* **162**:553–556.

93. **Tesh, V. L., B. Ramegowda, and J. E. Samuel.** 1994. Purified Shiga-like toxins induce expression of proinflammatory cytokines from murine peritoneal macrophages. *Infect. Immun.* **62**:5085–5094.

94. **Tilden, J., Jr., W. Young, A. M. McNamara, C. Custer, B. Boesel, M. A. Lambert-Fair, J. Majkowski, D. Vugia, S. B. Werner, J. Hollingsworth, and J. G. Morris.** 1996. A new route of transmission for *Escherichia coli*: infection from dry fermented salami. *Am. J. Public Health* **86**:1142–1145.

95. **Tzipori, S., F. Gunzer, M. S. Donnenberg, L. deMontigny, J. B. Kaper, and A. Donohue-Rolfe.** 1995. The role of *eaeA* gene in diarrhea and neurological complications in a gnotobiotic piglet model of enterohemorrhagic *Escherichia coli* infection. *Infect. Immun.* **63**:3621–3627.

96. **Tzipori, S., H. Karch, L. K. Wachsmuth, R. M. Robins-Browne, A. D. O'Brien, H. Lior, M. L. Cohen, and M. Levine.** 1987. Role of a 60-megadalton plasmid and Shiga-like toxins in the pathogenesis of infection caused by enterohemorrhagic *Escherichia coli* O157:H7 in gnotobiotic piglets. *Infect. Immun.* **55**:3117–3125.

97. **Walterspiel, J. N., S. Ashkenazi, A. L. Morrow, and T. G. Cleary.** 1992. Effect of subinhibitory concentrations of antibiotics on extracellular Shiga-like toxin I. *Infection* **20**:25–29.

98. **Watanabe, H., A. Wada, Y. Inagaki, K. Itoh, and K. Tamura.** 1996. Outbreaks of enterohaemorrhagic *Escherichia coli* O157:H7 infection by two different genotype strains in Japan, 1996. *Lancet* **348**:831–832.

99. **Waters, J. R., J. C. M. Sharp, and V. J. Dev.** 1994. Infection caused by *Escherichia coli* O157:H7 in Alberta, Canada, and in Scotland: a five-year review, 1987–1991. *Clin. Infect. Dis.* **19**:834–843.

100. **Wells, J. G., B. R. Davis, I. K. Wachsmuth, L. W. Riley, R. S. Remis, R. Sokolow, and G. K. Morris.** 1983. Laboratory investigation of hemorrhagic colitis outbreaks associated with a rare *Escherichia coli* serotype. *J. Clin. Microbiol.* **18**:512–520.

101. **Zadik, P. M., P. A. Chapman, and C. A. Siddons.** 1993. Use of tellurite for the selection of verocytotoxigenic *Escherichia coli* O157. *J. Med. Microbiol.* **39**:155–158.

chapter 13

Malaria: A Reemerging Disease

Peter B. Bloland, Ronald C. Neafie, and Aileen M. Marty

The relationship between humans and malaria is as old as written history, and probably much older. The first account of a malaria-like illness is in an Egyptian papyrus dated 1600 B.C., and Hippocrates provided the first detailed clinical description in 400 B.C. (98). Today, malaria remains one of the most common and widespread infectious diseases. It is an important public health concern in countries where transmission is common as well as in areas where transmission has been largely eliminated. In this context, thinking of malaria as an emerging infection is difficult. Nonetheless, the development, intensification, and spread of drug resistance in malaria is emerging as one of the greatest challenges to public health in malarious areas today (59).

Peter B. Bloland, Malaria Epidemiology Section, Division of Parasitic Diseases, National Center for Infectious Diseases, Centers for Disease Control and Prevention, Mailstop F-22, 1600 Clifton Road, Atlanta, GA 30333. **Ronald C. Neafie,** Parasitic Disease Pathology Branch, Geographic Pathology Division, Department of Infectious and Parasitic Disease Pathology, Armed Forces Institute of Pathology, Washington, DC 20306-6000. **Aileen M. Marty,** Infectious Disease Pathology, Department of Infectious and Parasitic Disease Pathology, Armed Forces Institute of Pathology, Washington, DC 20406-6000.

Pathology of Emerging Infections 2
Edited by Ann Marie Nelson and C. Robert Horsburgh, Jr.
© 1998 American Society for Microbiology, Washington, D.C.

Malaria is indigenous in over 90 countries worldwide, and an estimated 2.5 billion people (40% of the world's population) are at risk of malaria

Malaria is indigenous in over 90 countries worldwide, and an estimated 2.5 billion people (40% of the world's population) are at risk of malaria (24, 80) (Fig. 13.1). Each year an estimated 300 to 500 million patients will develop clinical malaria and 1.5 to 2.7 million will die, making malaria one of the most prevalent infectious diseases. The World Health Organization estimates that more than 90% of the 1.5 to 2.0 million deaths in Africa attributed to malaria each year occur in children (106). The annual economic burden of malaria infection in Africa alone for 1995 was estimated at $1.7 billion (76). The heavy clinical and financial toll associated with malaria can hinder economic and community development.

Malaria transmission occurs primarily in tropical and subtropical regions in sub-Saharan Africa, Central and South America, the Caribbean island of Hispaniola, the Middle East, the Indian subcontinent, Southeast Asia, and Oceania (Fig. 13.2). In areas where malaria occurs, however, there is considerable variation in the intensity of transmission and risk of infection. Highland (>1,500 m) and arid (<1,000 mm of rainfall a year) areas typically have less malaria, although they are also prone to epidemic malaria when parasitemic individuals provide a source of infection and climatic conditions are favorable to mosquito development (106). Although urban areas have typically been at lower risk, explosive, unplanned population growth has contributed to the increasing problem of urban malaria transmission (46).

Malaria is an extremely complex condition that manifests differently in different parts of the world, depending on a range of variables that includes the infecting parasite species and their susceptibility to antimalarial drugs; the distribution and efficiency of insect vectors; climatic and environmental conditions; and the genetic composition, acquired immunity, and behavior of human populations. In some highly malarious areas, children, pregnant women, and nonimmune visitors are at greatest risk of severe or fatal infections; in less endemic areas, all age groups are affected. The clinical presentation of malaria can vary widely from area to area, from predominately acute, non-severe, febrile disease to large-scale epidemics with high mortality rates, and from chronic anemia to acute neurologic disease.

Malaria affects nonendemic areas as well. In the United States, more than 1,000 cases of malaria are reported each year (45). Nearly all of the malaria cases reported in the United States develop in immigrants, refugees, and travelers from parts of the world where ongoing transmission persists. A small number of malaria cases, however, are acquired within the United States. Some of these cases are congenitally acquired, while some are associated with blood transfusion, organ donation, or sharing needles with infected persons. Over the last 14 years, there have been 19 instances of malaria transmitted by local anopheline mosquitoes (26–28, 46, 62, 109; Centers for Disease Control and Prevention [CDC], unpublished data). These instances of mosquito-borne malaria in the United States are of concern because they demonstrate the potential for reintroduction of transmission, even in temperate climates where malaria has been eradicated.

Agent and Life Cycle

In humans, infection is caused by one or more of four species of malarial parasite: *Plasmodium falciparum*, *P. vivax*, *P. ovale*, and *P. malariae*. Each species differs in geographic distribution, microscopic appearance, clinical features (periodicity of infection, potential for severe or complicated disease, and tendency for clinical relapses or recrudescences), and immunogenic potential (Table 13.1). Although *P. vivax* infections are more commonly reported worldwide, *P. falciparum* malaria represents the most serious public health problem because of its tendency to severe or fatal infections.

Transmission and Classification of Malaria

Malaria is typically transmitted by the bite of an infective female *Anopheles* mosquito. The majority of malaria seen in the United States is acquired during travel to malaria-endemic areas (*imported malaria*), although occasionally local mosquitoes can become infected by gametocytemic individuals and pass the infection to nontravelers (*autochthonous* or *introduced malaria*). Malaria can be transmitted without mosquitoes as well. *Congenital malaria* refers to infection passed from mother to infant in utero or during birth (18). *Induced malaria* refers to infection that is passed directly from one individual to another, either intentionally (such as with malariotherapy) or accidentally, through contaminated blood or blood products, injection equipment, or organ transplant (22). Until the 1950s, malariotherapy was widely used as a treatment for late neurosyphilis (8, 99). Malariotherapy has resurfaced, primarily as an unproven alternative medicine practice for diseases as diverse as Lyme disease, HIV, and breast cancer (25). Finally, when a route of transmission cannot be established, even after careful investigation, a case is classified as *cryptic malaria*.

> *Malaria is typically transmitted by the bite of an infective female Anopheles mosquito*

Table 13.1 Clinical characteristics of the four species of human malaria[a]

Clinical features	P. falciparum	P. vivax	P. ovale	P. malariae
Exoerythrocytic cycle	6–7 days	6–8 days	9 days	14–16 days
Prepatent period	9–10 days	11–13 days	10–14 days	15–16 days
Incubation period (mean)	9–14 (12) days	12–17 (15) days to 6–12 months	16–18 (17) days or longer	18–40 (28) days or longer
Severity of primary attack	Severe	Mild to severe	Severe	Severe
Duration of primary attack[b]	16–36 h or longer	8–12 h	8–12 h	8–10 h
Duration of untreated infection[b]	1–2 yrs	1.5–5 yrs	1.5–5 yrs	3–50 yrs
Relapse	No	Yes	Yes	No
Central nervous system complications[b]	Frequent	Infrequent	Infrequent	Infrequent
Anemia[b]	Frequent	Common	Infrequent	Infrequent
Renal insufficiency[b]	Common	Infrequent	Infrequent	Infrequent
Effects on pregnancy[b]	Frequent	Infrequent	Unknown	Unknown
Hypoglycemia	Frequent	Unknown	Unknown	Unknown

[a]Adapted from reference 20a.
[b]Influenced by immunity. Documentation of complications for species other than *P. falciparum* is limited.

Life Cycle and Symptoms

Malaria infection begins when an infective female mosquito injects *Plasmodium* sp. sporozoites into the bloodstream while feeding. The sporozoites circulate only momentarily; those that survive host immune defenses infect cells of the liver parenchyma. There they undergo asexual reproduction (exoerythrocytic schizogony), producing hepatic schizonts.

In 6 to 14 days, these schizonts mature and rupture, releasing merozoites into the bloodstream. Merozoites then invade red blood cells (RBCs), where they undergo a second phase of asexual reproduction (erythrocytic schizogony), developing into rings, trophozoites, and finally erythrocytic schizonts. Once the parasites mature, the infected RBCs rupture, releasing still more merozoites into the bloodstream and starting another cycle of asexual development and multiplication.

The rupture of erythrocytic schizonts produces clinical symptoms which usually develop after several cycles of erythrocytic schizogony. Typical incubation periods range from 9 to 30 days, depending on infecting species, and can be prolonged in patients taking medicines with antimalarial properties or among patients who have developed a semi-immune status from repeated attacks. The classical clinical presentation of periodic fever occurs when the cycles of erythrocytic schizogony are synchronized and, in practice, only occurs occasionally.

Some merozoites differentiate into sexual forms called gametocytes. Both male and female gametocytes circulate without causing symptoms and can be ingested by a mosquito during a subsequent blood meal. Sexual reproduction occurs within the mosquito midgut. The fertilized zygote quickly transforms into an amoeboid ookinete that penetrates the midgut wall and forms an oocyst. After several days to weeks, the oocyst ruptures, releasing sporozoites that migrate through the coelomic cavity to the salivary glands. The life cycle starts again when the infective mosquito bites another human.

P. vivax and *P. ovale* can produce a dormant form (hypnozoites) which can persist in the liver from months up to 3 or 4 years, causing periodic relapses of parasitemia and illness. Hypnozoites result only from primary sporozoite inoculation in mosquito-borne infections and are not present after cases of induced or congenital malaria. While *P. falciparum* and *P. malariae* do not form hypnozoites, infection with these parasites can persist in the blood at subpatent or undetectable levels after resolution of symptoms. This very low-level parasitemia can result in recrudescence of clinical disease. Except in partially immune persons, *P. falciparum* rarely recrudesces more than several months after initial infection. However, recrudescent *P. malariae* infections can occur 40 years or longer after infection.

The classical clinical presentation of periodic fever occurs when the cycles of erythrocytic schizogony are synchronized and, in practice, only occurs occasionally

Clinical Manifestations

Typical symptoms include fever, chills, myalgias, arthralgias, headache, diarrhea, and other nonspecific signs. Other findings might include enlarged liver and spleen, anemia, thrombocytopenia, pulmonary or renal dysfunction, and neurologic involvement. The initial symptoms of a malaria infection can be modified by immunity or antimalarial drugs, causing the illness to intensify more slowly or to appear milder than would normally be expected. In the United States approximately four people die from malaria each year. Risk factors for mortality include delays in diagnosis and initiation of specific treatment, failure to adhere to malaria chemoprophylaxis recommendations during travel, and older age (CDC, unpublished data). Cerebral manifestations of malaria can develop at any peripheral parasite density. Falciparum malaria during pregnancy, particularly among nonimmune women, carries a high risk for both fetus and mother, potentially causing maternal and/or fetal death, acute pulmonary edema, prematurity, or low birth weight (104).

Pathogenesis

Malaria is a systemic disease. The parasites are in the circulatory system, and therefore every organ is affected (Table 13.2). The most direct effect by malarial parasites is RBC breakdown leading to loss of RBCs and release of endogenous pyrogens (tumor necrosis factor [TNF], macrophage inflammatory protein 1α [MIP-1α], and MIP-1β). These pyrogens mediate the induction of fever and other signs and symptoms of acute inflammation. In addition, *P. falciparum* organisms alter parasitized RBC (pRBC) membranes, causing pRBCs to clog blood vessels and produce more serious consequences. The remaining pathophysiologic repercussions are indirect and variable. Accordingly, the clinical symptoms of malaria are variable, depending on the species involved, the level of parasitemia, and host factors.

Congestion and edema develop in virtually all tissues of individuals killed by falciparum malaria. Patients usually die from cerebral involvement, renal failure, or pulmonary edema. Localization of parasites in tissue capillaries depends to an extent on the parasite load. Finding parasites in nonvital tissues such as skin, skeletal muscle, and adipose tissue probably represents an overwhelming parasitemia.

Cellular and Humoral Immunity

Overeager cellular and humoral immune responses produce a large part of the damage in patients with malaria. This is readily apparent in hyperreactive malarial splenomegaly (HMS) and renal complications, but is also a feature of cerebral malaria, anemia, and jaundice. T cells reactive against malaria parasites express a memory phenotype (CD45Ro$^+$, CD45Ra$^-$, CD4$^+$) (35). These T cells arise in two ways, (i) through stimulation with organisms that cross-react with malaria and (ii) through direct exposure to malaria parasites.

T cells induced by the parasite itself (unlike T cells produced to cross-reactive organisms) do not have an attraction for other organs and are more likely to circulate through the spleen. Parasite-reactive T cells release cytokines that contribute to the pathologic manifestations (44). In the spleen the cytokines released by parasite-reactive T cells tend to facilitate interactions between other T cells, monocytes, neutrophils, and parasites

Overeager cellular and humoral immune responses produce a large part of the damage in patients with malaria

Table 13.2 Interrelated processes that lead to clinical illness

Fever and its physiologic consequences
    Delirium or unconsciousness
    Febrile convulsions
    Nutritional and metabolic changes
    Alterations in liver metabolism
Hemolysis
    Anemia
    Hyperkalemia
    Unconjugated hyperbilirubinemia
Hypersplenism
    Anemia
    Clotting defects
Anemia
    Tissue hypoxia
    Tachycardia
Tissue hypoxia
    Liver injury
    Cerebral anoxia
    Intestinal injury
    Pulmonary damage
Host immune response
    Hyperreactive malarial splenomegaly (tropical splenomegaly syndrome)
        Increased reticulocytes
        Thrombocytopenia
        Leukopenia, but increased proportion of villous lymphocytes or lymphocytosis
        Hyperglobulinemia (polyclonal IgM with cryoglobulinemia, reduced C3, and rheumatoid factor)
    Renal disease
    Clotting defects
    Elevated serum euglobulin (IgG, IgM)
    False-positive VDRL
Liver injury
    Prothrombin deficiency
    Hypoglycemia
    Cholesterol and lecithin alterations
    Disturbed glycogenic function
    Decreased production of albumin and other plasma proteins
    Elevated conjugated bilirubinemia
    ALT (SGPT) elevations during fever spikes
Renal disease
    Elevated BUN and creatinine
    Hemoglobinemia and hemoglobinuria (in blackwater fever)
    Proteinuria
Pulmonary damage
    Cough
    Pulmonary edema
Gastrointestinal injury
    Malabsorption leading to diarrhea
    Erosion, ulceration
    Blood in stools

and directly contribute to parasite death. The sharp increase in immunity and decline in pathologic changes in later childhood in endemic areas are attributed to an increase in the number of T cells induced by the parasite itself (41).

Symptoms may be severe with any *Plasmodium* species, but life-threatening disease is common only in *P. falciparum* infection. The rare fatal outcome in patients with *P. vivax*, *P. ovale*, or *P. malariae* is generally the result of traumatic or spontaneous splenic rupture. Malarial parasites of nonhuman primates (*P. inui*, *P. eylesi*, *P. simium*, *P. brasilianum*, *P. shorttii*, *P. cynomolgi*, *P. cynomolgi-bastianelli*, and *P. knowlesi*) (67, 96, 99) can, in rare instances, infect humans; these infections cause a relatively mild disease.

Fever

Plasmodium species cause fever, and the fever periodicity varies with the interval of release of merozoites. There is a direct temporal correlation between the release of merozoites from infected RBCs and the febrile paroxysm. For *P. falciparum*, *P. vivax*, and *P. ovale*, merozoite populations erupt out of pRBCs approximately every 48 h; with *P. malariae* they erupt about every 72 h. Thus, classically, the fever is intermittent and the pattern varies with the species.

What confuses the clinical picture is that more than one population of merozoites may exit RBCs at dysynchronous times. In primary infection, fever is usually irregular and has no distinct pattern; the pattern becomes intermittent when (and if) the exodus of merozoites becomes synchronized. During the early phase of *P. vivax* infection it is common for merozoite populations to exit pRBCs dysynchronously, with a corresponding dyssynchronous fever periodicity. Likewise, patients with *P. falciparum* with high parasitemia often experience a continuous fever with intermittent elevations of temperature but without a resting stage. Finally, the fever in patients with mixed infections (infection with more than one species of malaria) may have no discernible pattern (17).

The rupture of pRBCs releases merozoites and other plasmodial antigens (42) such as hemozoin (malarial pigment). Hemozoin is apparently one of the key substances that induce the production of the pyrogenic cytokines (TNF, cachectin), MIP-1α, and MIP-1β (77). The precise mechanism is uncertain but probably involves the following sequence:

1. Plasmodial antigens activate T cells in various ways (53), leading to release of IL-2.
2. IL-2 stimulates T-helper cell production of gamma interferon, which activates monocytes that produce IL-1 and TNF (35, 61).
3. TNF and IL-1 synergistically help mediate the host response to acute inflammation leading to fever.

This rise in TNF and IL-1 also causes leukocytosis, increased muscle proteolysis, modifications in carbohydrate, lipid, and trace mineral metabolism, and profound changes in the plasma concentrations of liver-derived plasma proteins. TNF and IL-1 induce the expression of phospholipase A_2,

More than one population of merozoites may exit RBCs at dysynchronous times

a proinflammatory enzyme (91, 92). Phospholipase A_2 rises in direct relation with the severity of malaria and may be largely responsible for the physiologic complications of severe malaria (respiratory distress, acute renal failure, disseminated intravascular coagulation, and sometimes shock) (90).

These cytokines act as pyrogens on the hypothalamus, causing the release of prostaglandins. The prostaglandins act on the posterior hypothalamus to stimulate sympathetic nerves to contract blood vessels and decrease heat loss. This leads to the three stages of malarial fever:

1. *Cold stage.* The patient experiences a feeling of intense cold that stimulates shivering and rigor. This can last 30 min to an hour.
2. *Hot stage.* The patient experiences an intense dry heat. This stage lasts 2 to 6 h and is often accompanied by headache, nausea, and vomiting.
3. *Perspiration stage.* Profuse sweating leads to a rapid drop in fever. The patient experiences a sense of well-being.

Anemia

Anemia is a common complication of malaria and can cause death

Anemia is a common complication of malaria and can cause death. The two predominant clinical presentations are severe acute malaria, and severe anemia in patients with repeated attacks of malaria. The degree of anemia correlates with parasitemia, schizontemia, serum bilirubin, and serum creatinine. Anemia can lead to secondary bacterial infection and retinal hemorrhage. Pregnancy increases the risk of anemia. HLA-associated genetic factors, common in areas endemic for malaria, may protect against the development of anemia (63).

Anemia results from both decreased production and increased destruction of RBCs (102). Increased destruction is caused by (i) extensive hemolysis (loss of pRBCs by rupture during schizogony [55] or phagocytosis of uninfected RBCs from antibody sensitization or physiochemical membrane changes) and (ii) splenic sequestration of pRBCs. Decreased production results from (i) marrow hypoplasia (acute infections) and (ii) ineffective erythropoiesis leading to a decrease in the peripheral reticulocytes needed to compensate for hemolytic anemia (97).

Grossly, the bone marrow is slightly pigmented. Red and white cell hyperplasia, pRBCs, and phagocytic cells filled with pigment are observed under the microscope. There may be evidence of dyserythropoiesis, the morphological expression of ineffective erythropoiesis. TNF is implicated as the cause of dyserythropoiesis (30, 31).

Rarely, massive hemolysis develops in *P. falciparum* malaria, leading to extensive hemoglobinuria, a condition known as blackwater fever. Blackwater fever is rare in patients native to endemic areas. The risk is greater in nonimmune persons with high parasitemia or with an atypical immune response during reinfection. Sometimes, hypersensitivity to quinine or ingestion of oxidant antimalarial agents in patients with glucose-6-phosphate dehydrogenase (G6PD) deficiency seems to stimulate blackwater fever.

Liver Damage

Jaundice is common in adult patients, particularly those with severe falciparum malaria, but rare in African children. The jaundice is mainly a manifestation of unconjugated bilirubinemia secondary to hemolysis, but there is also some degree of hepatocyte damage. In severe falciparum malaria the hepatocyte damage can be marked and coupled with cholestasis; this is reflected as an increase in the percentage of conjugated bilirubinemia. Tender enlargement of the liver is a common finding in malaria, especially in young children and nonimmune adults. Hepatomegaly in acute malaria is mainly the result of congestion. In chronic malaria, chronic enlargement of the liver results from an increase in malarial pigment and some fine fibrosis of the portal tracts.

Gross. In patients dying with a primary attack of falciparum malaria the liver is markedly congested. If malaria is more chronic the liver is slightly enlarged and soft, usually with a slate-gray to black discoloration, but it can be dark chocolate-red.

Microscopic. Hyperplasia and hypertrophy of Kupffer cells containing pRBCs and birefringent malarial pigment are observed. Parasitized RBCs are also found in sinusoids and centrilobular veins. In severe infections, centrilobular necrosis occurs. Some livers show fatty infiltration, possibly caused by malarial toxins (10).

Alterations to the Spleen

Hypersplenism is nearly universal in acute malaria (107). The spleen enlarges early in infection with *P. vivax* and *P. falciparum* but later in *P. malariae*. Splenic size varies with duration and degree of exposure. Enlargement results primarily from impeded blood flow but also from the aggregation of phagocytes. Splenic rupture is most likely in the acute stage, especially during the primary attack. *P. vivax* is the most frequent cause of spontaneous rupture, but all four species can cause splenic rupture (39). Lack of prior immunity to malaria may be a major predisposing factor (108).

Acutely, the spleen is enlarged, soft, and diffusely pigmented, with rounded edges and a thin capsule. Chronically, the capsule is thickened and the enlargement is more solid. Microscopically there is congestion and reticuloendothelial hyperplasia. Pigment-filled phagocytic cells and pRBCs line the sinusoids. Immature forms of parasites are preferentially phagocytosed (65). The malpighian corpuscles are relatively small. On occasion there are hemorrhages and infarcts. In chronic malaria, fibrosis, Gamna-Gandy bodies, and a concentration of pigment along arterioles are observed. Malaria can cause other damage to the spleen such as hematoma, torsion, cyst formation, and hyperreactive malarial splenomegaly.

HMS (hyperreactive malarial splenomegaly, tropical splenomegaly syndrome) refers to a combination of splenomegaly, high antimalarial antibodies, and high serum immunoglobulin M (IgM) content. HMS is mainly a disease of adult residents of endemic areas of tropical and sub-Saharan

Hypersplenism is nearly universal in acute malaria

Africa and parts of New Guinea and Vietnam. Only a small percentage of adults develop HMS, mainly those with a high malarial antibody titer. It is twice as common in women as in men. Hereditary factors may play a role since it is extremely rare in European Caucasians despite long-term residency in endemic areas (only six reported cases) (36, 93). The cause relates to an abnormal immunological response to prolonged *Plasmodium* exposure. In these patients, *Plasmodium* organisms inhibit T-suppressor cells, allowing for an increase in B-cell production of IgM and, consequentially, immune complex formation. The condition is usually benign and chronic; however, there is an increased risk of secondary infection, and some patients develop severe anemia. The spleen is massively enlarged, with dilated sinusoids lined with phagocytic cells containing parasitized RBCs. There is lymphocytic infiltration of the pulp and, often, characteristic changes in the liver and peripheral blood. The liver shows sinusoidal dilation, lymphocytic infiltration, and hyperplasia of pigment-laden Kupffer cells. Also observed are a normocytic, normochromic anemia, increased numbers of reticulocytes, leukopenia (although in some patients there is a prominent lymphocytosis), thrombocytopenia, and hyperglobulinemia due to polyclonal IgM with cryoglobulinemia, reduced C3, and the presence of rheumatoid factor.

Lymphoproliferative Disorders and HMS

A study in Ghana revealed that patients with a clinical diagnosis of HMS had significant numbers of villous lymphocytes in their peripheral blood. These patients had over 30% villous lymphocytes but no leukocytosis. The discovery of uncommon villous lymphocytes in both nonmalignant and malignant disorders in the same geographical area suggested that HMS may increase the risk for B-cell splenic lymphoma with villous lymphocytes. Specifically, the excessive proliferation of polyclonal B lymphocytes, driven by frequent exposure to *Plasmodium*, may predispose to the emergence of a malignant lymphoma in tropical West Africa (13). In another study from Ghana, some patients with HMS had a prominent lymphocytosis in blood and bone marrow that clinically resembled chronic lymphocytic leukemia. Clonal rearrangement studies of the Jh region in these patients revealed that some of these patients had developed clonal lymphoproliferation and had clinical features intermediate between HMS and chronic lymphocytic leukemia, supporting the hypothesis that HMS may evolve into a malignant lymphoproliferative disorder (12).

Gastrointestinal Damage

Impaired blood flow can cause malabsorption. Patients with *P. falciparum* can develop an impediment to the blood flow from the clogging of capillaries by altered RBCs. Patients present with intense diarrhea. If severe tissue anoxia develops there can be necrosis leading to erosion and ulceration of the mucosa. The damaged mucosa leads to intestinal bleeding with occult blood in the stool. Microscopic examination reveals that RBCs in the stool contain malarial parasites. In severe infections, patients may have bright red blood per rectum.

*P*atients with P. falciparum can develop an impediment to the blood flow from the clogging of capillaries by altered RBCs

On gross examination any portion of the gastrointestinal tract may be edematous and congested, with or without hemorrhagic foci. Microscopically, the mucosa is edematous and small vessels may contain parasitized RBCs and pigment. In severe cases there is erosion and ulceration of the mucosa.

Renal Damage

A high percentage of patients demonstrate elevated serum creatinine and blood urea nitrogen, but the cause is usually pre-renal. Only a small percentage of patients develop true renal lesions. Falciparum malaria may cause immunological renal disease (acute and transient proliferative glomerulonephritis) and/or ischemic renal lesions (that range from mild proteinuria with urinary sediment changes to acute renal failure). Quartan malaria (*P. malariae*) may cause an immune complex nephritis with clinical and biochemical features of a childhood nephrotic syndrome, but with distinct changes under light, electron, and immunofluorescence microscopy. Renal damage in patients with *P. vivax* and *P. ovale* is very rare and generally mild and nonspecific.

Renal disease in falciparum malaria. Acute and transient proliferative glomerulonephritis is generally mild. Patients have mild hematuria and proteinuria. The symptoms usually disappear with treatment but can develop into a persistent nephritic syndrome. Glomerulonephritis is proliferative and varies from mesangial to segmental to mildly diffuse. Repeat biopsy after treatment generally reveals no residual pathology, and the lesion is reversible (70).

Less commonly, patients may develop malaria-associated renal failure. The majority of these patients develop the clinical and biochemical features of acute tubular necrosis, often accompanied by liver dysfunction (87). Uncommonly, the cause is acute cortical necrosis (78). Heavy parasitemia (>5% parasitized RBCs) and excessive intravascular hemolysis are risk factors for malaria-associated renal failure. Renal hyperfusion, oxygen-free radicals, complement activation, and hyperpyrexia contribute to the renal injury.

Patients may develop malaria-associated renal failure

Renal disease in quartan malaria. Chronic progressive glomerulonephritis is most common in children and presents as a nephrotic syndrome. Eventually the edema disappears, but the proteinuria persists with gradual development of hypertension and renal failure which does not respond to antimalarial therapy. Proliferative changes are common in some countries (e.g., Uganda), especially in adults, but rare in others (e.g., Nigeria). Renal histology is distinctive and does not conform to any of the categories included in the conventional classification of the nephrotic syndrome in childhood. The basic lesion consists of thickening of glomerular capillary walls (which can be plexiform), leading to eventual obliteration of capillary lumina and accompanying mesangial sclerosis (focal segmental sclerosis) that ultimately develops into total glomerular sclerosis (43). In addition to the progressive loss of glomeruli, there is tubular atrophy.

Electron microscopy reveals variable degrees of cellular proliferation, mesangial matrix formation, and electron-dense deposits in mesangial cells. The capillaries have thickened basement membranes along with subepithelial and intramembranous deposits and occasionally subendothelial deposits. The combination of mesangial proliferation with subepithelial and intramembranous deposits can mimic the membranous and proliferative glomerulonephritis of systemic lupus erythematosus. In other patients, the changes resemble those of mesangiocapillary (membranoproliferative) glomerulonephritis.

Early on, in patients that usually respond to treatment, immunofluorescence is coarsely granular, but later, in patients who are unresponsive to treatment, immunofluorescence tends to be diffuse. Immunofluorescence reveals immunoglobulins (IgM, IgG), C3, and occasionally C1q and C4 in the glomeruli. One-third to one-fourth of patients also have malarial antigens in the glomeruli, suggesting the deposition of immune complexes. Usually, in acute disease the deposits are mesangial and lie along the capillary wall as fine or coarse granules, while in chronic disease the deposits are in short linear stretches.

In patients with P. vivax and P. ovale infection, benign tertian malaria can occasionally cause a nephrotic syndrome

In patients with *P. vivax* and *P. ovale* infection, benign tertian malaria can occasionally cause a nephrotic syndrome. Renal biopsy reveals generalized mesangial cell proliferation, matrix expansion, and basement membrane thickening, sometimes accompanied by tubular atrophy and focal interstitial inflammation and fibrosis. Immunohistochemical stains reveal fine granular staining along the capillary loops and glomeruli basement membrane for IgM and IgA and sometimes IgG (15).

Thrombocytopenia and Clotting Defects

Loss of platelets may result from an immune mechanism (56) or hypersplenism. Decreased platelets can cause prothrombin deficiency, leading to coagulation defects and, in severe infections, disseminated intravascular coagulation.

Pulmonary Damage

Many patients experience cough and mild bronchitis in the early stages of malaria. Only a small percentage develop the dreaded complication of malarial lung. Malarial lung is an acute, noncardiogenic pulmonary insufficiency that presents as pulmonary edema.

Acute malarial lung manifests 2 to 3 days after chills and fever in approximately 3.5 to 7% of patients with *P. falciparum* infection (4, 48). Usually, pulmonary edema begins abruptly and progresses rapidly to death despite intensive treatment, often within a day after the diagnosis (66). The cause of the acute pulmonary distress is not known (34), but it is not secondary to heart failure. Increased capillary permeability may be the mechanism (29, 72). Cytoadherence of malarial parasites could cause increased capillary permeability (32), but pulmonary symptoms can progress even after drug therapy has eliminated parasitemia. Delay in chemotherapy appears to contribute to the development of pulmonary complications. Some patients suffer from injury to septal capillaries with resulting microinfarcts as a consequence of increased release of TNF (82).

A milder, nonfatal, atypical pulmonary malaria develops in some patients (23). These patients have pleural effusions, interstitial edema, and lobar consolidation. Symptoms resolve with antimalarial chemotherapy.

Grossly, the lungs are generally unremarkable, except in patients with malarial lung. In malarial lung there is brown-red pleural effusion and the lungs are heavy and edematous. These lungs are congested and have petechial hemorrhages. Microscopically, alveolar walls become thickened by swollen endothelial cells and an infiltrate of chronic inflammatory cells. There are scattered pRBCs in capillaries. Cytoadherence of pRBCs within capillaries is thought to cause septal interstitial edema (32). In more severe cases, capillary congestion, hyaline membranes, thickened alveolar septa, alveolar and interstitial edema, and hemozoin-laden macrophages can be found. Additionally, there can be injury to septal capillaries with resulting microinfarcts. Numerous trophozoites of *P. falciparum* are found within RBCs in septal capillaries (37). There may be evidence of disseminated intravascular coagulation.

Cerebral Injury

The high fevers caused by malaria can lead to delirium or unconsciousness, and some patients experience febrile convulsions. Alterations in liver metabolism and immunologic factors also contribute to some degree of neurologic damage, but the most profound cerebral injury is cerebral malaria. Cerebral malaria is the most common and most deadly complication of falciparum malaria. There is now some evidence that cerebral sequestration is not specific to falciparum malaria but also manifests in the brain and eyes of some patients with *P. vivax* infection (5, 74, 86).

Blockage of cerebral microvasculature by infected RBCs (cerebral sequestration) is the proximate cause of cerebral malaria. There is significantly more sequestration in the brains of patients with clinical cerebral malaria than in patients without cerebral malaria. Knobs form on *P. falciparum*-infected RBC membranes, which adhere to the endothelium and cause obstruction of cerebral microvessels. The knobs consist of malarial adherence ligands which vary in their ability to bind, depending on the isolate (40). PfEmp1 (*P. falciparum* erythrocyte membrane protein 1) is a very large malarial protein that gathers on the surface of the infected RBCs and binds to the host receptors (11). Protein molecules of endothelial cell membranes such as CD36 (platelet glycoprotein IV), ICAM-1 (intercellular adhesion molecule-1, CD-54), VCAM-1 (adhesion molecule of the immunoglobulin superfamily expressed on endothelial cells), E-selectin (endothelial cell selectin adhesion molecule), and TSP (thrombospondin) act as receptors for attachment (1, 2, 60, 88). CD36 of endothelial cells helps bind monocytes. ICAM-1 binds infected RBCs to monocytes (89).

The pathogenesis of cerebral malaria remains a mystery. Adhesion of parasitized RBCs to cerebral endothelial cells does not always cause destruction (88). Several factors including sludging (leading to hypoxia), modifications

The pathogenesis of cerebral malaria remains a mystery

of blood-brain barrier permeability, mechanical phenomena (vasculitis or intraluminal deposition of fibrin-platelet thrombi), immunological processes (intravascular complement activation), and metabolic phenomena (metabolite competition or local parasite toxin) may be responsible (3). Several cytokines, mainly TNF and IL-1, seem to be involved. Congenital host factors (as suggested by HLA group) as well as acquired immunologic/nutritional deficiencies can alter the consequences of infection. In addition, parasite factors such as strain characteristics can also modify the outcome.

Survivors rarely have any residual neurologic defects, and therefore a reduction in blood flow, microthrombus formation, inflammation, and cerebral edema as the pathogenic mechanism of cerebral malaria are unlikely. It is more plausible that the syndrome represents a metabolic encephalopathy. Sequestration of infected RBCs in cerebral microvasculature leads to marked glucose use and lactate production by the parasite, which may result in local disturbances in brain metabolism (104). The concept of metabolic alterations is supported by studies revealing that antioxidants can prevent experimental cerebral malaria in mice (50, 85).

Grossly the brain is edematous and heavy, with broad flattened gyre, grooving of uncinate and cingulate gyre, and flattening of the cerebellar tonsils. There is selective congestion of white matter. Congestion of arachnoid vessels produces "pink brain." Microscopically, pRBCs stick to the endothelium, causing occlusion (Fig. 13.3). If the patient survives at least 9 days with clinical malaria, then the following three changes can be seen: (i) ring hemorrhages, frequently with a central capillary, surrounded by necrotic neural parenchyma (Fig. 13.4); (ii) perivascular glial proliferations (Dürck's granulomas); and (iii) focal demyelinations. In addition, focal areas of endothelial cell degeneration, hyperplasia, and necrosis are present. The ring hemorrhages consist of concentric rings surrounding a central necrosed cerebral vessel. The outermost ring contains a mixture of parasitized RBCs, free pigment, and monocytes; the inner layer shows uninfected RBCs and gliosis. Birefringent malarial pigment is present within the capillaries. The distinctive pattern suggests that ring hemorrhages may result from re-perfusion to a cerebral microvessel previously filled with sequestered parasitized RBCs. Perivascular and ring hemorrhages are more frequent in the white matter than in the cortex (58). Rarely, a few ring hemorrhages are present in the brains of malaria patients who did not have clinical evidence of cerebral malaria. Dürck's granulomas consist of perivascular patchy gliosis with extravasated monocytes. Some monocytes contain phagocytized malarial pigment. Most likely the ring hemorrhages and Dürck's granuloma represent a temporal spectrum of the same lesion (88). Even patients who survive cerebral malaria long enough to receive treatment may remain in coma and die with little histological evidence of cerebral sequestration of parasitized RBCs, but they will certainly have malaria pigment in cerebral vessels.

Ultrastructurally, a progressive deterioration of the blood-brain barrier leads ultimately to endothelial lesions and hemorrhage. First there is adherence of blood cells, singularly and in clusters, to the endothelium. The infected cells interdigitate with the vascular endothelial lining. Endothelial

The distinctive pattern suggests that ring hemorrhages may result from re-perfusion to a cerebral microvessel previously filled with sequestered parasitized RBCs

cells become activated, exhibiting pseudopodia formation, increased pinocytotic activity with lipid droplet accumulation, and phagocytic activity. Endothelial cells phagocytize parasitized RBCs and contain ghosts and membrane remnants. Frequently, white cells migrate between endothelial cells, causing them to lift off and die. These changes are associated with degenerative changes in the basement membrane, where swelling with deposition of collagenlike fibers and loss of fragments is observed. In some places fingerlike extensions of pericytes pass through the basement membrane and bulge into the cytoplasm of endothelial cells. Ballooning and coalescence of perivascular astrocytes contribute to the appearance of a perivascular edematous space (64).

The eyes of patients with malarial infection may show multiple superficial blotchy retinal hemorrhages over the posterior pole, or acute bilateral panuveitis with changes caused by secondary glaucoma that may resolve with antimalarial therapy to multiple blotchy superficial retinal hemorrhages with perivasculitis, or subconjunctival and retinal hemorrhages (mainly in the posterior pole). Microscopically there is cytoadherence of parasitized RBCs (16).

The placenta is usually unremarkable grossly, but microscopically there is accumulation of parasitized RBCs, pigment, and occasional mononuclear cells in the maternal blood space (49, 84). On electron microscopy there is thickening and duplication of the trophoblastic basement membrane (83).

Diagnosis

Malaria Infections

Thick and thin blood films should be prepared from any patient suspected of having malaria (6, 7). The thick film is for establishing the diagnosis of malaria, and the thin film helps in determining the species. The thick film permits a fairly rapid examination of a large amount of blood and often reveals light infections. It is estimated that the thick film is 25 times better than the thin film for diagnosis because 16 to 30 times as much blood could be examined in the same time. Thick blood films should be studied using the oil-immersion objective, and the examiner should search for at least 5 min (100 fields) before reporting "no parasites seen." Thin blood films best demonstrate the morphologic features of the parasite and permit an evaluation of the size of the parasitized erythrocyte.

For best results all blood smears should be stained with a good-quality Giemsa stain that has been diluted with distilled water buffered to pH 7.0–7.2. It is essential that the blood films be carefully prepared and meticulously stained. The slides should be scrupulously clean, free from chemicals, grease, dust, and scratches. Since blood loses its affinity for stain, all blood films should be stained within 72 h and preferably within 24 h. If the first blood film is negative, additional thick and thin films should be obtained every 6 h for 2 days.

The morphologic features of the parasite and the characteristics of the infected erythrocyte are best seen in thin blood films. It should be emphasized

Thick and thin blood films should be prepared from any patient suspected of having malaria

that malarial parasites are almost always found within the erythrocyte. Three basic stages of the malarial parasite are observed in peripheral blood, trophozoites (growing forms), schizonts (dividing forms), and gametocytes (sexual forms). A table describing the common features of the four species, as seen in thin peripheral blood films, is included (Table 13.3).

Mixed infections are probably more common in highly infected areas than are diagnosed by the microscopist. Technicians usually look no further after identifying one species. There also seems to be a tendency in mixed infections for one species to predominate over others, thus making the rarer species more difficult to identify. The diagnosis of a mixed infection is made cautiously.

Exflagellated parasites, a form (microgametocyte) normally present in the mosquito's stomach, have been observed in thin peripheral blood smears made from humans. This occurs through a series of events probably unnoticed by the laboratory technician. The exflagellated parasite is usually composed of one large mass or two closely related central masses from which four to six cytoplasmic flagellum-like processes protrude. Each of these may contain a chromatin dot somewhere along its length. These have been erroneously interpreted as spirochetes.

In the process of identifying malarial parasites, one must consider changes that take place in erythrocytes, changes the parasite makes during maturation, variations between species at any specific stage, and the reaction by the patient to the particular infection. A process of elimination can be useful in the identification of the various species, since it is often easier to proceed

Exflagellated parasites, a form (microgametocyte) normally present in the mosquito's stomach, have been observed in thin peripheral blood smears made from humans

Table 13.3 Microscopic and morphologic features of human malaria parasites

Feature	P. falciparum	P. vivax	P. ovale	P. malariae
Size of infected erythrocyte	Normal	Enlarged	Enlarged	Normal to smaller
Morphology/ microscopic characteristics	Maurer's dots present	Schüffner's dots present	Schüffner's dots present	Ziemann's dots rarely present
	Frequent multiply-infected cell	Occasional multiply-infected cell	Occasional multiply-infected cell	Rare multiply-infected cell
	Frequent double chromatin dots	Occasional double chromatin dots	Occasional double chromatin dots	Rare double chromatin dots
	Pigment brown-black	Pigment yellow-brown	Pigment yellow-brown	Pigment black
	Usually ring forms only	All stages present	All stages present	All stages present
	Frequent appliqué trophozoites	Ameboid trophozoites	Fimbriation of erythrocyte	Band-form trophozoites
Number and size of merozoites in mature schizont	8–24, very small	12–24, small, grape-like cluster	4–16, very large, rosette pattern	6–12, large, rosette pattern
Shape of gametocytes	Crescent shaped	Round	Round	Round

when one determines first what the species in question *cannot* be, rather than what it can be. Of course, to do this one must be sure of what one is seeing and the proper interpretation. Sometimes, if parasites are rare and only ring forms are present, the species may not be determined. It should also be emphasized that pigment cannot always be observed in ring trophozoites of malaria, and although babesiosis may be considered, malaria is not excluded.

Artifacts frequently may be mistaken for malarial parasites. This is especially true for the inexperienced microscopist who does not realize the structures in question lie above the blood plane, or they may be refractile and focus out of the microscopic field unevenly. Bacteria, dirt from skin, dust particles, vegetable spores, yeast cells or fungi, and other protozoans can all be mistaken for malarial parasites. The stain itself may precipitate and appear as a parasite. Sometimes red dots appear without any cytoplasm, but one should never call a slide positive on the basis of these dots alone. Several erythrocyte abnormalities can be mistaken for parasites. Platelets are frequently confused with malarial parasites. Malarial parasites occurring outside erythrocytes in thin blood films should be diagnosed carefully.

The definitive diagnosis of malaria, during life, is usually made by identifying the parasite in thick or thin films of peripheral blood. This is time-consuming and subject to error in unskilled hands. Newer technologies have been developed which aid the diagnosis of malaria, especially in settings where skilled, experienced microscopists are unavailable.

The most promising of the existing new techniques are based on an antigen-capture dipstick methodology using a monoclonal antibody to *P. falciparum* histidine-rich protein (HRPII). In various trials, this test has proven to be highly sensitive (85 to 95%) and specific (81 to 99%), as well as easy to use, even by minimally trained personnel (105). Disadvantages include being only semiquantitative at best, being able to detect only *P. falciparum*, and poor sensitivity for identifying low parasite densities. The fact that persistent antigenemia can produce a positive test for days to weeks after successful treatment, creating the possibility of incorrectly identifying treatment failure, is also of concern.

Similar tests are currently in development which are enzyme based (parasite lactic acid dehydrogenase or pLDH) rather than antigen based, which should remove the concerns about lingering false-positivity among treated patients (51). This test is also highly sensitive and specific and has the advantage of identifying *P. falciparum* infections from non-falciparum infections, although they cannot distinguish between *P. vivax*, *P. ovale*, and *P. malariae*.

A third technology, based on examination of acridine orange-stained parasites in a proprietary capillary tube under UV light (Quantitative Buffy Coat or QBC) (21), has also been evaluated in a variety of settings. While this test requires less training than normal light microscopy of Giemsa-stained thick smears, it requires far more than the dipstick methods to achieve reliable results (33). In trained hands, it is sensitive, but species diagnosis is unreliable (71). Other molecular technologies such as PCR (47, 79) and flow cytometry (95) are used as research tools only.

Newer technologies have been developed which aid the diagnosis of malaria, especially in settings where skilled, experienced microscopists are unavailable

Babesiosis is a tick-transmitted infection caused by protozoans of the genus Babesia

Babesia Infections

Babesiosis is a tick-transmitted infection caused by protozoans of the genus *Babesia*. Babesia, also called piroplasms, are malaria-like parasites that invade and destroy erythrocytes. *Babesia* spp. differ from *Plasmodium* spp. in that they lack pigment and have no sexual stages. Although there are many differences between the two genera, a ring trophozoite of *Babesia* can be virtually indistinguishable from a ring trophozoite of *Plasmodium*.

There are about 100 known species of *Babesia*, and these infect a great variety of mammals. Babesiosis was once an extremely important, often fatal disease of cattle in the United States, but it has now been eliminated. Important species include *B. bovis*, *B. argentina*, *B. bigemina*, and *B. divergens* in cattle, *B. caballi* and *B. equi* in horses, *B. canis* in dogs, and *B. microti* and *B. rodhaini* in rodents. The identification of species is based primarily on their morphologic features and the vertebrate host in which the parasite is found. A single species of *Babesia* may have different morphologic features depending on the vertebrate host infected.

Occasionally *Babesia* spp. infect humans. Most infections in humans in the New World are caused by *B. microti*, whereas *B. divergens* causes most infections in humans in the Old World. *B. bovis* and a newly recognized *Babesia* sp. called the WA1 piroplasm can also cause human infections.

The diagnosis of babesiosis is usually made by identifying parasites in Giemsa- or Wright's-stained thick or thin peripheral blood films. *Babesia* trophozoites consist of a mass of blue cytoplasm and a single red chromatin dot. They can be very pleomorphic and vary considerably in size, appearing from less than 1 μm to 5 μm or more in diameter. Multiple chromatin dots may be common. Multiple parasites per erythrocyte, 16 or more in *B. canis*, are common. *Babesia* organisms appear in pyriform, ameboid, spherical, rod-shaped, or bizarre configurations. Maltese-cross formations and paired, attached trophozoites may be readily observed. Parasitized erythrocytes are of normal size and there is no stippling. *Babesia* parasitemias can be heavy, and parasites can frequently be seen extracellularly.

Treatment

See Table 13.4 for a listing of drugs used to treat malaria.

The development of antimalarial drug resistance has had a tremendous impact on malaria control. Drug resistance has been implicated in the spread of malaria to new areas and reemergence of malaria in areas where the disease had been eradicated. Drug resistance has also played a significant role in the occurrence and severity of epidemics in some parts of the world. Population movement has introduced resistant parasites to areas previously free of drug resistance. Currently, at a time when fewer and fewer resources are being invested in developing new drugs, malaria parasites have demonstrated some level of resistance to almost every existing antimalarial drug, significantly increasing the cost and complexity of case management. Finally, the increasing number of travelers who are visiting malarious areas for reasons of tourism, business, or humanitarian or peacekeeping activities

Table 13.4   Drugs used to treat malaria[a]

Disease condition	Drug	Adult dosage	Pediatric dosage
Uncomplicated *P. falciparum* in areas WITHOUT chloroquine resistance; *P. malariae*	Chloroquine phosphate	600 mg (base) immediately, followed by 300 mg (base) in 6–8 h, then 300 mg (base) daily for 2 days (total of 1,500 mg base)[b]	10 mg/kg (base) immediately, followed by 5 mg/kg (base) in 6–8 h, then 5 mg/kg (base) daily for 2 days (total of 25 mg/kg base)[b]
P. vivax[c] or *P. ovale*	Chloroquine phosphate AND	As above	As above
	Primaquine phosphate[d, e, f]	15 mg (base) daily for 14 days	0.3 mg/kg (base) daily for 14 days
Uncomplicated *P. falciparum* acquired in areas WITH chloroquine resistance	Quinine sulfate AND Tetracycline[h]	650 mg (salt) three times daily for 3 to 7 days[g] 250 mg qid orally for 7 days	10 mg/kg (salt) three times daily for 3 to 7 days[g] 5 mg/kg qid for 7 days[i]
	Sulfadoxine/ pyrimethamine (SP)	3 tablets, single dose	<4 mos: 1/4 tablet 4–11 mos: 1/2 tablet 1–2 yrs: 3/4 tablet 3–4 yrs: 1 tablet 5–9 yrs: 1 1/2 tablets 10–11 yrs: 2 tablets 12–13 yrs: 2 1/2 tablets >14 yrs: 3 tablets
	Mefloquine[j]	15 mg/kg, single dose[k]	Same
	Artesunate[l, m]	4 mg/kg stat, followed by 2 mg/kg once daily for 3 days (total of 10 mg/kg over 3 days)	Same
	AND Mefloquine	15 mg/kg, single dose	Same
Severe *P. falciparum* malaria	Quinidine gluconate[n]	10 mg/kg (salt) loading dose i.v. over 1–2 h, then 0.02 mg/kg/min continuous infusion until p.o. therapy can be started	Same
	AND Tetracycline[h]	As above	As above[i]

[a]Adapted from reference 17a.

[b]A standard dosing option: adults, 600 mg (base) once daily for 2 days, followed by 300 mg (base) once on day 3; children, 10 mg/kg (base) once daily for 2 days, followed by 5 mg/kg once on day 3.

[c]Some *P. vivax* parasites from Southeast Asia (Burma, Thailand, Indonesia), India, and South America (Guyana) have been shown to be resistant to chloroquine.

[d]Primaquine is used to eradicate hypnozoites from the liver of infected individuals. Because of the probability of reinfection, routine use of primaquine in endemic areas is generally not recommended. Primaquine is also gametocidal; for this reason, some malaria control programs use primaquine therapy to help decrease transmission. The overall efficacy of this practice in most areas is questionable.

[e]Some experts recommend primaquine used at 30 mg/kg daily for 14 days, especially for *P. vivax* infections acquired in Southeast Asia and Oceania.

[f]Patients who require primaquine should be screened for G6PD deficiency prior to therapy. Patients with mild G6PD deficiency (A variant, with 10% to 60% residual enzyme activity) can be treated with 45 mg (adult dose) once per week for 8 weeks. Severely deficient patients (B variant, with <10% residual enzyme activity) should not be treated with primaquine because of risk of severe and potentially fatal hemolysis. Primaquine should not be used during pregnancy.

[g]Quinine sulfate given for 3 days should be used in conjunction with a second drug such as tetracyline for 7 days, or SP. *P. falciparum* infections from some areas of Southeast Asia, most notably Thailand, should be treated with 7 days of quinine sulfate and 7 days of tetracycline.

[h]Preferred regimen for nonimmune patients. Possible alternatives for very young children or pregnant women include SP (dose as described above), trimethoprim-sulfamethoxazole, or clindamycin. SP or trimethoprim-sulfamethoxazole regimens may fail in infections from areas with SP resistance. Clindamycin use in nonimmune patients has been associated with high rates of recrudescence. qid, four times daily.

[i]The benefits of using tetracycline must be weighed against the known risks of adverse effects in children under 9 years old. Alternatives include SP, trimethoprim-sulfamethoxazole, mefloquine, or clindamycin.

[j]Mefloquine at treatment doses has been associated with a high incidence of serious neuropsychiatric side effects (1/2,000 to 1/1,200). Incidence was higher among patients treated with 25 mg/kg, and much higher (1/173) among patients receiving 25 mg/kg after failing 15 mg/kg. Splitting the dose (15 mg/kg on the first day followed by 10 mg/kg 24 h later) may reduce side effects of high-dose mefloquine.

continued

Table 13.4 *continued*

[k]In Thailand, response to treatment with 15 mg/kg mefloquine is poor, and even treatment with 25 mg/kg results in low-grade resistance in about 50% of cases and high-grade resistance in about 15%.

[l]Artesunate and related compounds should not be used except as an adjunct therapy in the treatment of cerebral malaria and treatment of multidrug-resistant *P. falciparum* (such as occurs in Thailand).

[m]Artesunate given for 5 to 7 days appears to be an effective treatment of multidrug-resistant *P. falciparum* malaria. Courses shorter than 5 to 7 days have a high rate of recrudescence and should be used only in conjunction with a second drug (mefloquine). Single-day therapy of 10 mg/kg artesunate and 15 mg/kg mefloquine has recently been shown to be highly effective, although less so than the 3-day regimen given, and improves compliance and reduces risk of adverse reactions associated with high-dose mefloquine therapy.

[n]Quinine dihydrochloride can also be used, if available (it is not available in the United States). Adults: 600 mg diluted in 300–500 ml of normal saline, infused intravenously (i.v.) over 1–2 h. Dose is repeated every 8 h until the patient is able to take oral (p.o.) quinine sulfate (as described for p.o. quinine sulfate). Children: 25 mg/kg divided into three doses per day, infused over 1–2 h until the patient is able to take p.o. quinine sulfate (as described for p.o. quinine sulfate).

not only require effective prophylaxis, but also bring resistant parasites back with them, requiring clinicians in nonendemic areas to be prepared to deal with drug-resistant malaria infections.

Antimalarial drug resistance has traditionally been defined as the "ability of a parasite strain to survive and/or multiply despite the administration and absorption of a drug given in doses equal to or higher than those usually recommended but within the tolerance of the subject"; this definitions was later modified to specify that the drug in question must "gain access to the parasite or the infected red blood cell for the duration of the time necessary for its normal action" (103). It is exceedingly important to distinguish drug resistance from treatment failure and prophylaxis failure. Drug resistance, per se, is primarily a laboratory-defined entity based on the presence or absence of parasites in the face of known drug concentrations. Treatment or prophylaxis failure is primarily a clinical phenomenon resulting from a wide variety of causes including true drug resistance, poor drug quality, poor compliance, inadequate dosage, poor absorption, rapid or aberrant metabolism, rapid excretion, and interfering concurrent treatments. Importantly, many antimalarial drugs may cause significant pathologic changes (14, 38).

The extent and geographic distribution of antimalarial drug resistance have complicated formulation of treatment and prophylaxis recommendations. Since no simple and rapid bedside in vitro assay exists to determine whether any particular malaria infection is drug resistant or not, clinical decisions on treatment must be based on the infecting species and the resistance patterns of the geographic region where the person acquired the infection. Similarly, although drug resistance is not an all-or-nothing phenomenon in endemic areas, decisions about appropriate chemoprophylaxis regimens must be based on potential exposure to drug-resistant malaria.

Currently, chloroquine resistance occurs in all areas where *P. falciparum* is transmitted except for the island of Hispaniola, Central America northwest of the Panama Canal, and limited areas of the Middle East. *P. falciparum* infections from all other areas should be considered resistant to chloroquine. Mefloquine prophylaxis failure and in vitro mefloquine resistance have been reported sporadically in West Africa (54), and there is increasing evidence of high-level sulfadoxine-pyrimethamine (SP) resistance in Tanzania (73). In Southeast Asia, specifically border areas of Thailand, Cambodia, and Myanmar, *P. falciparum* resistance to SP, mefloquine, halofantrine, and quinine has been reported (100). Chloroquine-resistant *P. vivax* has been

Decisions about appropriate chemoprophylaxis regimens must be based on potential exposure to drug-resistant malaria

reported to occur sporadically in parts of Southeast Asia, Oceania, Myanmar, India, and Guyana. On the island of New Guinea, chloroquine-resistant *P. vivax* now occurs frequently enough to be of public health significance (9). New rapidly acting and effective antimalarial drugs, such as artemisinin and its derivatives, may serve as alternative therapies in areas with chloroquine and mefloquine resistance (101).

In the United States, patients suspected of having a malaria infection should be evaluated, at minimum, for the following factors: infecting species, parasite density, geographic area of acquisition, coexistent medical complications (especially cerebral involvement and pregnancy), and ability to take oral medications. Cerebral manifestations of malaria can occur at any peripheral parasite density. *P. falciparum* infection during pregnancy carries a high risk for both the fetus and mother, potentially causing maternal or fetal death, acute pulmonary edema, prematurity, or low birth weight (104).

In general, parasite density can be used to judge severity of infection and need for aggressive therapy. Low- to moderate-density infections (<5% of RBCs infected) can be treated with oral medications, typically a combination of quinine sulfate and tetracycline for *P. falciparum* infections and chloroquine for non-falciparum infections. Patients with *P. vivax* or *P. ovale* infections should also receive primaquine to reduce risk of relapse (provided they have been screened for G6PD deficiency). Therapeutic efficacy should be monitored by repeated blood smears, if indicated, as often as every 6 to 12 h. Significant decreases in parasite density should be observed within 24 to 48 h after therapy is initiated. Fever typically resolves within 36 to 48 h, and most patients will be cleared of visible parasites within 5 days.

> *In general, parasite density can be used to judge severity of infection and need for aggressive therapy*

Patients with higher-density infections (>5% of RBCs infected) are at increased risk of life-threatening complications and death. The majority of these patients, and all patients with altered mental status, should be treated with intravenous quinidine gluconate until the parasite density drops below 1% of RBCs infected. At this time, patients able to take oral medications can be given oral quinine sulfate for a total of 3 days of combined quinidine/quinine therapy (7 days for falciparum infections acquired in Thailand). Seven days of tetracycline or a single treatment dose of SP (depending on likelihood of SP resistance and age or pregnancy status of patient) should be given with the quinine/quinidine (94).

The use of exchange transfusions should be considered for persons with very high-density infections (>10% of RBCs infected), altered mental status (at any density infection), pulmonary edema not due to fluid overload, or renal complications. Typically, 8 to 10 U of blood are required in an adult to decrease parasite density to below 1%.

Prevention

See Table 13.5 for a listing of drugs used in malaria chemoprophylaxis.

Successful prevention of malaria requires the use of appropriate chemoprophylactic drugs as well as avoidance and personal protection methods (19, 20, 52, 57, 59, 69, 75). The choice of an appropriate chemoprophylactic regimen is determined by the exact itinerary of the traveler, the length of

Table 13.5 Drugs used for chemoprophylaxis of malaria

Purpose	Drug	Adult dosage	Pediatric dosage
Travel in areas with chloroquine-sensitive *P. falciparum*	Chloroquine phosphate	300 mg base (500 mg salt) orally, once a week	5 mg/kg base (8.3 mg/kg salt) orally, once a week; up to maximum adult dose of 300 mg base/week
	Hydroxychloroquine sulfate	310 mg base (400 mg salt) orally, once a week	5 mg/kg base (6.5 mg/kg salt) orally, once a week; up to maximum adult dose of 310 mg base/week
Travel in areas with chloroquine-resistant *P. falciparum*[b]	Mefloquine[c]	228 mg base (250 mg salt) orally, once a week	15–19 kg: 1/4 tablet weekly 20–30 kg: 1/2 tablet weekly 31–45 kg: 3/4 tablet weekly >45 kg: 1 tablet weekly
	Doxycycline	100 mg orally, once a day	>8 years of age: 2 mg/kg orally, once a day, up to maximum adult dose of 100 mg/day
	Chloroquine phosphate	300 mg base (500 mg salt) orally, once a week	5 mg/kg base (8.3 mg/kg salt) orally, once a week; up to maximum adult dose of 300 mg base/week
	AND Proguanil[d]	200 mg orally, once a day	<2 yrs: 50 mg daily 2–6 yrs: 100 mg daily 7–10 yrs: 150 mg daily >10 yrs: 200 mg daily
Prevention of relapses	Primaquine[e]	15 mg base (26.3 mg salt) orally, once a day for 14 days	0.3 mg/kg base (0.5 mg/kg salt) orally, once a day for 14 days

[a]Adapted from reference 17a.

[b]Chemoprophylaxis should begin 1 to 2 weeks before travel (1–2 days for doxycycline) and continued while in the malarious area and for 4 weeks after leaving the malarious area.

[c]Mefloquine is contraindicated for persons with known hypersensitivity to the drug and is not recommended for persons with a history of serious psychiatric or seizure disorder. Small children who are given mefloquine for prophylaxis should receive a weekly dose of 5 mg/kg.

[d]Proguanil is not available in the United States.

[e]Primaquine can cause hemolytic anemia in patients with G6PD deficiency. Primaquine should not be given during pregnancy.

stay in malarious areas, the estimated intensity or risk of exposure, and pre-existing conditions such as age, pregnancy, allergies or hypersensitivities (81), or concurrent medication. Exact quantification of risk for any given traveler is difficult. In many areas of Asia and South America, a risk of malaria is confined to rural areas, and travelers to urban areas are at little or no risk and would not require any specific chemoprophylaxis. On the other hand, most travelers to sub-Saharan Africa are at high risk.

For most travelers to most areas of the world, mefloquine would be the prophylactic drug of choice. Currently, mefloquine prophylaxis is also recommended for very young children, pregnant women insisting on travel to malarious areas (although only a small amount of data is available regarding its safety in the first trimester), and for long-term prophylaxis. People who should not take mefloquine include patients with preexisting epilepsy or psychiatric problems (including clinical depression) and people with known hypersensitivity to mefloquine. Based on available data, previous concerns about its use in patients using beta-blocking drugs or those involved in activities requiring fine coordination appear to be unwarranted. Nonetheless, patients with underlying cardiac conduction abnormalities, particularly bradyarrhythmias, should avoid taking mefloquine.

The best alternative to mefloquine, and the drug of choice for the few travelers to areas with a high incidence of mefloquine resistance (Thai-Cambodian and Thai-Myanmar border areas), is daily doxycycline. Doxycycline's short half-life requires a high degree of compliance with the daily regimen; failure to take doxycycline, even for a day or two, can compromise its efficacy. Chloroquine can be used in the few areas where chloroquine resistance has not been reported and for patients unable to take either mefloquine or doxycyline, although the efficacy of this strategy can be low in many areas. In chloroquine-resistant areas, the addition of daily proguanil to the weekly chloroquine regimen offers a marginal increase in efficacy (proguanil is not available within the United States). Patients using chloroquine in areas of chloroquine resistance should be counseled about the need to seek medical assistance promptly if a febrile illness occurs and should carry a treatment dose of SP for self-treatment if medical care is not immediately available.

Avoidance of mosquitoes during evening hours and the use of personal protection measures can further reduce the risk of malaria while traveling. Personal protection measures include the use of mosquito nets, preferably impregnated with pyrethroid insecticides, mosquito repellents such as DEET (*N,N*-diethyl-*m*-toluamide), sleeping in screened rooms, and wearing protective clothing. Vaccine research continues, but the growing realization of the difficulty of creating an effective vaccine emphasizes the importance of alternative preventive measures (68).

Current malaria prophylaxis advice may be obtained from the CDC at (888) 232-3288 or (888) 232-3299 (fax), or on the Internet (www.cdc.gov). Physicians requesting advice on the treatment of patients with malaria can call (770) 488-7788.

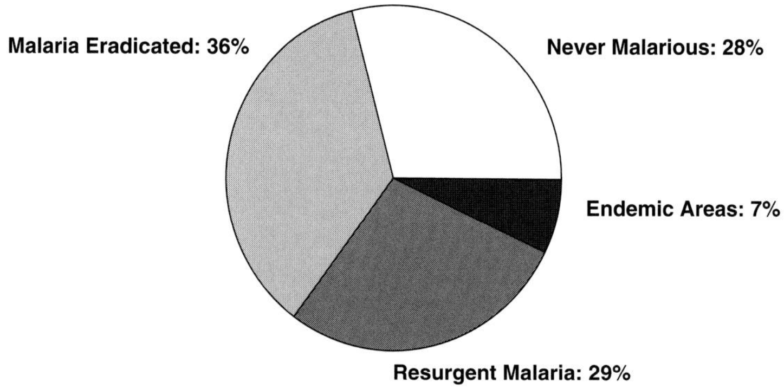

Figure 13.1 Percentage of the world's population exposed to malaria. Endemic areas are those where malaria has never been under significant control. Resurgent areas are those where malaria was once eradicated or under significant control, but where the disease has become a significant public health problem again. (Data from WHO, 1996.)

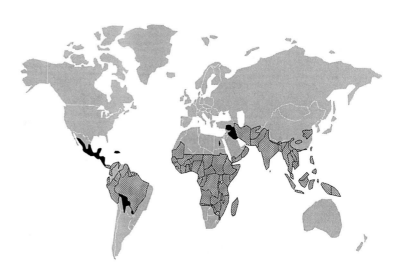

Malaria Eradicated: 36%

Never Malarious: 28%

Endemic Areas: 7%

Resurgent Malaria: 29%

Figure 13.2 Geographic distribution of chloroquine-resistant (cross-hatched areas) and chloroquine-susceptible (solid black areas) *P. falciparum* malaria. Significant SP resistance occurs in the Amazon basin, Southeast Asia, and limited areas of East Africa (primarily Tanzania). Significant mefloquine and halofantrine resistance occurs along the Thailand-Cambodia and Thailand-Myanmar borders. Reduced susceptibility to quinine has been reported in Thailand. Mefloquine prophylaxis failures and in vitro mefloquine resistance have been reported sporadically in Africa and South America.

Figure 13.3 Villus of small intestine with edema and many malarial parasites in congested blood vessel. Note schizonts, trophozoites, and malarial pigments. Hematoxylin and eosin (H&E) stain; ×250.

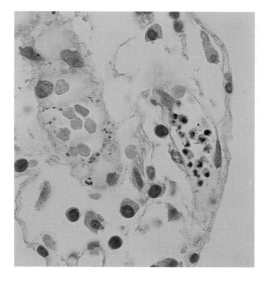

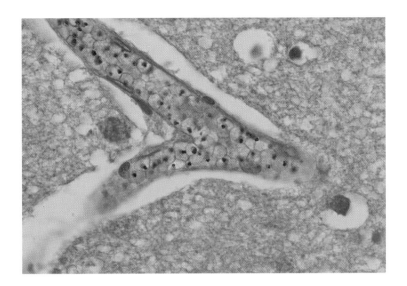

Figure 13.4 Brain of patient with acute, severe cerebral malaria. Note numerous malarial parasites in RBCs of congested blood vessel. ×250.

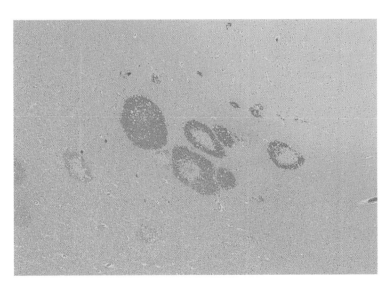

Figure 13.5 Brain of patient who died after 9 days of suffering with cerebral malaria. Note the numerous ring hemorrhages. H&E; ×10.

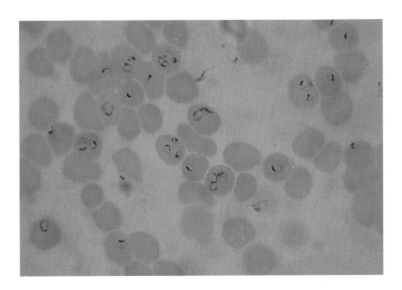

Figure 13.6 Giemsa-stained thin blood film of *P. falciparum*. The erythrocytes are of normal size, some erythrocytes contain multiple parasites, and parasites with double chromatin dots are common. ×330.

Figure 13.7 Giemsa-stained thin blood film demonstrating banana-shaped female gametocytes of *P. falciparum*. The chromatin and pigment are compact and centered in the parasite. ×450.

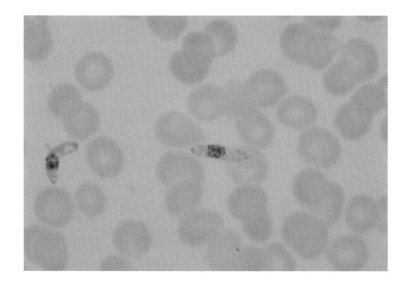

Figure 13.8 Giemsa-stained thin blood film illustrating an ameboid trophozoite of *P. vivax*. The erythrocyte is greatly enlarged and contains Schüffner's dots. The parasite has a large chromatin dot and its cytoplasm extends throughout the erythrocyte. ×290.

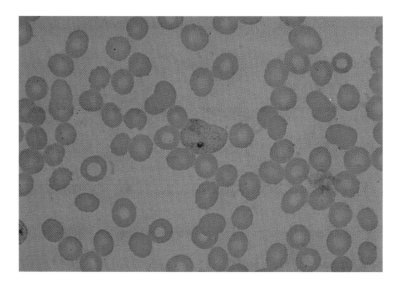

Figure 13.9 Giemsa-stained thin blood film demonstrating a band form of *P. malariae*. The erythrocyte is smaller than normal. ×330.

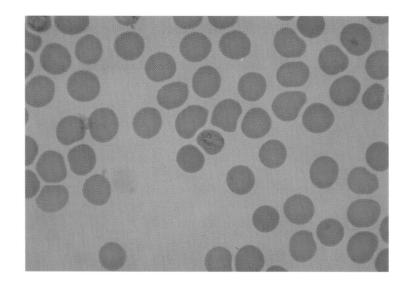

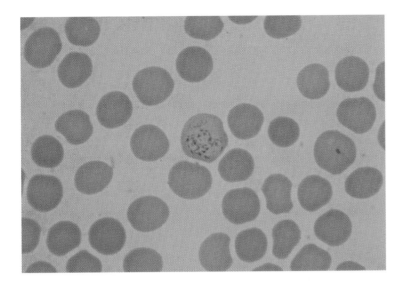

Figure 13.10   Giemsa-stained thin blood film demonstrating a mature female gametocyte of *P. ovale*. The parasite occupies most of the enlarged erythrocyte and is composed of blue cytoplasm, scattered pigments, and an eccentric mass of red chromatin. ×290.

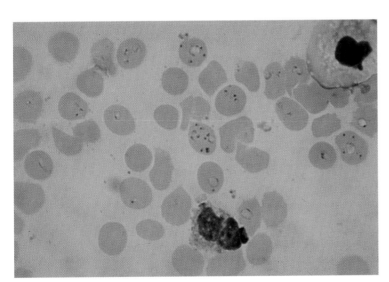

Figure 13.11   Giemsa-stained thin blood film of *Babesia microti*. The erythrocytes are of normal size, but many contain multiple parasites. The parasites are pleomorphic. ×330.

References

1. **Aikawa, M.** 1988. Human cerebral malaria. *Am. J. Trop. Med. Hyg.* **39:**3–10.

2. **Aikawa, M., M. Iseki, J. W. Barnwell, D. Taylor, M. M. Oo, and R. J. Howard.** 1990. The pathology of human cerebral malaria. *Am. J. Trop. Med. Hyg.* **43:**30–37.

3. **Ambroise-Thomas, P., S. Picot, and H. Pelloux.** 1992. Pathophysiology of malaria. The current issue. *Bull. Soc. Pathol. Exot.* **85:**150–155.

4. **Appelbaum, I. L., and J. Shrager.** 1944. Pneumonitis associated with malaria. *Arch. Intern. Med.* **74:**155.

5. **Arora, R. C., R. K. Garg, N. Agarwal, P. Sood, and R. B. Mangal.** 1988. Cerebral malaria caused by *Plasmodium vivax*. *J. Assoc. Physicians Ind.* **36:**564.

6. **Ash, L. R., and T. C. Orihel.** 1987. Examination of blood, p. 99–116. *In Parasites: a Guide to Laboratory Procedures and Identification.* ASCP Press, Chicago.

7. **Ash, L. R., and T. C. Orihel.** 1990. *Atlas of Human Parasitology,* 3rd ed., p. 103–113. ASCP Press, Chicago.

8. **Austin, S. C., P. D. Stolley, and T. Lasky.** 1992. The history of malariotherapy for neurosyphilis. Modern parallels. JAMA **268:**516–519.

9. **Baird, J. K., M. F. S. Nalim, H. Basri, S. Masbar, B. Leksana, E. Tjitra, R. M. Dewi, M. Khairani, and F. S. Wignall.** 1996. Survey of resistance to chloroquine by *Plasmodium vivax* in Indonesia. *Trans. R. Soc. Trop. Med. Hyg.* **90:**409–411.

10. **Bajpai, R., and G. P. Dutta.** 1990. Role of fatty infiltration in pathology of malaria. *Life Sci.* **47:**25–28.

11. **Baruch, D. I., J. A. Gormely, C. Ma, R. J. Howard, and B. L. Pasloske.** 1996. *Plasmodium falciparum* erythrocyte membrane protein 1 is a parasitized erythrocyte receptor for adherence to CD36, thrombospondin, and intercellular adhesion molecule 1. *Proc. Natl. Acad.Sci.* **93:**3497–3502.

12. **Bates, I., G. Bedu-Addo, D. H. Bevan, and T. R. Rutherford.** 1991. Use of immunoglobulin gene rearrangements to show clonal lymphoproliferation in hyper-reactive malarial splenomegaly. *Lancet* **337:**505–507.

13. **Bates, I., G. Bedu-Addo, T. R. Rutherford, and D. H. Bevan.** 1997. Circulating villous lymphocytes—a link between hyperreactive malarial splenomegaly and splenic lymphoma. *Trans. R. Soc. Trop. Med. Hyg.* **91:**171–174.

14. **Begbie, S., and K. R. Burgess.** 1993. Maloprim-induced pulmonary eosinophilia. *Chest* **103:**305–306.

15. **Bircan, A., M. Kervanciolu, M. Soran, G. Gönlüen, and I. Tuncer.** 1997. Two cases of nephrotic syndrome and tertian malaria in south-eastern Anatolia. *Pediatr. Nephrol.* **11:**78–79.

16. **Biswas, J., R. Fogla, P. Srinivasan, S. Narayan, K. Haranath, and V. Badrinath.** 1996. Ocular malaria. A clinical and histopathologic study. *Ophthalmology* **103:**1471–1475.

17. **Black, J., M. Hommel, G. Snounou, and M. Pinder.** 1994. Mixed infections with *Plasmodium falciparum* and *P. malariae* and fever in malaria. *Lancet* **343:**1095. (Letter.)

17a. **Bloland, P. B., and C. C. Campbell.** 1992. Malaria, p. 82–88. *In* R. E. Rakel (ed.), *Conn's Current Therapy.* W. B. Saunders, Philadelphia.

18. **Boukari, B. S., G. Napo-Koura, N. Kampatibe, K. Kpodzro, D. Rabineau, and M. Vovor.** 1991. Congenital malaria: clinical, parasitological and histological considerations. Apropos of 200 observations collected at the Lome University Teaching Hospital and Kpalime Hospital. *Bull. Soc. Pathol. Exot. Filiales* **84:**448–457.

19. **Bradley, D.** 1993. Prophylaxis against malaria for travellers from the United Kingdom. *Br. Med. J.* **306:**1247–1252.

20. **Brown, G. V.** 1993. Chemoprophylaxis of malaria. *Med. J. Aust.* **159:**187–196.

20a. **Bruce-Chwatt, L. J.** 1985. *Essential Malariology*, 2nd ed. John Wiley & Sons, New York.

21. **Cabezos, J., and J. Bada.** 1993. The diagnosis of malaria by the thick film and the QBC: a comparative study of both technics. *Med. Clin.* (Barcelona) **101:**91–94.

22. **Cantarovichm, F., M. Vazquez, W. D. Garcia, M. Abbud Filho, C. Herrera, and A. Villegas Hernandez.** 1992. Special infections in organ transplantation in South America. *Transplant. Proc.* **24:**1902–1908.

23. **Cayea, P. D., E. Rubin, and H. S. Teixidor.** 1981. Atypical pulmonary malaria. *Am. J. Roentgenol.* **137:**51–55.

24. **Centers for Disease Control and Prevention.** 1988. *Malaria Surveillance Annual Summary 1987.* Centers for Disease Control and Prevention, Atlanta, Ga.

25. **Centers for Disease Control and Prevention.** 1990. Imported malaria associated with malariotherapy for Lyme disease—New Jersey. *Morbid. Mortal. Weekly Rep.* **39:**667–668.

26. **Centers for Disease Control and Prevention.** 1995. Local transmission of *Plasmodium vivax* malaria—Houston, Texas, 1994. *Morbid. Mortal. Weekly Rep.* **44:**295, 301–303.

27. **Centers for Disease Control and Prevention.** 1996. Mosquito-transmitted malaria—Michigan, 1995. *Morbid. Mortal. Weekly Rep.* **45:**398–400.

28. **Centers for Disease Control and Prevention.** 1997. Probable locally acquired mosquito-transmitted *Plasmodium vivax* infection—Georgia, 1996. *Morbid. Mortal. Weekly Rep.* **46:**264–267.

29. **Charoenpan, P., S. Indraprasit, S. Kiatboonsri, O. Suvachittanont, and S. Tanomsup.** 1990. Pulmonary edema in severe falciparum malaria. Hemodynamic study and clinicophysiologic correlation. *Chest* **97:**1190.

30. **Chulay, J. D., and C. F. Ockenhouse.** 1990. Host receptors for malaria-infected erythrocytes. *Am. J. Trop. Med. Hyg.* **43**(Suppl.):6–14.

31. **Clark, I. A., and G. Chaudhri.** 1988. Tumor necrosis factor may contribute to the anaemia of malaria by causing dyserythropoiesis and erythrophagocytosis. *Br. J. Haematol.* **70:**99–103.

32. **Corbett, C. E., M. I. Duarte, C. L. Lancellotti, M. A. Silva, and H. F. Andrade.** 1989. Cytoadherence in human falciparum malaria as a cause of respiratory distress. *J. Trop. Med. Hyg.* **92:**112–120.

33. **Craig, M. H., and B. L. Sharp.** 1997. Comparative evaluation of four techniques for the diagnosis of *Plasmodium falciparum* infections. *Trans. R. Soc. Trop. Med. Hyg.* **91:**279–282.

34. **Deaton, J. G.** 1970. Fatal pulmonary edema as a complication of acute falciparum malaria. *Am. J. Trop. Med. Hyg.* **19:**196.

35. **Dick, S., M. Waterfall, J. Currie, A. Maddy, and E. Riley.** 1996. Naive human alpha beta T cells respond to membrane-associated components of malaria-infected erythrocytes by proliferation and production of interferon-gamma. *Immunology* **88:**412–420.

36. **Dluzewski, A. R., G. B. Nash, R. J. Wilson, D. M. Reardon, and W. B. Gratzer.** 1992. Invasion of hereditary ovalocytes by *Plasmodium falciparum* in vitro and its relation to intracellular ATP concentration. *Mol. Biochem. Parasitol.* **55:**1–7.

37. **Duarte, M. I. S., C. E. P. Corbett, M. Boulos, and V. A. Neto.** 1985. Ultrastructure of the lung in falciparum malaria. *Am. J. Trop. Med. Hyg.* **34:**31.

38. **Easterbrook, M.** 1992. Long-term course of antimalarial maculopathy after cessation of treatment. *Can. J. Ophthalmol.* **27:**237–239.

39. **Falk, S., H. Protz, U. Kobrich, and H. J. Stutte.** 1992. Spontaneous splenic rupture in acute malaria tropica. *Dtsch. Med. Wochenschr.* **117**(22)**:**854–857.

40. **Goldring, J. D., M. E. Molyneux, T. Taylor, J. Wirima, and M. Hommel.** 1992. *Plasmodium falciparum*: diversity of isolates from Malawi in their cytoadherence to melanoma cells and monocytes in vitro. *Br. J. Haematol.* **81:**413–418.

41. **Good, M. F., and J. Currier.** 1992. The importance of T cell homing and the spleen in reaching a balance between malaria immunity and immunopathology: the molding of immunity by early exposure to cross-reactive organisms. *Immunol. Cell. Biol.* **70:**405–410.

42. **Hedstrom, R. C., J. R. Campbell, M. L. Leef, M. Charoenvit, M. Carter, M. Sedegah, R. L. Beaudoin, and S. L. Hoffman.** 1990. A malaria sporozoite surface antigen distinct from the circumsporozoite protein. *Bull. W.H.O.* **68**(Suppl.)**:**152–157.

43. **Hendrickse, R. G.** 1976. The quartan malarial nephrotic syndrome. *Adv. Nephrol. Necker Hosp.* **6:**229–247.

44. **Hommel, M.** 1996. Physiopathology of symptoms of malaria. Role of cytokines, cytoadherence, and premunition. *Presse Med.* **25:**70–76.

45. **Kachur, S. P., M. E. Reller, A. M. Barber, L. M. Barat, E. H. A. Koumans, M. E. Parise, J. Roberts, T. K. Ruebush, and J. R. Zucker.** 1997. Malaria surveillance—United States, 1994. *In* CDC Surveillance Surveillance Summaries, October 17, 1997 (no. SS-5). *Morbid. Mortal. Weekly Rep.* **46:**1–18.

46. **Knudsen, A. B., and R. Slooff.** 1992. Vector-borne disease problems in rapid urbanization: new approaches to vector control. *Bull. W.H.O.* **70:**1–6.

47. **Liu, K. Y., B. C. Huang, H. H. Zhang, Y. B. Liu, R. Q. Kong, and Y. L. Cheng.** 1993. Cloning of a DNA probe and its application in the detection of *Plasmodium falciparum*. A preliminary report. *Chin. Med. J.* **106:**31–34.

48. **Lutalo, S. K., and C. Mabuwa.** 1990. Complications of seasonal adult malaria at a central hospital. *Centr. Afr. J. Med.* **36:**268.

49. **Macleod, C. L.** 1988. Malaria, p. 9–42. *In* C. L. Macleod (ed.), *Parasitic Infections in Pregnancy and the Newborn.* Oxford Medical Publications, London.

50. **Mahdi, A. A., R. Chander, N. K. Kapoor, and S. Ahmad.** 1992. Role of free radicals in *Plasmodium berghei* infected *Mastomys natalensis* brain. *Indian J. Exp. Biol.* **30:**1193–1196.

51. **Makler, M. T., and D. J. Hinrichs.** 1993. Measurement of the lactate dehydrogenase activity of *Plasmodium falciparum* as an assessment of parasitemia. *Am. J. Trop. Med. Hyg.* **48:**205–210.

52. **Martin, G. J., J. L. Malone, and E. V. Ross.** 1993. Exfoliative dermatitis during malarial prophylaxis with mefloquine. *Clin. Infect. Dis.* **16:**341–342. (Letter.)

53. **Melancon-Kaplan, J., and W. P. Weidanz.** 1989. Role of cell-mediated immunity in resistance to malaria, p. 37–63. *In* M. M. Stevenson (ed.), *Malaria: Host Responses to Infection.* CRC Press, Boca Raton, Fla.

54. **Mockenhaupt, F. P.** 1995. Mefloquine resistance in *Plasmodium falciparum. Parasitol. Today* **11:**248–253.

55. **Mohan, K., N. K. Ganguly, M. L. Dubey, and R. C. Mahajan.** 1992. Oxidative damage of erythrocytes infected with *Plasmodium falciparum.* An in vitro study. *Ann. Hematol.* **65:**131–134.

56. **Mohanty, D., N. Marwaha, K. Ghosh, S. Sharma, G. Garewal, S. Shah, S. Devi, and K. C. Das.** 1988. Functional and ultrastructural changes of platelets in malarial infection. *Trans. R. Soc. Trop. Med. Hyg.* **82:**369–375.

57. **Murphy, G. S., H. Basri, Purnomo, E. M. Andersen, M. J. Bangs, D. L. Mount, J. Gordon, A. A. Lal, A. R. Purwokusumo, S. Harjosuwarno, K. Sorensen, and S. L. Hoffman.** 1993. Vivax malaria resistant to treatment and prophylaxis with chloroquine. *Lancet* **341:**96–100.

58. **Nagatake, T., V. T. Hoang, T. Tegoshi, J. Rabbege, T. K. Ann, and M. Aikawa.** 1992. Pathology of falciparum malaria in Vietnam. *Am. J. Trop. Med. Hyg.* **47:**259–264.

59. **Nakajima, H.** 1992. Press Release WHO/66: Opening of Ministerial Conference on Malaria Towards a New Global Partnership. 26 October. World Health Organization, Geneva.

60. **Nakamura, K., T. Hasler, K. Morehead, R. J. Howard, and M. Aikawa.** 1992. *Plasmodium falciparum*-infected erythrocyte receptor(s) for CD36 and thrombospondin are restricted to knobs on the erythrocyte surface. *J. Histochem. Cytochem.* **40:**1419–1422.

61. **Ockenhouse, C. F., and H. L. Shear.** 1983. Malaria-induced lymphokines: stimulation of macrophages for enhanced phagocytosis. *Infect. Immun.* **42:**733–739.

62. **Oliveira-Ferreira, J., R. Lourenco-De-Oliveira, A. Teva, L. M. Deane, and C. T. Daniel-Ribeiro.** 1990. Natural malaria infections in anophelines in Rondonia State, Brazilian Amazon. *Am. J. Trop. Med. Hyg.* **43:**6–10.

63. **Phillips, R. E., and G. Pasvol.** 1992. Anaemia of *Plasmodium falciparum* malaria. *Baillieres Clin. Haematol.* **5:**315–330.

64. **Polder, T. W., W. M. Eling, J. H. Curfs, C. R. Jerusalem, and M. Wijers-Rouw.** 1992. Ultrastructural changes in the blood-brain barrier of mice infected with *Plasmodium berghei. Acta Leiden* **60:**31–46.

65. **Pongponratn, E., M. Riganti, T. Harinasuta, and D. Bunnag.** 1989. Electron microscopic study of phagocytosis in human spleen in falciparum malaria. *S. E. Asian J. Trop. Med. Public Health* **20:**31–39.

66. **Punyagupta, S., F. Srichaikul, P. Nitiyanat, and B. Petchclai.** 1974. Acute pulmonary insufficiency in falciparum malaria: summary of 12 cases with evidence of disseminated intravascular coagulation. *Am. J. Trop. Med. Hyg.* **23:**551.

67. **Qari, S. H., Y.-P. Shi, I. F. Goldman, V. Udhayakumar, M. P. Alpers, W. E. Collins, and A. A. Lal.** 1993. Identification of *Plasmodium vivax* like human malaria parasite. *Lancet* **341:**780–783.

68. **Ramasamy, M. S., and R. Ramasamy.** 1990. Effect of anti-mosquito antibodies on the infectivity of the rodent malaria parasite *Plasmodium berghei* to *Anopheles farauti*. *Med. Vet. Entomol.* **4:**161–166.

69. **Rangel-Frausto, M. S., and M. B. Edmond.** 1993. Malaria: protection of the international traveler. *Infect. Control Hosp. Epidemiol.* **14:**155–160.

70. **Rath, R. N., D. K. Patel, P. K. Das, B. K. Das, A. C. Mishra, R. N. Sahu, and C. Mohanty.** 1990. Immunopathological changes in kidney in Plasmodium falciparum malaria. *Indian J. Med. Res.* **91:**129–132.

71. **Rickman, L. S., G. W. Long, R. Oberst, A. Cabanban, R. Sangalang, J. I. Smith, J. D. Chulay, and S. L. Hoffman.** 1989. Rapid diagnosis of malaria by acridine orange staining of centrifuged parasites. *Lancet* **i:**68–71.

72. **Rioult, B., J. B. Merit, N. Varache, and M. Trichet.** 1990. Fatal pulmonary edema in a pernicious malaria attack. *Ann. Fr. Anesth. Reanim.* **9:**557.

73. **Ronn, A. M., H. A. Msangeni, J. Mhina, W. H. Wernsdorfer, and I. C. Bygbjerg.** 1996. High level of resistance of Plasmodium falciparum to sulfadoxine-pyrimethamine in children in Tanzania. *Trans. R. Soc. Trop. Med. Hyg.* **90:**179–181.

74. **Sachdev, H. S., and M. Mohan.** 1985. Vivax cerebral malaria. *J. Trop. Pediatr.* **31:**213–215.

75. **Sexton, J. D., T. K. Ruebush, II, A. D. Brandling-Bennett, J. G. Breman, J. M. Roberts, J. S. Odera, and J. B. O. Were.** 1990. Permethrin-impregnated curtains and bed-nets prevent malaria in Western Kenya. *Am. J. Trop. Med. Hyg.* **43:**11–18.

76. **Shepard, D. S., M. B. Ettling, U. Brinkmann, and R. Sauerborn.** 1991. The economic cost of malaria in Africa. *Trop. Med. Parasitol.* **42:**199–203.

77. **Sherry, B. A., G. Alava, K. J. Tracey, J. Martiney, A. Cerami, and A. F. Slater.** 1995. Malaria-specific metabolite hemozoin mediates the release of several potent endogenous pyrogens (TNF, MIP-1 alpha, and MIP-1 beta) in vitro, and altered thermoregulation in vivo. *J. Inflamm.* **45:**85–96.

78. **Singhal, M. K., P. Arora, V. Kher, R. Pandey, S. Gulati, and A. Gupta.** 1997. Acute cortical necrosis in falciparum malaria: an unusual cause of end-stage renal disease. *Renal Failure* **19:**491–494.

79. **Snounou, G., S. Viriyakosol, W. Jarra, S. Thaithong, and K. N. Brown.** 1993. Identification of the four human malaria parasite species in field samples by the polymerase chain reaction and detection of a high prevalence of mixed infections. *Mol. Biochem. Parasitol.* **58:**283–292.

80. **Stürchler, D.** 1989. How much malaria is there worldwide? *Parasitol. Today* **5:**39.

81. **Stürchler, D., M. L. Mittelholzer, and L. Kerr.** 1993. How frequent are notified severe cutaneous adverse reactions to Fansidar? *Drug Safety* **8:**160–168.

82. **Tatke, M., and G. B. Malik.** 1990. Pulmonary pathology in severe malaria infection in health and protein deprivation. *J. Trop. Med. Hyg.* **93:**377.

83. **Tegoshi, T., R. S. Desowitz, K. G. Pirl, Y. Maeno, and M. Aikawa.** 1992. Placental pathology in *Plasmodium berghei*-infected rats. *Am. J. Trop. Med. Hyg.* **47:**643–651.

84. **Testa, J., J. Awodabon, N. Lagarde, T. Olivier, and J. Delmont.** 1990. Plasmodial indices and malarial placentopathy in 299 parturients in Central Africa. *Med. Trop. (Mars)* **50:**85–90.

85. **Thumwood, C. M., N. H. Hunt, W. B. Cowden, and I. A. Clark.** 1989. Antioxidants can prevent cerebral malaria in *Plasmodium berghei*-infected mice. *Br. J. Exp. Pathol.* **70:**293–303.

86. **Tilluckdharry, C. C., D. D. Chadee, R. Doon, and J. Nehall.** 1996. A case of vivax malaria presenting with psychosis. *West Indian Med. J.* **45:**39–40.

87. **Trang, T. T., N. H. Phu, H. Vinh, T. T. Hien, B. M. Cuong, T. T. Chau, N. T. Mai, D. J. Waller, and N. J. White.** 1992. Acute renal failure in patients with severe falciparum malaria. *Clin. Infect. Dis.* **15:**874–880.

88. **Turner, G.** 1997. Cerebral malaria. *Brain Pathol.* **7:**569–582.

89. **Udomsangpetch, R., H. K. Webster, K. Pattanapanyasat, S. Pitchayangkul, and S. Thaithong.** 1992. Cytoadherence characteristics of rosette-forming *Plasmodium falciparum. Infect. Immun.* **60:**4483–4490.

90. **Vadas, P., W. Pruzanski, E. Stefanski, L. G. Ellies, J. E. Aubin, A. Sos, and A. Melcher.** 1991. Extracellular phospholipase A_2 secretion is a common effector pathway of interleukin-1 and TNF action. *Immunol. Lett.* **28:**187–194.

91. **Vadas, P., W. Pruzanski, E. Stefanski, B. Sternby, R. Mustard, H. Bohnen, I. Fraser, V. Farewell, and C. Bombardier.** 1988. The pathogenesis of hypotension in septic shock: correlation of circulating phospholipase A_2 levels with circulatory collapse. *Crit. Care Med.* **16:**1–7.

92. **Vadas, P., T. E. Taylor, L. Chimsuku, D. Goldring, E. Stefanski, W. Pruzanski, and M. E. Molyneux.** Increased serum phospholipase A_2 activity is associated with manifestations of severe falciparum malaria in children. *Am. J. Trop. Med. Hyg.*, in press.

93. **Van den Ende, J., A. Van Gompel, E. Van den Enden, and R. Colebunders.** 1994. Development of hyperreactive malarious splenomegaly in an 8-year-old Caucasian boy, 18 months after residence in Africa. *Ann. Soc. Belg. Med. Trop.* **74:**69–73.

94. **Van Hensbroek, M. B., D. Kwiatkowski, B. Van Den Berg, F. J. Hoek, C. J. Van Boxtel, and P. A. Kagier.** 1996. Quinine pharmacokinetics in young children with severe malaria. *Am. J. Trop. Med. Hyg.* **54:**237–242.

95. **van Vianen, P. H., A. van Engen, S. Thaithong, M. van der Keur, H. J. Tanke, H. J. van der Kaay, B. Mons, and C. J. Janse.** 1993. Flow cytometric screening of blood samples for malaria parasites. *Cytometry* **14:**276–280.

96. **Voler, A., and P. C. C. Garnham.** 1966. Cross immunity in monkey malaria. *J. Trop. Med. Hyg.* **69:**121–131.

97. **Weatherall, D. J., and S. Abdalla.** 1982. The anemia of *Plasmodium falciparum* malaria. *Brit. Med. Bull.* **38:**147–151.

98. **Wernsdorfer, W. H.** 1980. The importance of malaria in the world, p. 1–10. *In* J. P. Kreier (ed.), *Malaria,* vol. 1. Academic Press, Inc., New York.

99. **White, N. J.** 1993. Malaria parasites go ape. *Lancet* **341:**793.

100. **White, N. J.** 1996. The treatment of malaria. *N. Engl. J. Med.* **335:**800–806.

101. **White, N. J., and S. Pukrittayakamee.** 1993. Clinical malaria in the tropics. *Med. J. Aust.* **159:**197–203.

102. **Wickramasinghe, S. N., S. Looareesuwan, B. Nagachinta, and N. J. White.** 1989. Dyserythropoiesis and ineffective erythropoiesis in *Plasmodium vivax* malaria. *Br. J. Haematol.* **72:**91–99.

103. **World Health Organization.** 1986. Drug resistance in malaria, p. 102–118. *In* L. J. Bruce-Chwatt (ed.), *Chemotherapy of Malaria.* World Health Organization, Geneva.

104. **World Health Organization.** 1990. Severe and complicated malaria. *Trans. R. Soc. Trop. Med. Hyg.* **84**(Suppl. 2)**:**1–65.

105. **World Health Organization.** 1996. A rapid dipstick antigen capture assay for the diagnosis of falciparum malaria. WHO Informal Consultation on recent advances in diagnostic techniques and vaccines for malaria. *Bull W.H.O.* **74:**47–54.

106. **World Health Organization.** 1996. World malaria situation in 1993, part I. *Weekly Epidemiol. Rec.* **71:**17–22.

107. **Wyler, D. J., C. N. Oster, and T. C. Quinn.** 1983. The role of the spleen in malaria infections, p. 1–12. *In* G. Torrigiani (ed.), *The Role of the Spleen in the Immunology of Parasitic Diseases.* Tropical Disease Research Series, no 1. Schwabe & Co. AG, Basel.

108. **Zingman, B. S., and B. L. Viner.** 1993. Splenic complications in malaria case report and review. *Clin. Infect. Dis.* **16:**223–232.

109. **Zucker, J. R.** 1996. Changing patterns of autochthonous malaria transmission in the United States. *Emerg. Infect. Dis.* **2:**37–43.

chapter 14

Lymphatic Filariasis

Gerusa Dreyer, José Figueredo-Silva, Ronald C. Neafie, and David G. Addiss

Lymphatic filariasis is a tropical disease of global importance that affects an estimated 120 million persons in Africa, southern Asia, the western Pacific Islands, the Atlantic coast of South and Central America, and the Caribbean (66). The debilitating and socially stigmatizing sequelae of lymphatic filariasis make it the second leading cause of disability worldwide (67). After years of relative scientific and medical neglect, lymphatic filariasis has recently emerged as an increasingly important public health problem in many areas of the world and a focus of international attention. Large-scale water projects and uncontrolled urban growth, with its attendant environmental degradation and disruption in sanitary conditions, have expanded vector habitat and dramatically increased the numbers of infected persons and those at risk of

Gerusa Dreyer, Departamento de Parasitologia, Centro de Pesquisas Aggeu Magalhães-FIOCRUZ, Av. Moraes Rego S/N, Ciudade Universitaria, Recife, PE, Brazil, 52020-200. José Figueredo-Silva, Laboratorio de Immunopatologia Keiso Asami, Universidade Federal de Pernambuco, Recife, Brazil. Ronald C. Neafie, Parasitic Disease Pathology Branch, Geographic Pathology Division, Department of Infectious and Parasitic Disease Pathology, Armed Forces Institute of Pathology, Washington, DC 20306-6000. David G. Addiss, Division of Parasitic Diseases, National Center for Infectious Diseases, Centers for Disease Control and Prevention, Mailstop F-22, Atlanta, GA 30341.

Pathology of Emerging Infections 2
Edited by Ann Marie Nelson and C. Robert Horsburgh, Jr.
© 1998 American Society for Microbiology, Washington, D.C.

infection (4, 37). Our understanding of the host-parasite relationship and of treatment and control of lymphatic filariasis has also undergone major changes during the past few years as new approaches and tools have been developed for diagnosis, clinical investigation, and safe, effective mass treatment of persons infected with the parasite. In part because of these advances, the International Task Force for Disease Eradication has identified lymphatic filariasis as one of only six diseases that are eradicable or potentially eradicable (10). In May 1997, the World Health Assembly passed a resolution calling for global elimination of lymphatic filariasis as a public health problem. Thus, filariasis is considered, at the same time, both an emerging and a potentially eradicable infectious disease. This paradoxical juxtaposition highlights the current need for public health action.

Filariasis is considered, at the same time, both an emerging and a potentially eradicable infectious disease

The lymphatic filarial parasite is an elegant, threadlike nematode with two major species. *Wuchereria bancrofti* is responsible for approximately 90% of infections worldwide. *Brugia malayi*, which occurs in Southeast Asia and parts of the South Pacific, accounts for about 10%. The two species cause similar signs and symptoms, although urogenital involvement seems to occur only with *W. bancrofti* infection and lymphadenopathy tends to be a prominent feature of brugian filariasis. Adult female *W. bancrofti* measure 6 to 10 cm in length and 200 μm wide; the male worms are 4 cm in length and 100 μm in width. Adult *B. malayi* are somewhat smaller. Because of the greater global importance of *W. bancrofti* and the relative paucity of new diagnostic and epidemiologic tools for control of *B. malayi*, the focus of this chapter will be bancroftian filariasis.

The life cycle of both species requires a human host and a mosquito vector. When an infected mosquito takes a blood meal, third-stage filarial larvae (L3) are deposited on the skin; they penetrate the skin and migrate to the lymph nodes and, primarily, to the lymphatic vessels, where they develop into sexually mature adult worms. The mean estimated life span of the adult worm is approximately 5 to 10 years. Beginning 6 to 12 months after infection, millions of microfilariae (230 to 300 μm in length) are released by the fertile female worms and migrate to peripheral blood. In most areas where lymphatic filariasis is endemic, the concentration of microfilariae in the blood is much greater at night, especially between midnight and 2 a.m., than during the day. This phenomenon, which is known as nocturnal periodicity, facilitates transmission, since the peak biting period of the principal mosquito vector (*Culex quinquefasciatus* in many areas) is usually at night. The life cycle of the parasite is completed by the development within the mosquito of the larval stage (L3) that is infective for humans.

Epidemiology

In areas where lymphatic filariasis is endemic, the prevalence of microfilaremia increases during the childhood years and tends to plateau in adulthood. In some but not all studies, children born to infected mothers are more likely to become infected than are children born to uninfected mothers. During the childbearing years, prevalence of infection is often higher among men than among women. Recent data indicate that the prevalence of persons with circulating *W. bancrofti* antigen, which is associated both with microfilariae and with the adult worm, may be 10 to 50% higher than that of microfilaremia, and that in areas of intense transmission, filarial infection may frequently occur during the first 5 years of life. Within filariasis-endemic areas, transmission of the parasite may be quite focal, and prevalence may vary even within the same village. The prevalence of clinical disease tends to be correlated with the prevalence of microfilaremia and the intensity of transmission. A notable exception to this general rule can be found in parts of Papua New Guinea, where infection is almost universal but clinical disease is relatively uncommon.

Clinical manifestations of lymphatic filariasis are influenced not only by age and by gender, but by a number of cofactors, including the anatomic location and possibly the number of the adult worms, the immune response to the parasite, and secondary bacterial infections. Apart from the "acute attacks," which are described below, lymphedema and urogenital disease are the most common clinical manifestations of chronic disease. Lymphedema and elephantiasis of the leg affect an estimated 15 million persons worldwide (66); in most areas of the world, lymphedema of the leg is more common in women than in men (36, 44, 66). In contrast, in areas where *B. malayi* is endemic, men and women are affected to a similar extent.

Lymphedema and elephantiasis of the leg affect an estimated 15 million persons worldwide

Chronic urogenital manifestations, which principally affect men, have important social, economic, and psychological consequences (20, 57, 61). Hydrocele, the most frequent chronic manifestation of bancroftian filariasis, has a prevalence in men that increases with age and tends to approximate the prevalence of microfilaremia in the general population.

Tropical pulmonary eosinophilia (TPE) is a fascinating but relatively rare progressive pulmonary manifestation of lymphatic filariasis. It is found most frequently in men 20 to 40 years old.

Clinical Features and Pathogenesis

Asymptomatic and Subclinical Lymphatic Filariasis

Until recently, it was thought that as long as the adult worms remained alive, the human host was "in harmony" with the parasite. Damage to the lymphatic vessels and clinical disease were thought to occur when the host ceased to be immunologically tolerant of the parasite. Clear immunologic differences do exist between persons who are asymptomatically infected with the parasite and those with chronic lymphedema; microfilaria-positive persons have elevated levels of filaria-specific immunoglobulin G4 (IgG4), while those with chronic lymphedema characteristically are microfilaria negative and have elevated serum levels of IgG1 and IgG3 and enhanced lymphocyte proliferation to filarial antigens (43, 44, 55). However, the role of the immune system in the pathogenesis of filarial disease has not been clearly elucidated, with the exception of TPE.

> *A more recent but growing body of evidence indicates that virtually all persons with W. bancrofti infection have some degree of lymphatic damage and clinical or subclinical disease*

A more recent but growing body of evidence indicates that virtually all persons with *W. bancrofti* infection have some degree of lymphatic damage and clinical or subclinical disease. Lymphangiectasis is the central pathologic lesion in lymphatic filariasis; it can be detected even in persons with *W. bancrofti* infection who are asymptomatic and amicrofilaremic (25). The mechanisms that cause lymphangiectasis are, as yet, unknown. At the site of the adult worm in the spermatic cord of infected men, the lymphatic vessels may increase from the normal 1 mm in diameter to more than 20 mm (50; G. Dreyer, unpublished data). Dilated lymphatic vessels can be detected by ultrasound throughout the scrotal area only in men living in filariasis-endemic areas (50). Lymphoscintigraphy may reveal dilated and tortuous lymphatic vessels in the lower limbs in asymptomatically infected males (13, 33). However, these lymphoscintigraphic findings of the lower limbs are indistinguishable from those in some men from nonendemic areas (F. Marchetti, unpublished data).

Acute Manifestations

"Acute attacks" associated with lymphatic filariasis cause considerable pain, suffering, and loss of work. The etiology of these episodes has been the subject of confusion and controversy for more than half a century. They have been attributed to bacterial infections, immunologic responses to a variety of filarial antigens, and release of substances from, or death of, the adult worm (1, 28, 48, 54, 65). It is now clear that the syndrome of acute attacks comprises two distinct clinical entities: "true" filarial adenolymphangitis (FADL) and acute dermatolymphangioadenitis (ADLA) (19, 23).

Filarial Adenolymphangitis (FADL)

FADL is caused by death of the adult worm, either spontaneously or as a result of treatment with a macrofilaricidal drug such as diethylcarbamazine (DEC). This "classical" filarial adenolymphangitis was extensively described and investigated in American and European soldiers in the South Pacific during World War II (e.g., reference 65), but it is also observed among life-long residents of areas in which lymphatic filariasis is endemic.

When death of an adult worm occurs, the clinical findings depend on the location of the worm and the extent of the inflammatory reaction. Undoubtedly, many spontaneous adult worm deaths go unrecognized. When the initial inflammatory response is clinically apparent, it is manifested as adenitis or lymphangitis, depending on whether the worm is located in the lymph node or lymphatic vessel, respectively. Lymphangitis progresses distally, i.e., in a "retrograde" fashion, producing a palpable "cord" (see Fig. 14.1), and is frequently accompanied by mild fever, headache, and malaise. Occasionally, lymphedema of the extremities occurs; in most cases, this resolves spontaneously.

In adult men, where the lymphatic vessels of the intrascrotal area appear to be a preferred site, the picture may be one of orchidalgia, epididymitis, or funiculitis. The inflammatory reaction may cause a palpable thickening of the spermatic cord, and development of a granuloma at the site of the adult worm produces a palpable nodule. Similar findings may occur in infected men after treatment with DEC (12, 24, 30). Acute hydroceles sometimes occur; in most cases, they seem to resolve spontaneously.

Acute Dermatolymphangioadenitis (ADLA)

Dilation of the lymphatic vessels induced by the presence of the adult worm eventually leads to lymphatic dysfunction. The lower limbs, in particular, become predisposed to recurrent bacterial infections. Trauma, interdigital fungal infections, and onychomycosis provide entry sites for these bacteria, which multiply rapidly and cause inflammation of the small collecting vessels (ADLA) (23). Beta-hemolytic streptococci (48) and organisms which are generally regarded as commensal or saprophytic have been isolated from the blood or tissues during the acute attacks (52; Dreyer, unpublished data).

The clinical pattern of ADLA is distinctly different from that of FADL (19, 48). The lymphangitis develops in a reticular rather than a linear pattern (see Fig. 14.2), and the local and systemic symptoms, including edema, pain, fever, and chills, are frequently more severe. Biopsies reveal acute and chronic inflammation but no evidence of adult *W. bancrofti*. In Recife, Brazil, where bancroftian filariasis is endemic, ADLA occurs much more frequently than FADL. Recurrent ADLA is a major risk factor for the development of elephantiasis, regardless of whether the initial cause of lymphatic dysfunction is filarial infection, congenital malformation, mastectomy, radiotherapy, or adenectomy. Thus, appropriate treatment and prevention of ADLA are key components of lymphedema and elephantiasis prevention.

Chronic Manifestations of Lymphatic Filariasis

The chronic manifestations of lymphatic filariasis include adenopathy, lymphedema, urogenital manifestations, and TPE.

The chronic manifestations of lymphatic filariasis include adenopathy, lymphedema, urogenital manifestations, and TPE

Adenopathy

When the adult worms live in the lymphatic vessels of a lymph node, the node may become enlarged. Lymph node enlargement is usually painless, and it may be the only clinical sign in infected persons, whether or not they are microfilaria positive. Most commonly involved are the inguinal, epitrochlear, and axillary nodes (30). The lymph nodes may attain considerable size, but they usually remain discrete and do not become fused.

Lymphedema

Dilatation of the lymphatic vessels induced by the presence of the adult worm eventually leads to lymphatic dysfunction. Patients often report that the initial episode of clinical lymphedema begins at the time of an injury, infection, or other event that stresses the lymphatic system, such as pregnancy. Lymphedema most frequently occurs in the lower extremities, but it also can involve the arms, breast, scrotal wall, penis, and, rarely, the vulva.

The differential diagnosis for edema of the leg includes lymphedema, chronic venous insufficiency, deep vein thrombophlebitis, lipedema, tumors, and a variety of other conditions (49, 56, 62). No clinical or laboratory marker currently exists that reliably distinguishes filarial from non-filarial etiology of lymphedema for an individual patient.

Although not all patients with elephantiasis report episodes of acute attacks, recurrent bacterial infections hasten the progression of lymphedema to elephantiasis by accelerating the process of fibrosis and sclerosis of the subcutaneous tissues and further damaging existing lymphatic vessels. These changes lead to the characteristic features of elephantiasis, including skin fold thickening, pachydermia, epidermal nodules, and pigmentary changes (8).

Urogenital Manifestations of Lymphatic Filariasis

The chronic urogenital manifestations of lymphatic filariasis include hematuria, hydrocele, chylocele, chyluria, lymphedema and elephantiasis of the scrotal wall and penis, and lymph scrotum.

Hematuria. Microscopic, or occasionally macroscopic, hematuria or proteinuria can be found in approximately 45% of persons who have *W. bancrofti* microfilaremia (22). The specific mechanisms underlying these abnormalities are not well defined, but it is thought that filaria-related circulating immune complexes are involved in producing renal damage. The hematuria and proteinuria are associated with microfilaria; clearing microfilariae from the peripheral blood results in complete resolution, even if the live adult worms remain (22).

Hydrocele. The pathogenesis and natural history of hydrocele in filariasis-endemic areas are not well understood. In most cases, onset of hydrocele is silent; i.e., it is not usually accompanied by an acute episode of FADL. These hydroceles are probably caused by lymphatic dysfunction secondary to lymphangiectasia induced by living worms. Death of adult worms following treatment with DEC can also provoke acute hydrocele. Most of these resolve spontaneously, but some require surgery.

When men with hydrocele in filariasis-endemic areas are examined by ultrasound, lymphangiectasia and adult worms can often be detected in the lymphatic vessels of the scrotal area. The location of the adult worms does not, by itself, explain the occurrence of hydrocele (50). Microfilaria may be found in the peripheral blood. When microfilariae are found in the hydrocele fluid, it is usually a result of fluid being contaminated by blood during the collection procedure (J. Noroes, unpublished data).

Chylocele. Chylocele occurs when dilated lymphatic vessels from the intrascrotal area rupture, causing leakage of lymph into the cavity of the testicular tunica vaginalis. The fluid may be milky white in color or reddish due to the presence of blood (hematochylocele). In filariasis-endemic areas, the presence of chylous fluid in the vaginal space is almost always associated with lymphatic filariasis. Chylocele cannot be reliably distinguished from

Microscopic, or occasionally macroscopic, hematuria or proteinuria can be found in approximately 45% of persons who have W. bancrofti microfilaremia

hydrocele on clinical examination or by ultrasound or transillumination. For this reason, aspiration and examination of fluid is the way to discriminate between these two conditions.

Chyluria.   Chyluria occurs when dilated lymphatic vessels of the urinary excretory system rupture, causing leaking of lymphatic fluid and chyle into the urine. The urine may be milky white in color, particularly after a fatty meal; red blood cells are often found. Chyluria is often intermittent. The diagnosis of filarial etiology is a process of exclusion, except when microfilariae are found in the urine.

Scrotal and penile lymphedema.   Dysfunction of the lymphatic vessels that drain the scrotal wall and penis occurs as a result of the presence of living worms. As occurs in the legs, secondary bacterial infections play an important role in the development of urogenital lymphedema and elephantiasis.

Lymph scrotum (acquired lymphangioma).   The pathogenesis of lymph scrotum is unclear, but previous surgery for hydrocele, and mainly chylocele, may be an important risk factor (2). Delicate vesicles on the surface of the skin that are formed by dilated lymphatic vessels may rupture, leak lymphatic fluid, and predispose the patient to secondary bacterial infection.

Tropical Pulmonary Eosinophilia (TPE)
TPE, a syndrome characterized by symptoms of bronchial asthma with paroxysmal nocturnal cough and anorexia, is a relatively unusual manifestation of infection with the filariae *W. bancrofti* or *B. malayi*. Patients usually have peripheral hypereosinophilia and high titers of IgE and antifilarial IgG4 antibodies. The chest X-ray can be normal or show diffuse pulmonary infiltrates. Although patients with TPE are amicrofilaremic by routine diagnosis, living adult worms may be seen on ultrasound (21).

Diagnosis

Blood and Serum
The standard of diagnosis of filarial infection is detection of microfilaria in peripheral blood (27). Samples of 20 to 60 μl of capillary blood are dried on a slide, stained with Giemsa or hematoxylin/Carrazzi stain, and examined under a microscope. A more sensitive method is to filter at least 1 ml of venous blood through a 3- to 5-μm Nuclepore filter (Nuclepore Corp., Pleasanton, Calif.) (27). In most areas where lymphatic filariasis is endemic, peak microfilarial densities occur at night; thus, blood must be collected at night to enhance test sensitivity. The microfilariae of *W. bancrofti* can be distinguished from those of other filarial nematodes by size, the presence of a sheath, the shape of the tail, and the pattern of the nuclei (Table 14.1).

Highly sensitive and specific assays that detect circulating *W. bancrofti* antigen are now commercially available. A major advantage of these

The standard of diagnosis of filarial infection is detection of microfilaria in peripheral blood

Table 14.1 Morphologic features of microfilariae commonly found in humans

Organism	Length (μm)	Diameter (μm)	Sheath	Length of cephalic space (μm)	The most anterior nuclei	Terminal nucleus	Length of caudal space (μm)	Shape of tail
Wuchereria bancrofti[a]	230–300	7–10	Yes[b]	5–7	Side by side	Elongate	5–15	Pointed
Brugia malayi[c]	175–260	4–6	Yes[b]	6–11	Side by side	Round	0	Terminal and subterminal nuclei, with constriction
Brugia timori[d]	290–340	6–7	Yes[b]	10–14	Side by side	Elongate to oval	0	Terminal and subterminal nuclei, without constriction
Loa loa[e]	175–300	5–8	Yes[b]	3–6	Side by side	Elongate	0–1	Pointed
Onchocerca volvulus	220–360	5–9	No	7–13	Side by side	Elongate	9–15	Finely pointed
Mansonella perstans	100–200	3.5–4.5	No	1–3	Side by side	Round	0	Bluntly rounded
Mansonella streptocerca	180–240	2.5–5.0	No	3–5	First four staggered but not overlapping	Oval or round	0	Bluntly rounded, "shepherd's crook"
Mansonella ozzardi	170–240	3–5	No	2–6	Side by side	Oval	3–8	Pointed

[a]See Fig. 14.10.
[b]Sheath may or may not stain with Giemsa.
[c]See Fig. 14.11.
[d]See Fig. 14.12.
[e]See Fig. 14.14 and 14.15.

assays is that circulating filarial antigen remains diurnally constant; therefore, blood for diagnosis can be collected during the day. The sensitivity of these assays tends to exceed that of examination of night blood for microfilaria, although sensitivity decreases in persons with ultra-low levels of microfilaremia (59).

Although antifilarial antibodies (anti-Brugia IgG) are elevated in infected persons, their specificity, even for IgG4, is inadequate for diagnostic use (11). PCR-based assays have been developed that detect circulating DNA for both W. bancrofti (69) and B. malayi (45), but they are not yet commercially available. Peripheral eosinophilia is often observed in persons with W. bancrofti infection, but this is a nonspecific finding that can result from coinfections with other nematodes (29).

Ultrasound examination of the scrotal area of infected men provides a noninvasive method with which to identify and localize living adult worms. Ultrasonographic diagnosis is possible because the live adult worms have a distinctive pattern of movement (called the "filaria dance sign") (5) (see Fig. 14.3) and the location of the adult worm "nests" remains stable within the lymphatic vessels (15). In men, the lymphatic vessels of the spermatic cord appear to be a preferred site of the adult worm, being detectable in at least 80% of infected men. In women and children, the adult worms are detected by ultrasound less frequently, although they have been observed in the breast (17), limbs, and inguinal cord (Dreyer, unpublished data).

Tissue Biopsies

Biopsies of lymph nodes or nodules in patients with lymphatic filariasis may reveal degenerating or apparently intact adult worms (30, 40, 41). Adult *W. bancrofti* can be distinguished from other adult filariae by size, thickness, and other features of the cuticle, the number of uteri, and other features (Tables 14.2 and 14.3).

Table 14.2 Morphologic features of eight adult female filariae that infect humans and for which humans are the common definitive host

Organism	Length (mm)	Maximum diameter (µm)	Thickness of cuticle (µm)	Other features of cuticle	Lateral chords	Somatic muscle	Uteri	Other features
Wuchereria bancrofti[a]	60–100	250	1–2	Fine transverse striations, thicker in lateral chords	Usually inconspicuous	Slightly to moderately developed	Usually two fill body cavity	
Brugia malayi	50–60	160	1–2	Fine transverse striations, thicker in lateral chords	Inconspicuous to prominent	Slightly to moderately developed	Usually two fill body cavity	
Brugia timori	21–39	140	NA[b]	NA	NA	NA	Usually	
Loa loa[c]	40–70	600	4–10	Irregularly spaced bosses, thicker in lateral chords	Usually conspicuous	Well developed	Usually three or four fill body cavity	Portion of uterus anterior to vulva
Onchocerca volvulus	230–500	450	4–10	Regularly spaced annulations	Inconspicuous to prominent	Slightly to well developed	Usually two do not fill body cavity	Diameter of intestines may be larger than uterus
Mansonella perstans	60–80	150	1–2	Very fine transverse striations, thicker in lateral chords	Usually inconspicuous	Slightly to moderately developed	Usually two fill body cavity	Conspicuous to inconspicuous pigmented granules in lateral chords
Mansonella ozzardi	65–81	250	NA	Smooth	NA	NA	NA	NA
Mansonella streptocerca	27	85	1–2	Smooth, thicker in lateral chords	Usually inconspicuous	Slightly to moderately developed	Usually two fill body cavity	Conspicuous to inconspicuous pigmented granules in lateral chords

[a] See Fig. 14.4.
[b] NA, Not available.
[c] See Fig. 14.13.

Table 14.3 Morphologic features of eight adult male filariae that infect humans and for which humans are the common definitive host

Organism	Length (mm)	Maximum diameter (μm)	Thickness of cuticle (μm)	Other features of cuticle	Lateral chords	Somatic muscle
Wuchereria bancrofti	40	150	1–2	Fine transverse striations, thicker in lateral chords	Inconspicuous to prominent	Moderately to well developed
Brugia malayi	22–25	90	1–2	Fine transverse striations, thicker in lateral chords	Inconspicuous to prominent	Moderately to well developed
Brugia timori	13–23	80	NA[a]	NA	NA	NA
Loa loa	30–34	400	4–10	Irregularly spaced bosses, internal longitudinal ridges	Usually conspicuous	Well developed
Onchocerca volvulus	16–42	200	3–5	Regularly spaced annulations	Conspicuous to prominent	Moderately developed
Mansonella perstans	35–45	70	1–2	Smooth, internal longitudinal ridges	Usually inconspicuous, with pigmented granules	Moderately to well developed
Mansonella ozzardi	38[b]	200	NA	Smooth	NA	NA
Mansonella streptocerca	17–18	50	1–2	Smooth, thicker in lateral chords	Usually inconspicuous, with pigmented granules	Moderately to well developed

[a]NA, Not available.
[b]Incomplete worm.

Pathology

Asymptomatic and Subclinical Lymphatic Filariasis

The mechanisms that cause lymphangiectasis, the earliest and most common lesion in lymphatic filariasis, are unknown. As long as the adult worms are alive, no inflammatory response occurs within the wall or lumen of the dilated lymphatic vessel, even at the site of the adult worm (see Fig. 14.4). Although distended, the endothelial lining remains well preserved as seen by light microscopy.

Acute Manifestations

Filarial Adenolymphangitis (FADL)

Both in American soldiers during World War II and in residents of endemic areas, biopsies of FADL reveal dead adult *W. bancrofti* and a local inflammatory response. The presence of a granulomatous reaction at the site of the adult worm is consistently observed, although the precise histologic pattern varies from case to case and even within the same patient.

In the initial phases of this inflammatory response, the endothelial lining of the lymphatic vessel is damaged and the lymphatic wall shows a diffuse infiltration of neutrophils, eosinophils, and mononuclear cells. In the lumen of the vessel, the degenerating worms are entrapped in a network of fibrin-like material and leukocytes (see Fig. 14.5). The characteristic detail of the worms is lost, and the usual contour of the surface becomes distorted. As the process of adult worm disruption progresses, a granulomatous reaction takes place, consisting of variable numbers of macrophages, lymphocytes, plasma cells, and eosinophils (see Fig. 14.6). The adult worm splits into several fragments, each with its own local clusters of inflammatory cells. At this stage, in some patients the lumen of the lymphatic vessel becomes obstructed and the inflammatory process spreads into the adjacent tissues. In some cases, a rim of eosinophilic and fibrinoid material around the parasite is observed, the so-called Splendore-Hoeppli phenomenon (see Fig. 14.7). Occasionally, neutrophils accumulate and form microabscesses in the center of the granulomas. Eosinophils are particularly abundant in biopsies from persons who have been treated with DEC. In other cases, an intramural nodule develops and the vessel remains patent. This explains the absence of obstruction in most cases of FADL.

The period for which an adult worm, once dead, remains recognizable in the tissues and the time course of its complete digestion are unknown. In time, however, the granulomas are dominated by giant cells, fibroblasts, and concentric collagen deposition; debris from the dead worms remains in the center (see Fig. 14.8). Before the adult worms have been completely destroyed and phagocytosed, they not rarely undergo calcification (see Fig. 14.9), which halts further shedding of parasite antigens and is a significant factor in terminating the inflammatory response.

Characteristically, FADL tends to recur at the same site. This can be explained by the occasional death of some, but not all, worms in the same nest. Indeed, ultrasound examinations have shown that the filaria dance sign may persist at the site of nodules that develop after treatment with DEC (51). When biopsied, these nodules reveal adult worms in various phases of degeneration side by side with apparently intact ones (24, 30). The factors that lead to death of some, but not all, worms within the same nest are unknown.

The period for which an adult worm, once dead, remains recognizable in the tissues and the time course of its complete digestion are unknown

Acute Dermatolymphangioadenitis (ADLA)

In marked contrast to FADL, biopsies of ADLA reveal acute and chronic inflammation but no evidence of adult *W. bancrofti*. In the early phases of lymphedema there is edema of the dermis, especially of the reticular areas without prominent epidermal alterations. In elephantiasis, the surface of the skin shows a verrucose pattern due to fibrotic protuberances and epidermal alterations such as hyperkeratosis, acanthosis, and papillomatosis. The dermal fibrosis may be extensive and usually presents dilated lymphatics and foci of perivascular chronic inflammation.

Chronic Manifestations

Adenopathy

Lymphadenopathy secondary to lymphatic filariasis is characterized by follicular and paracortical hyperplasia and reactive histiocytosis. The afferent and efferent lymphatic vessels are dilated. Apart from the presence of the adult parasite within the afferent or efferent lymphatic vessel, the histologic pattern is nonspecific, and no true lymphadenitis is observed. Even when eosinophilia of the peripheral blood occurs, eosinophils may not be present in the tissue sections when the adult worms are alive (29).

During episodes of FADL, the reactions evoked by dead adult worms in lymphatics reverberate secondarily in the draining lymph nodes. In biopsies of lymph nodes, living worms may be localized in the afferent or efferent lymphatics or, rarely, within the lymph node itself. When these worms die, the inflammatory response produces a true filarial adenitis. The inflammatory process is similar to that observed in the lymphatic vessels.

Treatment

The recent development of sensitive diagnostic tools and changes in understanding of the disease have led to opportunities for improved treatment of lymphatic filariasis. In the past, all patients have been treated with antiparasitic drugs, regardless of their clinical manifestations or infection status. However, for many of the acute and chronic manifestations of lymphatic filariasis, supportive or other forms of clinical care may be much more important than antiparasitic medication.

For many of the acute and chronic manifestations of lymphatic filariasis, supportive or other forms of clinical care may be much more important than antiparasitic medication

Diethylcarbamazine (DEC)

Fifty years after it was first introduced for lymphatic filariasis, DEC remains the drug of choice for treatment of persons infected with *W. bancrofti* or *B. malayi*. When given in conventional World Health Organization-recommended doses of 6 mg/kg/day for 12 consecutive days, microfilariae are rapidly cleared from the peripheral blood, although in a small percentage of infected persons, clearance of microfilariae is incomplete (53). A single 6-mg/kg dose produces a somewhat less rapid reduction in microfilaremia, although microfilaria levels for both regimens are similar 6 to 12 months after treatment (6, 63).

The degree to which DEC kills adult *W. bancrofti* or *B. malayi* appears to vary. Evidence for adult worm death after treatment includes prolonged suppression of microfilaremia, development of local nodules, and identification of degenerating adult worms in biopsies of these nodules (24, 30, 53). In Brazil, ultrasound has recently been used to directly monitor the effect of DEC on the adult worm in vivo (16, 51). After treatment with DEC, the characteristic movement of the adult worms became undetectable in 22 (42%) of 53 worm nests in 31 men (51). The efficacy of a single 6-mg/kg dose of DEC against the adult worm now appears to be comparable to that of the full 12-day course of treatment (30, 51). Furthermore, adult *W. bancrofti* that are not susceptible to low- or standard-dose DEC do not appear to be susceptible to higher doses of the drug (51).

Side effects, i.e., signs and symptoms associated with DEC per se, are mild or absent when the drug is given in daily doses of 6 mg/kg or less. Adverse reactions, i.e., signs and symptoms that are triggered by DEC in persons with filarial infections, can be either localized (associated with death of the adult worm) or systemic (associated with death of microfilariae). Local adverse reactions, which usually begin 1 to 3 days after the first dose of DEC (24), may include localized pain and inflammation, tender nodules, adenitis, and retrograde lymphangitis (12, 24). Systemic adverse reactions include fever, headache, malaise, myalgias, and hematuria (12, 24, 53). The occurrence of these reactions in a given individual is not predictable, but when they occur, their severity is directly related to the concentration of circulating microfilaria. They generally begin a few to 48 h after treatment with DEC is begun and last 1 to 3 days.

Because the inflammatory reaction against dying microfilariae can cause severe Mazzotti reactions and worsen ocular manifestations in persons with *Onchocerca volvulus* infection, DEC is contraindicated in persons with onchocerciasis. DEC may also cause severe adverse reactions, including encephalitis, in patients with loaiasis who have high levels of microfilariae. For these reasons, an attempt should be made to rule out *Loa loa* and *O. volvulus* infection before treating persons for lymphatic filariasis if they also may have been exposed to these parasites.

DEC appears to have no effect on lymphatic function (13, 34) and little or no effect on long-standing lymphedema or hydrocele. This is not surprising since most persons with long-standing lymphedema are no longer infected with the parasite. Therefore, DEC is not recommended for treatment of chronic manifestations of the disease, but as an antiparasitic drug.

Wyeth-Ayerst, the sole supplier of DEC in the United States, discontinued manufacture of the drug in 1997. The Centers for Disease Control and Prevention Drug Service plans to provide the drug to licensed United States physicians under an investigational new drug protocol. The drug will be available for treatment of persons with confirmed *W. bancrofti* or *B. malayi* infection.

> DEC is contraindicated in persons with onchocerciasis

Other Antifilarial Drugs

Ivermectin profoundly suppresses the concentration of *W. bancrofti* and *B. malayi* microfilariae in the peripheral blood for periods of 6 to 24 months when given in a single 200- to 400-µg/kg dose (3, 18, 26, 42, 58). However, the adult worms are not killed, even at high doses (14). For this reason, ivermectin is not used to treat individual patients with *W. bancrofti* or *B. malayi* infection, although it may play a very important role in community-based control programs. Ivermectin is commercially available in the United States as Stromectol (Merck and Co., Inc.). It is licensed by the Food and Drug Administration for treatment of onchocerciasis and strongyloidiasis.

Jayakody and colleagues have reported that repeat high-dose albendazole may have a macrofilaricidal effect against *W. bancrofti* (39). The efficacy of a single 400-mg dose has not been established. However, when given in combination with single-dose ivermectin or DEC, albendazole appears to enhance the microfilarial suppression of these other drugs. This feature has led Smith Kline Beecham to donate albendazole for control and elimination of lymphatic filariasis worldwide.

Specific Conditions

Persons with Active Filarial Infection

To prevent further lymphatic damage in infected individuals, treatment with DEC is recommended regardless of whether the individual has symptoms. In microfilaria-positive individuals, efficacy of treatment can be assessed by retesting for microfilaria 6 to 12 months after treatment. In men, the effect of DEC on the adult worm can be monitored by ultrasound of the scrotal area 2 to 4 weeks after treatment and by the appearance of nodules detected by physical examination. Periodic monitoring of circulating filarial antigen levels may be useful, although criteria have not been established for posttreatment monitoring using the antigen assays. Repeat treatment may be required.

Counseling should be provided on how to avoid overloading the capacity of the lymphatic vessels and thereby provoking clinical signs and symptoms. Secondary bacterial infections can be avoided through fastidious attention to hygiene, care of the skin and nails, prompt treatment of interdigital fungal infections, and wearing proper shoes to protect the feet from injury. Lymph stasis should be avoided through regular exercise, movement, and elevation of the limbs, especially at night.

Acute Filarial Adenolymphangitis (FADL)

Supportive treatment is recommended for acute FADL, including rest, postural drainage (particularly if the lower limb is affected), cold compresses at the site of inflammation, and antipyretics and analgesics for symptomatic relief. Hygiene of the affected area is also advised. During the acute episode, treatment with antifilarial drugs is not recommended because it may provoke additional adult worm death and exacerbate the inflammatory response. After the acute attack has resolved, if microfilaremia, circulating filarial antigen, or the filaria dance sign persist, a single dose of DEC can be given to kill the remaining adult worms. Because it is not always possible to rule out the possibility of living worms, treatment with DEC may still be indicated even if these diagnostic tests are negative.

Acute Dermatolymphangioadenitis (ADLA)

Treatment with DEC appears to have no effect on the outcome of ADLA. Instead, cold compresses, antipyretics, and analgesics are recommended. The patient should remain at rest with the affected limb elevated. If facilities are available, specimens of blood, tissue swabs, or tissue aspirates can be collected for bacterial culture, but antibiotic therapy must be initiated promptly. The bacteria isolated during these attacks are susceptible to most systemic antibiotics, including penicillin. Hygiene of the affected area and cure of entry lesions are essential.

Treatment with DEC appears to have no effect on the outcome of ADLA

Lymphedema

Extensive experience in Brazil (23; Dreyer, unpublished data), as well as preliminary data from Haiti and India, now indicates that elephantiasis and lymphedema of the leg are reversible with a treatment regimen that emphasizes hygiene, prevention of secondary bacterial infections, and physiotherapy. The degree of reversibility is dependent on the severity of the disease. This regimen is similar to that now recommended for treatment of lymphedema in Europe, Australia, and the United States (7, 9, 31, 32), where it is known by a variety of names including complex decongestive physiotherapy and complex lymphedema therapy.

Patient education is a critical feature of lymphedema treatment, both to alter fatalistic beliefs about the inevitable progression of the disease and to foster motivation. In filariasis-endemic areas where hygienic conditions are often substandard, the most important component in preventing acute bacterial attacks is meticulous attention to hygiene and skin care and treatment of skin lesions and fungal infections. Prompt antibiotic treatment of acute bacterial attacks, when they occur, is also important (see treatment of ADLA, above). Measures to reduce and manage chronic lymphedema also include range-of-motion exercises and elevation of the limb. Compressive bandaging and gentle massage may be used under medical supervision in selected cases. In filariasis-endemic areas, the role of surgery in the treatment of lymphedema of the limbs is limited.

Hydrocele
Recurrence rates are high following simple puncture and aspiration of hydrocele fluid. Results are somewhat better following injection of a sclerosing agent, a procedure that can be done on an outpatient basis, but the relapse rate is still high. The definitive treatment for hydrocele is surgical; a variety of techniques have been recommended.

The definitive treatment for hydrocele is surgical

Chylocele
The treatment for chylocele is surgical. Complete excision of the affected tunica vaginalis is recommended (Norões, unpublished data).

Chyluria
Treatment for chyluria includes rest and a diet rich in protein but low in fat (68). Improvement has been reported when medium-chain triglyceride was the only source of dietary fat (38). Adequate hydration is recommended to increase the frequency of micturition and decrease the risk of clot formation within the bladder. Surgical treatment for chyluria is controversial, but it is sometimes recommended for severe or intractable cases.

Lymphedema of the External Genitalia
Treatment of men with scrotal and penile lymphedema and lymph scrotum is similar to that described above for lymphedema of the leg, although the prognosis is much more guarded. Attention to hygiene and skin care is essential to prevent secondary bacterial infections. Additional treatment for fungi, especially candidiasis, is particularly important. Methods of surgical repair of these conditions need to be improved in filariasis-endemic areas.

Hematuria
Treatment with DEC usually clears microfilariae from the blood and produces resolution of microscopic or gross hematuria and proteinuria within 2 weeks (22). Patients should be followed after treatment to confirm that

microfilariae have been cleared from the blood; if microfilaremia persists, repeat treatment is indicated. In microfilaria-positive persons who have no hematuria or proteinuria before treatment, these findings may appear transiently 2 to 3 days after the start of treatment (24).

Tropical Pulmonary Eosinophilia (TPE)

DEC is the drug of choice for treatment of TPE. Characteristically, respiratory symptoms rapidly resolve following treatment with DEC. A 21- to 30-day course of DEC is recommended. Despite dramatic initial improvement following conventional treatment with DEC, symptoms recur in approximately 20% of patients 12 to 24 months after treatment (64), and a majority of patients continue to have subtle clinical, radiographic, and functional abnormalities 5 to 40 months after treatment (60). Repeat treatment may be necessary since DEC may kill only a proportion of adult worms (51) and microfilaria may again be released by the remaining female worms.

Prevention

Filarial infection can be prevented by reducing exposure to the parasite through use of insect repellent, bed nets, and appropriate clothing

For the individual traveler, filarial infection can be prevented by reducing exposure to the parasite through use of insect repellent, bed nets, and appropriate clothing. The effectiveness of DEC as a prophylactic agent has not been adequately demonstrated for bancroftian filariasis.

For persons with lymphedema or preclinical lymphatic damage, secondary prevention of ADLA and elephantiasis can be accomplished through scrupulous attention to hygiene and skin care. Interdigital fungal infections should be treated with topical antifungal agents. Some patients with advanced disease may benefit from prophylactic penicillin as given for prevention of rheumatic fever (46, 52; Dreyer, unpublished data).

It is believed that profound suppression of microfilaremia, through annual or semiannual community-based mass treatment with DEC, ivermectin, or a combination of the two drugs, can interrupt transmission (66). Alternatively, cooking or table salt can be fortified with DEC (35). Community use of DEC-fortified salt has been shown to dramatically reduce microfilarial density with no apparent adverse reactions (47).

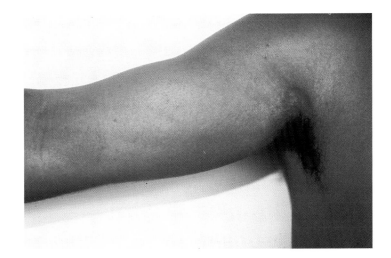

Figure 14.1 Characteristic linear cordlike lesion of filarial adenolymphangitis (FADL).

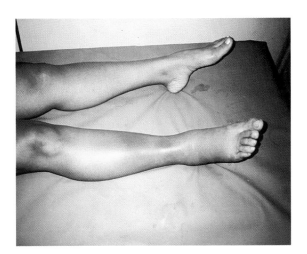

Figure 14.2 Acute dermatolymphangioadenitis (ADLA) of the lower limb. Note reticular pattern of inflammation.

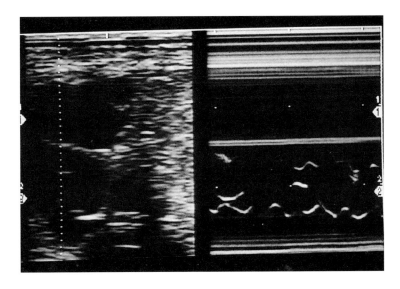

Figure 14.3 Characteristic pattern of movement within the lymphatic vessel, known as the filarial dance sign, seen on ultrasound of the scrotal area in a man infected with *W. bancrofti*.

Figure 14.4 Dilated lymphatic vessel containing several transverse sections of a male *W. bancrofti*, which is small and has a single reproduction tube. The single large section is of a gravid female *W. bancrofti* and demonstrates two uteri containing microfilariae. There is no inflammatory reaction in the vessel wall. Masson's trichrome stain; ×50.

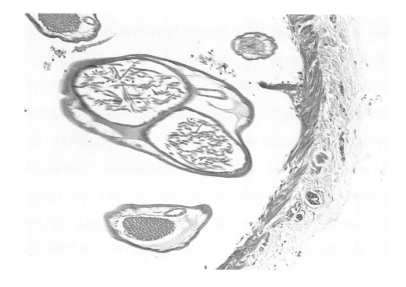

Figure 14.5 Lymphatic vessel containing degenerated adult worms entrapped in a fibrinous and leukocytic network. The vessel wall is thickened by a diffuse inflammatory infiltration. H&E stain, ×10.

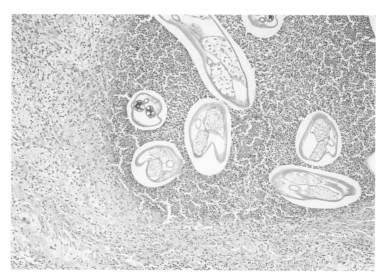

Figure 14.6 Granulomas composed of macrophages, lymphocytes, and eosinophils around transverse sections of degenerate adult worms; slender, elongate cells are embracing the parasite. H&E stain; ×50.

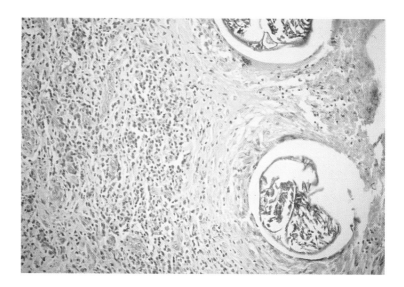

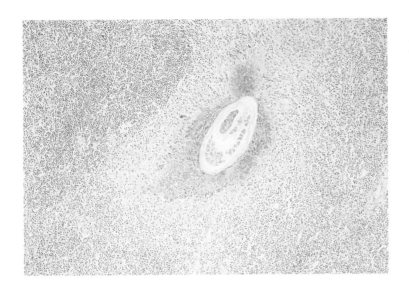

Figure 14.7 Granulomatous reaction around a degenerating adult worm within a lymph node. Note the rim of eosinophilic material (Splendore-Hoeppli phenomenon). H&E stain; ×25.

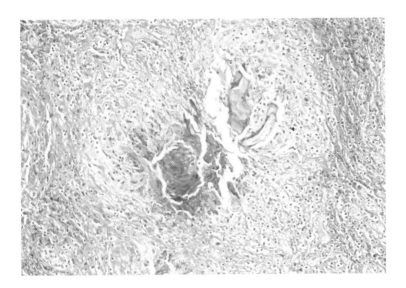

Figure 14.8 Concentric collagen deposition in a granuloma centered by remnants of dead adult worm. Masson's trichrome stain; ×50.

Figure 14.9 Fibrotic granulomas around calcified worms. H&E stain; ×25.

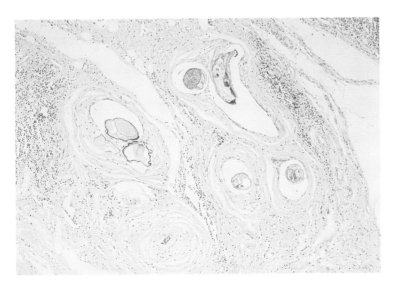

Figure 14.10 Microfilaria of *W. bancrofti* in thick blood film. The sheath is visible at both ends, and the terminal elongate nucleus does not extend to the tip of the tail. Delafield's hematoxylin stain; ×180.

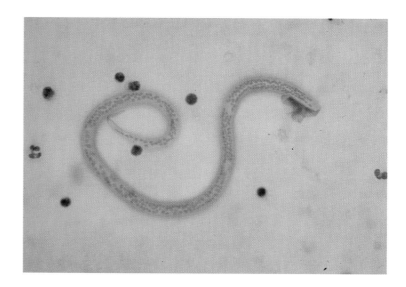

Figure 14.11 Microfilaria of *B. malayi* in thick blood film. The sheath and subterminal and terminal nuclei are demonstrated. Giemsa stain; ×250.

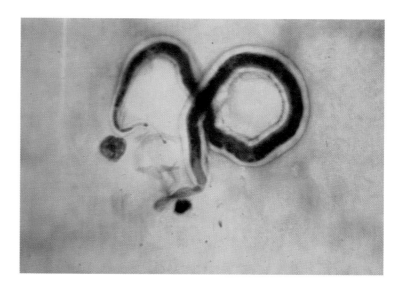

Figure 14.12 Microfilaria of *B. timori* in thick blood film. The sheath does not stain with Giemsa. The "innenkorper" and subterminal and terminal nuclei are observed. Giemsa stain; ×100.

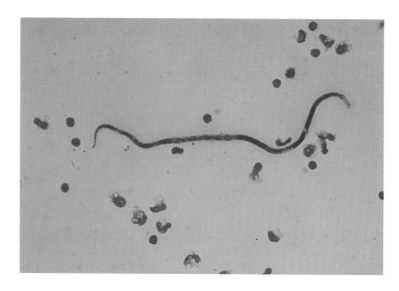

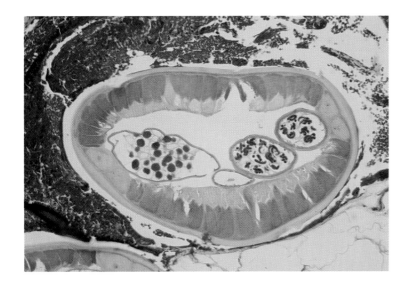

Figure 14.13   Transverse section of gravid *L. loa* in subcutaneous abscess. The worm has a thick cuticle, conspicuous lateral chords, prominent coelomyarian musculature, an intestine, and three sections of uteri containing microfilariae in various stages of development. Movat stain; ×45.

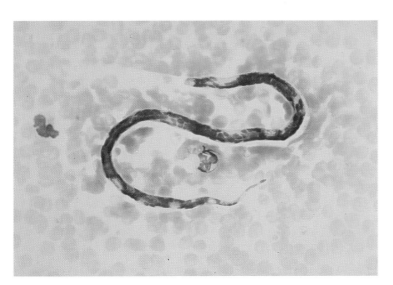

Figure 14.14   Microfilaria of *L. loa* in thin blood film. The sheath does not stain with Giemsa. The terminal elongate nucleus is at the tip of the tail. ×180.

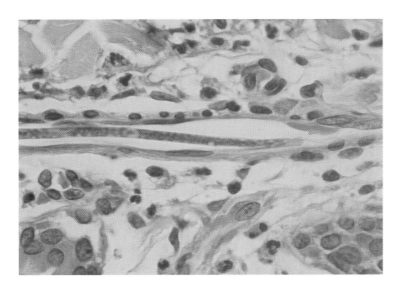

Figure 14.15   Microfilaria of *L. loa* in dermal capillary. Microfilariae of *L. loa* are usually 5 μm in diameter and sheaths are rarely observed. The cephalic space is 6 μm long. ×250.

References

1. **Acton, W. H., and S. S. Rao.** 1929. The importance of secondary infections in the causation of filarial lymphangitis. *Indian Med. Gaz.* **64:**421–423.

2. **Acton, W. H., and S. S. Rao.** 1930. The causation of lymph-scrotum. *Indian Med. Gaz.* **65:**541–546.

3. **Addiss, D. G., M. L. Eberhard, P. J. Lammie, M. B. McNeeley, S. H. Lee, D. M. McNeeley, and H. C. Spencer.** 1993. Comparative trial of clearing-dose and single high-dose ivermectin and diethylcarbamazine against *Wuchereria bancrofti* microfilaremia. *Am. J. Trop. Med. Hyg.* **48:**178–185.

4. **Albuquerque, M. F. M., M. C. Marzochi, P. C. Sabroza, M. C. Braga, T. Padilha, M. C. M. Silva, M. R. F. Silva, H. C. Schindler, M. A. Maciel, W. Souza, and A. F. Furtado.** 1995. Bancroftian filariasis in two urban areas of Recife, Brazil: pre-control observations on infection and disease. *Trans. R. Soc. Trop. Med. Hyg.* **89:**319–321.

5. **Amaral, F., G. Dreyer, J. Figueredo-Silva, J. Noroes, A. Cavalcanti, S. C. Samico, A. Santos, and A. Coutinho.** 1994. Adult worms detected by ultrasonography in human bancroftian filariasis. *Am. J. Trop. Med. Hyg.* **50:**753–757.

6. **Andrade, L. D., Z. Medeiros, L. Pires, A. Pimentel, A. Rocha, J. Figueredo-Silva, A. Coutinho, and G. Dreyer.** 1995. Comparative efficacy of three different diethylcarbamazine regimens in lymphatic filariasis. *Trans. R. Soc. Trop. Med. Hyg.* **89:**319–321.

7. **Boris, M., S. Weindorf, B. Lasinski, and G. Boris.** 1994. Lymphedema reduction by noninvasive complex lymphedema therapy. *Oncology* **8:**95–106.

8. **Burri, H., L. Loutan, V. Kumaraswami, and V. Vijayasekaran.** 1996. Skin changes in chronic lymphatic filariasis. *Trans. R. Soc. Trop. Med. Hyg.* **90:**671–674.

9. **Casley-Smith, J. R., and J. R. Casley-Smith.** 1992. Modern treatment of lymphoedema. I. Complex physical therapy: the first 200 Australian limbs. *Australas. J. Dermatol.* **33:**61–68.

10. **Centers for Disease Control and Prevention.** 1993. Recommendations of the International Task Force for Disease Eradication. *Morbid. Mortal. Weekly Rep.* **42**(RR-16):1–38.

11. **Chanteau, S., P. Glaziou, C. Moulia-Pelat, C. Plichart, P. Luquiaud, and J. L. Cartel.** 1994. Low positive predictive value of anti-*Brugia malayi* IgG and IgG4 serology for the diagnosis of *Wuchereria bancrofti*. *Trans. R. Soc. Trop. Med. Hyg.* **88:**661–662.

12. **Ch'en, T. T.** 1964. Demonstration of macrofilaricidal action of hetrazan, antimony, and arsenic preparations in man. *Chinese Med. J.* **83:**625–640.

13. **Dissanyake, S., L. Watawana, and W. F. Piessens.** 1995. Lymphatic pathology in *Wuchereria bancrofti* microfilaremic infections. *Trans. R. Soc. Trop. Med. Hyg.* **89:**517–521.

14. **Dreyer, G., D. Addiss, J. Norões, F. Amaral, A. Rocha, and A. Coutinho.** 1996. Direct assessment of the adulticidal efficacy of repeat high-dose ivermectin in bancroftian filariasis. *Trop. Med. Int. Health* **1:**427–432.

15. **Dreyer, G., F. Amaral, J. Norões, and Z. Medeiros.** 1994. Ultrasonographic evidence for stability of adult worm location in bancroftian filariasis. *Trans. R. Soc. Trop. Med. Hyg.* **88:**558.

16. **Dreyer, G., F. Amaral, J. Norões, Z. Medeiros, and D. Addiss.** 1995. A new tool to assess *in vivo* the adulticidal efficacy of antifilarial drugs for bancroftian filariasis. *Trans. R. Soc. Trop. Med. Hyg.* **89:**225–226.

17. **Dreyer, G., A. C. Brandao, F. Amaral, Z. Medeiros, and D. Addiss.** 1996. Detection by ultrasound of living adult *Wuchereria bancrofti* in the female breast. *Mem. Inst. Oswaldo Cruz* **91:**95–96.

18. **Dreyer, G., A. Coutinho, D. Miranda, J. Norões, J. A. Rizzo, E. Galdino, A. Rocha, Z. Medeiros, L. D. Andrade, A. Santos, J. Figueredo-Silva, and E. A. Ottesen.** 1995. Treatment of bancroftian filariasis in Recife, Brazil: a two-year comparative study of the efficacy of single treatment with ivermectin or diethylcarbamazine. *Trans. R. Soc. Trop. Med. Hyg.* **89:**98–102.

19. **Dreyer, G., and J. Norões.** 1997. Filariose bancroftiana, p. 399–421. *In* F. Militao, T. M. de Andrade Lima, T. F. Silva, and V. G. de Lucen (ed.), *Condutas em Clinica Medica.* Editora Universitaria, Recife, Brazil.

20. **Dreyer, G., J. Norões, and D. Addiss.** 1997. The silent burden of sexual disability associated with lymphatic filariasis. *Acta Trop.* **63:**57–60.

21. **Dreyer, G., J. Norões, A. Rocha, and D. Addiss.** 1996. Detection of living adult *Wuchereria bancrofti* in a patient with tropical pulmonary eosinophilia. *Brazilian J. Med. Biol. Res.* **29:**1005–1008.

22. **Dreyer, G., E. A. Ottesen, E. Galdino, L. Andrade, A. Rocha, Z. Medeiros, I. Moura, M. I. Cassimiro, M. F. Beliz, and A. Coutinho.** 1992. Renal abnormalities in microfilaremic patients with bancroftian filariasis. *Am. J. Trop. Med. Hyg.* **46:**745–751.

23. **Dreyer, G., and W. Piessens.** Worms and microorganisms can cause lymphatic disease in residents of filariasis-endemic areas. *In* S. Hoffman and G. Pasvol (ed.), *Tropical Medicine: Science and Practice.* Imperial College Press, London, in press.

24. **Dreyer, G., M. L. Pires, L. D. Andrade, E. Lopes, Z. Medeiros, J. Tenorio, A. Coutinho, J. Norões, and J. Figueredo-Silva.** 1994. Tolerance of diethylcarbamazine by microfilaraemic and amicrofilaraemic individuals in an endemic area of bancroftian filariasis, Recife, Brazil. *Trans. R. Soc. Trop. Med. Hyg.* **88:**232–236.

25. **Dreyer, G., A. Santos, J. Norões, A. Rocha, and D. Addiss.** 1996. Amicrofilaremic carriers of adult *Wuchereria bancrofti*. *Trans. R. Soc. Trop. Med. Hyg.* **90:**288–289.

26. **Eberhard, M. L., A. W. Hightower, D. F. McNeeley, and P. J. Lammie.** 1992. Long-term suppression of microfilaraemia following ivermectin treatment. *Trans. R. Soc. Trop. Med. Hyg.* **86:**287–288.

27. **Eberhard, M. L., and P. J. Lammie.** 1991. Laboratory diagnosis of filariasis. *Clin. Lab. Med.* **11:**977–1010.

28. **Edwards, E. A.** 1963. Recurrent febrile episodes and lymphedema. *JAMA* **184:**858–862.

29. **Figueredo-Silva, J., G. Dreyer, K. Guimaraes, C. Brandt, and Z. Medeiros.** 1994. Bancroftian lymphadenopathy: absence of eosinophils in tissues despite peripheral blood hypereosinophilia. *J. Trop. Med. Hyg.* **97:**55–59.

30. **Figueredo-Silva, J., P. Jungmann, J. Norões, W. F. Piessens, A. Coutinho, C. Brito, A. Rocha, and G. Dreyer.** 1996. Histological evidence for adulticidal effect of low doses of diethylcarbamazine in bancroftian filariasis. *Trans. R. Soc. Trop. Med. Hyg.* **90:**192–194.

31. **Foldi, E., M. Foldi, and L. Clodius.** 1989. The lymphedema chaos: a lancet. *Ann. Plast. Surg.* **22:**505–515.

32. **Foldi, E., M. Foldi, and H. Weissleder.** 1985. Conservative treatment of lymphoedema of the limbs. *Angiol. J. Vascul. Dis.* **3:**171–180.

33. **Freedman, D. O., P. J. Almeida Filho, S. Besh, M. C. Maia e Silva, C. Braga, and A. Maciel.** 1994. Lymphoscintigraphic analysis of lymphatic abnormalities in symptomatic and asymptomatic human filariasis. *J. Infect. Dis.* **170:**927–933.

34. **Freedman, D. O., T. Bui, P. J. De Almeida Filho, C. Braga, M. C. M. Silva, A. Maciel, and A. F. Furtado.** 1995. Lymphoscintigraphic assessment of the effect of diethylcarbamazine treatment on lymphatic damage in human bancroftian filariasis. *Am. J. Trop. Med. Hyg.* **52:**258–261.

35. **Gelband, H.** 1994. Diethylcarbamazine salt in the control of lymphatic filariasis. *Am. J. Trop. Med. Hyg.* **50:**655–662.

36. **Gyapong, J. O., P. Magnussen, and F. N. Binka.** 1994. Parasitological and clinical aspects of bancroftian filariasis in Kassena-Nankana District, Upper East Region, Ghana. *Trans. R. Soc. Trop. Med. Hyg.* **88:**555–557.

37. **Harb, M., R. Faris, A. M. Gad, O. N. Hafez, R. Ramzy, and A. A. Buck.** 1993. The resurgence of lymphatic filariasis in the Nile delta. *Bull. W. H. O.* **71:**49–54.

38. **Hashim, S. A.** 1964. Treatment of chyluria and chylothorax with medium chain triglycerides. *N. Engl. J. Med.* **270:**756–761.

39. **Jayakody, R. L., C. S. S. DeSilva, and W. I. Weerasinghe.** 1993. Treatment of bancroftian filariasis with albendazole: evaluation of efficacy and adverse reactions. *Trop. Biomed.* **10:**19–24.

40. **Jungmann, P., J. Figueredo-Silva, and G. Dreyer.** 1991. Bancroftian lymphadenopathy: a histopathologic study of fifty-eight cases from northeastern Brazil. *Am. J. Trop. Med. Hyg.* **45:**325–331.

41. **Jungmann, P., J. Figueredo-Silva, and G. Dreyer.** 1992. Bancroftian lymphangitis in northeastern Brazil: a histopathological study of 17 cases. *J. Trop. Med. Hyg.* **95:**114–118.

42. **Kazura, J., J. Greenberg, R. Perry, G. Weil, K. Day, and M. Alpers.** 1993. Comparison of single-dose diethylcarbamazine and ivermectin for treatment of bancroftian filariasis in Papua New Guinea. *Am. J. Trop. Med. Hyg.* **49:**804–811.

43. **Lal, R. B., and E. A. Ottesen.** 1988. Enhanced diagnostic specificity in human filariasis by IgG4 antibody assessment. *J. Infect. Dis.* **158:**1034–1037.

44. **Lammie, P. J., D. G. Addiss, G. Leonard, A. W. Hightower, and M. L. Eberhard.** 1993. Heterogeneity in filarial-specific immune responsiveness among patients with lymphatic obstruction. *J. Infect. Dis.* **167:**1178–1183.

45. **Lizotte, M. R., T. Supali, F. Partono, and S. A. Williams.** 1994. A polymerase chain reaction assay for the detection of *Brugia malayi* in blood. *Am. J. Trop. Med. Hyg.* **51:**314–321.

46. **Martin, W. J.** 1969. Antibiotic therapy in the management of lymphangitis. *Mod. Treat.* **6:**391–395.

47. **Meyrowitsch, D. W., P. E. Simonsen, and W. H. Makunde.** 1996. Mass diethylcarbamazine chemotherapy for control of bancroftian filariasis through community participation: comparative efficacy of a low monthly dose and medicated salt. *Trans. R. Soc. Trop. Med. Hyg.* **90:**74–79.

48. **Montestruc, E., E. Courmes, and R. Fontan.** 1960. Endemic lymphangitis in French Guiana and its relation to *W. bancrofti* filariasis. *Indian J. Malariol.* **14:**637–650.

49. **Mortimer, P. S.** 1990. Investigation and management of lymphoedema. *Vas. Med. Rev.* **1:**1–20.

50. **Norões, J., D. Addiss, A. Santos, Z. Medeiros, A. Coutinho, and G. Dreyer.** 1996. Ultrasonographic evidence of abnormal lymphatic vessels in young men with adult *Wuchereria bancrofti* infection in the scrotal area. *J. Urol.* **156:**409–412.

51. **Norões, J., G. Dreyer, A. Santos, V. G. Mendes, Z. Medeiros, and D. Addiss.** 1997. Assessment of the efficacy of diethylcarbamazine on adult *Wuchereria bancrofti in vivo. Trans. R. Soc. Trop. Med. Hyg.* **91:**78–81.

52. **Olszewski, W. L., S. Jamal, G. Manokaran, S. Pani, V. Kumaraswami, U. Kubicka, B. Lukomska, A. Dworczynski, E. Swoboda, and F. Meisel-Mikolajczyk.** 1997. Bacteriologic studies of skin, tissue fluid, lymph, and lymph nodes in patients with filarial lymphedema. *Am. J. Trop. Med. Hyg.* **57:**7–15.

53. **Ottesen, E. A.** 1985. Efficacy of diethylcarbamazine in eradicating infection with lymphatic-dwelling filariae in humans. *Rev. Infect. Dis.* **7:**341–356.

54. **Ottesen, E. A.** 1989. Filariasis now. *Am. J. Trop. Med. Hyg.* **41:**S9–S17.

55. **Ottesen, E. A., F. Skvaril, S. P. Tripathy, R. W. Poindexter, and R. Hussain.** 1985. Prominence of IgG4 in the IgG antibody response to human filariasis. *J. Immunol.* **134:**2707–2712.

56. **Pflug, J. J.** 1976. Diagnosis and management of the chronically swollen leg, p. 128–141. *In* J. Calnan (ed.), *Recent Advances in Plastic Surgery.* Churchill Livingstone, Edinburgh.

57. **Ramu, K., K. D. Ramaiah, H. Guyatt, and D. Evan.** 1996. Impact of lymphatic filariasis on the productivity of male weavers in a south Indian village. *Trans. R. Soc. Trop. Med. Hyg.* **90:**669–670.

58. **Richards, F. O., M. L. Eberhard, R. T. Bryan, D. F. McNeeley, P. J. Lammie, M. B. McNeeley, Y. Bernard, A. W. Hightower, and H. C. Spencer.** 1991. Comparison of high-dose ivermectin and diethylcarbamazine for activity against bancroftian filariasis in Haiti. *Am. J. Trop. Med. Hyg.* **44:**3–10.

59. **Rocha, A., D. Addiss, M. E. Ribiero, J. Norões, M. Baliza, Z. Medeiros, and G. Dreyer.** 1996. Evaluation of the Og4C3 ELISA in *Wuchereria bancrofti* infection: infected persons with undetectable or ultra-low microfilarial densities. *Trop. Med. Int. Health* **1:**859–864.

60. **Rom, W. N., V. K. Vijayan, M. J. Cornelius, V. Kumaraswami, R. Prabhakar, E. A. Ottesen, and R. G. Crystal.** 1990. Persistent lower respiratory tract inflammation associated with interstitial lung disease in patients with tropical pulmonary eosinophilia following conventional treatment with diethylcarbamazine. *Am. Rev. Respir. Dis.* **142:**1088–1092.

61. **Rome, H. P., and R. H. Fogel.** 1943. The psychosomatic manifestations of filariasis. *J. Am. Med. Assoc.* **123:**944–946.

62. **Ruschhaupt, W. F., and R. A. Graor.** 1985. Evaluation of the patient with leg edema. *Postgrad. Med.* **78:**132–139.

63. **Simonsen, P. E., D. W. Meyrowitsch, W. H. Makunde, and P. Magnussen.** 1995. Selective diethylcarbamazine chemotherapy for control of bancroftian filariasis in two communities of Tanzania: compared efficacy of a standard dose treatment and two semi-annual single dose treatments. *Am. J. Trop. Med. Hyg.* **53:**267–272.

64. **Udwadia, F. E.** 1967. Tropical eosinophilia. *Prog. Respir. Res.* **7:**35–155.

65. **Wartman, W. B.** 1947. Filariasis in American armed forces in World War II. *Medicine* **26:**333–394.

66. **World Health Organization.** 1994. Strategies for control of lymphatic filariasis infection and disease: report of a WHO/CTD/TDR consultative meeting held at the Universiti Sains, Malaysia, Penang, Malaysia, 22–24 August 1994.

67. **World Health Organization.** 1995. World Health Report, 1995. World Health Organization, Geneva.

68. **Yu, H. Y. Y.** 1984. Chyluria, p. 296–304. *In* I. Husain (ed.), *Tropical Urology and Renal Disease.* Churchill Livingstone, Edinburgh.

69. **Zhong, M., J. McCarthy, L. Bierwert, M. R. Lizott-Waniewski, S. Chanteau, T. B. Nutman, E. A. Ottesen, and S. A. Williams.** 1996. A PCR assay for the detection of the parasite *Wuchereria bancrofti* in human blood samples. *Am. J. Trop. Med. Hyg.* **54:**357–363.

chapter 15

Epidemiology and Molecular Biology of Antimicrobial Resistance in Bacteria

Fred C. Tenover and John E. McGowan, Jr.

The list is growing of emerging infectious diseases and traditional nosocomial and community-acquired infections that exhibit new or increased resistance to multiple antimicrobial agents (5). This change has suggested the possibility of a post-antibiotic era (13). *Enterococcus faecium, Streptococcus pneumoniae,* and *Staphylococcus aureus* (9, 36) are just a few of the organisms that have become considerably more difficult to treat due to increasing drug resistance. Examples of the types of resistant bacteria that have emerged around the world are shown in Fig. 15.1, while specific examples of emerging resistance problems in the United States are shown in Fig. 15.2. Clearly, the emergence of resistant organisms has been a global phenomenon. This article explores the development and spread of drug-resistant bacteria.

Fred C. Tenover, Nosocomial Pathogens Laboratory Branch, Hospital Infections Program, Centers for Disease Control and Prevention, Mailstop G-08, 1600 Clifton Road, Atlanta, GA 30333. **John E. McGowan, Jr.,** Department of Epidemiology, Rollins School of Public Health, and Department of Pathology and Laboratory Medicine, Emory University, Atlanta, GA 30322.

Pathology of Emerging Infections 2
Edited by Ann Marie Nelson and C. Robert Horsburgh, Jr.
© 1998 American Society for Microbiology, Washington, D.C.

A Brief History of Antimicrobial Resistance

Resistance to antimicrobial agents is not a new phenomenon in bacteria. The first resistance mechanism was recorded in 1940 by Abraham and Chain, who isolated and characterized an enzyme from *Escherichia coli* (then called *Bacterium coli*) that was capable of hydrolyzing penicillin (1). In 1944, Kirby reported the presence of a similar penicillinase-type enzyme in *S. aureus* (32). Thus, even before the widespread use of penicillin around the globe, resistance had already been detected in both gram-positive and gram-negative organisms. Furthermore, studies by Gardner and colleagues indicated that strains of bacteria resistant to tetracycline and streptomycin could be isolated from soil and human stool samples from the Solomon Islands even though antimicrobial agents had never been used in the population (19), indicating that resistance was not simply a consequence of use, but an integral part of a bacterium's own defense system enhancing its ability to survive in hostile environments.

In 1959, resistance to multiple drugs was recognized in strains of *Shigella dysenteriae* in Japan, and it was soon discovered that all of the resistance traits in that organism could be transferred to a recipient strain of *E. coli* via cell-to-cell matings (2). The implications of transferable drug resistance were of concern to many scientists, but others felt that this was only a unique laboratory phenomenon.

In the late 1960s and early 1970s, multiresistance again emerged, first in *S. aureus*, then in a variety of gram-negative bacilli, particularly those causing nosocomial outbreaks (45, 52, 69). Concerns regarding increased resistance in community-acquired pathogens were raised by the recognition of strains of *Haemophilus influenzae* and *Neisseria gonorrhoeae* that had acquired the genetic information required to produce ß-lactamase (18, 57). These events required physicians to alter the empiric therapy for these infections, thus making the threat of resistance more tangible. Fears of outbreaks of untreatable organisms were allayed by the hope that newer anti-infective agents, including extended-spectrum cephalosporins in the 1980s (50) and the fluoroquinolones in the 1990s (51), would be effective against even multiply resistant organisms. Yet, resistance to these classes of drugs also appeared. Some strains of several species of bacteria, including *Acinetobacter baumannii*, *Burkholderia* (*Pseudomonas*) *cepacia*, and *Enterococcus faecium*, are now resistant to essentially all approved antimicrobial agents (17, 39, 64). Unfortunately, there are very few new classes of antibacterial agents to look forward to at this time, as many pharmaceutical manufacturers had abandoned antibacterial drug discovery programs for several years, preferring to focus on identifying antifungal and antiviral drugs (72). Although new antibacterial compounds continue to appear in the literature, many will prove to be too toxic for human use, and those that appear suitable may take 7 to 10 years to receive final approval from the Food and Drug Administration (21). This has led some physicians to reconsider the use of older antimicrobial agents, such as novobiocin, colistin, and polymyxin, that had been abandoned due to their inherent toxicity problems, as possible therapeutic agents for these multiply resistant pathogens.

Unfortunately, there are very few new classes of antibacterial agents to look forward to at this time

Pathways by Which Resistance Appears

Several pathways have been described for the appearance or spread of resistance in bacteria (42). Each of these conceivably may have a role in the appearance or increase of resistant organisms in several different settings of the health care system.

First, new strains may be introduced into a new setting from an outside source, by way of a patient from the outside, a health care worker from outside or another institution, or a contaminated commercial product. Introduction of resistant strains into hospitals from nursing homes and extended care facilities, as well as transfer in the opposite direction from hospital to nursing home, has become common for certain pathogens (53). Resistant organisms may be more difficult to eradicate in certain parts of the health care system than in others. For example, extensive resources have been needed to eradicate methicillin-resistant *S. aureus* (MRSA) strains once they have been introduced (29).

Second, resistance can be acquired by a previously susceptible strain from another species or genus (61). Both genetic mutation and transfer of genetic material can produce this. Changes in only a few base pairs, causing substitution of one or a few amino acids in a crucial target (enzyme, cell structure, or cell wall), can affect chromosomal structural or control genes and lead to new resistant strains. The changed defense often is able to inactivate whole groups of antimicrobial agents. Many of the antibacterial resistance genes are on plasmids that can, and do, transfer themselves to another genus or species of bacteria. This pathway is presumed to be the means by which enterococci exchange genes with other gram-positive organisms. This exchange has not occurred in the past because the organisms seldom encounter each other in nature (61). However, both organisms are an important part of the ecosystem of the acute care hospital, and this is where glycopeptide-resistant as well as ß-lactamase-producing enterococci were first observed (46). Other resistance emerging by mutation or transfer has first been detected in the ambulatory care setting. For example, strains of *Shigella dysenteriae* that are resistant to all antibiotics except fluoroquinolones are being recovered with increasing frequency in Africa, particularly in Burundi (60). Transfer of such strains to ambulatory care clinics in the United States could have grave repercussions for health care systems.

Third, chromosomal determinants for resistance to a given drug may not be expressed until the organism comes in contact with it or similar compounds. When permissive conditions appear (e.g., new antibiotics in use, introduction of new conjugative plasmids), the resistance can be manifested rapidly (11). The trigger for emergence may be the antimicrobial agent to which resistance is directed. In some cases, exposure to another antimicrobial results in induction or derepression of a determinant (enzyme, etc.) that stimulates resistance as well to the studied drug (63). Likewise, exposure to a stimulus that inhibits or kills the susceptible majority of a population allows a resistant subset of strains to grow at the expense of susceptible organisms. The factor in this selection process usually is the antibiotic to which the subpopulation is resistant, but on occasion a related agent can have a great

Strains of S. dysenteriae that are resistant to all antibiotics except fluoroquinolones are being recovered with increasing frequency in Africa, particularly in Burundi

Health care systems must examine the use of all antimicrobial agents in all settings

impact as well; non-drug factors such as those stimulating activity of reactions like acetylation or glucuronylation also can provide a selective advantage to organisms (41). This explains why health care systems must examine the use of all antimicrobial agents in all of the settings that are part of the system, rather than looking only at use of the drug to which resistance has occurred or is feared. Yet, for certain organism-drug combinations use of the drug itself seems closely linked to resistance (38).

Fourth, organisms can be spread in clonal fashion from patient to patient, from one patient to another via a health care worker (e.g., on the hands of ward personnel), in contaminated commercial products (e.g., antiseptics), on other inanimate objects, or by widespread transfer of genetic material from the initial organism to others. The importance of cross-transmission varies from one health system to another. For example, a study from a medical center in Indianapolis found that endemic bacterial cross-transmission was uncommon in an intensive care unit setting, and that a variety of organisms were involved in the episodes of dissemination that were identified (10). In contrast, a more recent study from France found "a ubiquitous and prevalent clone" to be responsible for more than half of the clinical isolates of *Enterobacter aerogenes* in two intensive care units (15). This suggested a major role for cross-infection.

Most current outbreaks of resistance in hospital or community settings, and virtually all endemic occurrences of resistance, involve a number of these pathways, each to a greater or lesser degree (75). Risk determinants associated with each have been defined (Table 15.1). Sorting out the multiple and concurrent elements that lead to appearance and spread of resistance is an important but difficult problem (42). Control measures to deal with each of these resistance pathways vary considerably (Table 15.2), so efforts to prevent or control resistance problems depend in part on determining which pathways are operative in a given situation.

Table 15.1   Pathways[a] by which resistance appears or is spread and risk determinants for operation of each pathway

Pathway 1. Introduction of resistant organism from outside source
- Transfer of patient from other institutions in health care system (acute care, extended care, etc.)
- Transfer of patient from outside system
- Entry of patient from community
- Use of contaminated commercial product

Pathway 2. Mutation, genetic transfer
- Reservoirs with high organism concentration (increased chance for random mutation or transfer; lung abscess, abdominal abscess, etc.)

Pathway 3. Emergence, selection
- Selective pressures from antimicrobial use (whether prescribed appropriately or not)

Pathway 4. Clonal dissemination within an institution or setting
- Improper or insufficient barrier isolation
- Lack of attention to major vectors of transmission (intravenous catheters, transducers, respiratory therapy equipment, etc.)

[a]Described in detail in reference 42.

Table 15.2 Interventions to deal with resistant organisms, according to the pathway by which resistance appears or is spread

Pathway 1. Introduction of resistant organism from outside source
- Surveillance and empiric isolation
- Survey for resistance in patients coming from known reservoirs of resistant organisms (chart flagged, etc.)
- Implement barrier isolation precautions for patients from known sites within or outside the health care system (discontinue precautions only after cultures are negative)

Pathway 2. Mutation, genetic transfer
- Decrease reservoirs of organisms with potential for mutation (proper care of instruments, fluids, selective decontamination, etc.)

Pathway 3. Emergence, selection
- Decrease antibiotic selective pressures

Pathway 4. Clonal dissemination within an institution or setting
- Institute barrier isolation precautions to contain resistant organisms (by attention to reservoirs and pathways of spread)
- Maintain proper use of equipment and procedures (major risk determinants for spread)

Critical Factors in Emergence of Resistance

Among the factors above that have contributed to the emergence and spread of multiply resistant organisms, three are of key importance: mutations in common resistance genes that have extended their spectrum of resistance; exchange of genetic information among microorganisms, transferring well-known genes into new hosts; and the increase in selective pressures in hospitals, other institutional settings, and communities that allows resistant organisms to proliferate. The first two reflect the ability of bacteria to adapt to changing environments, while the last emphasizes that environmental conditions often enhance the emergence of novel phenotypes. All three are clearly interrelated (45, 52).

Mutations in Common Genes

One example of the role of mutations in emerging resistance concerns changes in ß-lactamases that extend their spectrum of activity. ß-Lactamases are enzymes that inactivate ß-lactam drugs such as penicillin, ampicillin, and cephalothin (7). Until recently, these enzymes were not able to hydrolyze newer extended-spectrum cephalosporins such as cefotaxime and ceftazidime. However, in 1982, mutant forms of ß-lactamases were reported that were capable of inactivating the extended-spectrum cephalosporins and monobactams such as aztreonam (34). The enzymes, called extended-spectrum ß-lactamases or ESBLs, have now been isolated from organisms throughout Europe, Japan, and the United States. At least 60 such ESBLs have now been reported (28, 56). When the amino acid sequences of the first ESBLs were examined (66), only three differences were found between the ESBL and the wild-type ß-lactamase that is found in 70% of *E. coli* strains that are ampicillin resistant but extended-spectrum cephalosporin susceptible (62). These amino acid changes were the reflection of point mutations in the coding sequence of the ß-lactamase gene. Recent experience suggests

In 1982, mutant forms of ß-lactamases were reported that were capable of inactivating the extended-spectrum cephalosporins and monobactams such as aztreonam

that under the selective pressure of high cephalosporin usage in a hospital ward, organisms with mutations that extend the spectrum of activity of β-lactamases can emerge and disseminate (43). The development and spread of ceftazidime-resistant *Klebsiella pneumoniae* is perhaps the best example of this phenomenon (59). These organisms, which contain variations of common bla_{TEM} or bla_{SHV} β-lactamase genes (*bla* for β-lactamase), have caused a number of outbreaks in the United States (6). Mutations in β-lactamase genes, however, are but one example of the many ways in which mutations can lead to resistance. Reduced membrane permeability limiting a drug's access into the cell, changes in a drug's target site, and blocking of drug uptake can all be a result of mutation.

Genetic Exchange

Bacteria can exchange genetic information by transformation (the uptake of naked DNA), transduction (transfer of DNA by bacteriophage), and conjugation (cell-to-cell contact) (16). Although conjugation was previously thought to be limited to gram-negative bacilli, extensive data now confirm the existence of a similar transfer process among gram-positive organisms whereby plasmids or independent transposable elements, often carrying multiple resistance genes, move from one organism to another (12). The transfer process extends even to highly unrelated groups of organisms, such as *Campylobacter coli* and enterococci (73), which have been shown to exchange aminoglycoside resistance genes.

Enterococci provide a prime example of how organisms can gradually accumulate resistance genes by genetic exchange and develop into multiresistant nosocomial pathogens causing untreatable infections. Enterococci accounted for 16,571 nosocomial infections in hospitals reporting to the National Nosocomial Infection Surveillance System (NNIS) during the period from January 1, 1989, to March 31, 1993 (8). Over the past decade, enterococci have become increasingly resistant to multiple antimicrobial agents. For example, the genes encoding resistance to gentamicin and the production of ß-lactamase were acquired from staphylococci (31, 47). When this development was added to resistance to streptomycin and vancomycin, it resulted in organisms that were very difficult, if not impossible, to treat (23, 44). Streptomycin resistance is mediated primarily by an aminoglycoside-modifying enzyme, ANT, although resistance due to ribosomal mutation has also been noted (55). Vancomycin resistance can be mediated by several genes, including *vanA*, *vanB*, *vanC1*, *vanC2*, and *vanD* (35, 49), that function in concert with other genetic loci frequently located on the same transposable element (35). The increase in the proportion of nosocomial enterococcal isolates resistant to vancomycin, particularly from intensive care unit patients, is alarming. It rose from 0.4% to 13.6% in the 4-year period from 1989 to 1993 (8) and continued to rise from 1994 to 1997.

Although resistance genes from gram-positive organisms may transfer into gram-negative organisms and vice versa, differences in the genetic control mechanisms present in various species may limit the ability of the new resistance genes to be expressed and to mediate resistance (14). Thus, there

The increase in the proportion of nosocomial enterococcal isolates resistant to vancomycin, particularly from intensive care unit patients, is alarming

appear to be some limits to the constellation of resistance genes that can be assembled and expressed in bacteria. Nonetheless, the ability of bacteria to acquire resistance genes from other members of the normal bacterial flora under the selective pressure of antimicrobial use should not be underestimated. It has been shown, for example, that the *vanA* vancomycin resistance gene cluster in *Enterococcus faecalis* can transfer to *S. aureus* via conjugation and can express high-level resistance (54). Although an *S. aureus* isolate with high-level vancomycin resistance has yet to be encountered in nature, the possibility clearly exists that the genetic unit that includes *vanA*, or perhaps one of the other vancomycin resistance genes, will be transferred under natural conditions to *S. aureus*. Such an occurrence would have serious patient and public health implications. MRSA strains, which may well be the recipient of the vancomycin resistance gene since they are most prevalent in hospitals, tend to be resistant to most clinically useful drugs (22). Strains of MRSA with reduced susceptibility to vancomycin (MIC = 8 µg/ml) have been isolated from patients on long regimens of vancomycin. The mechanisms of reduced susceptibility currently are unknown (24).

Selective Pressures in Institutional and Community Settings

The concept of selective pressure refers to the environmental conditions that encourage or enhance the proliferation of strains of bacteria that develop resistance to antimicrobial agents through spontaneous mutation or by acquisition of new DNA. It is hypothesized that organisms with new mutations or genes would likely not survive were it not for those environmental conditions that encouraged their emergence (16, 45). As noted above, resistant organisms can spread in communities or in hospital settings (13, 52). Expanded use of antimicrobial agents in sites outside of the hospital, e.g., nursing homes, day care centers, and animal feedlots, increases the selective pressure for resistant organisms to emerge in these settings (3). The use of broad-spectrum antimicrobial agents is increasing in outpatient settings (20, 40), and antimicrobial drugs are often used for common conditions for which their effectiveness is unclear (20).

S. pneumoniae serves as an example of a community-acquired organism that has become increasingly resistant to a wide variety of antimicrobial agents (33). A report from the metropolitan Atlanta area noted that 25% of invasive pneumococcal isolates from that region were no longer susceptible to penicillin and 9% were no longer susceptible to extended-spectrum cephalosporins (25). The development and spread of multiply resistant pneumococci can be a major problem among children in day care centers. In this setting, antimicrobial agent use is often high (58), in part because children have clinically confirmed, or suspected, otitis media (27). When children are on antimicrobial agents, the likelihood increases that multiresistant organisms will be found in their throats; these strains may disseminate to other children. Among three children with pneumococcal meningitis caused by strains resistant to cefotaxime and ceftriaxone, all had received prior cephalosporin therapy for otitis media (65). Thus, control of

> *S. pneumoniae serves as an example of a community-acquired organism that has become increasingly resistant to a wide variety of antimicrobial agents*

antimicrobials, particularly those used prophylactically in children attending day care centers, is an issue that must be reassessed and, hopefully, decreased.

Detection of Antimicrobial Resistance in the Clinical Laboratory

Several of the new resistance mechanisms recognized in gram-positive and gram-negative organisms are difficult to detect with current laboratory methods. For example, vancomycin resistance in enterococci can be difficult to detect by automated methods, such as Vitek and MicroScan Walk-Away, but is readily detected by most other broth- and agar-based methods (70). A vancomycin resistance agar screen test has been developed as a backup to traditional susceptibility testing methods for the detection of vancomycin-resistant enterococci (68).

With regard to resistance in gram-negative bacilli, a major problem noted recently is the detection of cefotaxime, ceftriaxone, and ceftazidime resistance in *K. pneumoniae* and *E. coli*, particularly when resistance is mediated by ESBLs (see above) (30). In part, the inability of the laboratory to recognize resistant strains is due to the minimal inhibitory concentration (MIC) breakpoints chosen by the National Committee for Clinical Laboratory Standards (NCCLS) to define "resistance" (48). The breakpoints, which for extended-spectrum cephalosporins are usually 32 or 64 µg/ml, were chosen based on population distributions of bacteria studied before ESBLs became widely disseminated. Depending on the antimicrobial agent tested in the laboratory, MICs for ESBL-containing strains may vary anywhere from 4 µg/ml (susceptible) to 256 µg/ml (highly resistant). Variation depends on the type of ESBL (of which there are over 60), the antimicrobial agent tested, and the method of testing. Given that the usual cefotaxime MIC of *K. pneumoniae* is 0.06 µg/ml, it is possible for the organism to achieve a 50-fold increase in MIC and still be in the "susceptible" MIC range. However, if ceftazidime were tested in lieu of cefotaxime, resistance might well be detected (30). New laboratory tests to confirm the presence of ESBLs in *K. pneumoniae* and *E. coli*, such as disk diffusion assays performed in parallel with and without the addition of the enzyme inhibitor clavulanic acid, may aid in the detection of such organisms. Other commercially prepared tests are under evaluation. NCCLS-sponsored studies also are currently under way to develop alternative testing procedures to detect ESBL-mediated resistance. Because laboratories need to screen a variety of bacterial pathogens that were once considered uniformly susceptible, a guide to appropriate susceptibility testing methods has been established (Table 15.3). While new testing methods may aid in identifying organisms with novel resistance genes, growing restraints on the personnel and supply budgets in hospital-based microbiology laboratories may hinder the widespread implementation of the tests. In fact, new laboratory information systems often mask important quantitative information, such as the actual MICs of antibiotics, in favor of reporting only the interpretive categories of susceptible,

New laboratory tests to confirm the presence of ESBLs in K. pneumoniae and E. coli may aid in the detection of such organisms

Table 15.3 Preferred antimicrobial susceptibility testing methods for emerging bacterial pathogens

Organism	Key drugs	Preferred method[a]	Alternate method	Screen test
Staphylococcus aureus	Oxacillin	Broth microdilution	(See screen test)	Oxacillin agar screen plate[b]
Enterococci	Vancomycin	Broth microdilution	Disk diffusion	Vancomycin agar screen plate[c]
Streptococcus pneumoniae	Penicillin, cefotaxime	Broth microdilution[d]	Etest	1-m g oxacillin disk for penicillin
Klebsiella pneumoniae (extended-spectrum β-lactamase producers)	Cefotaxime, ceftriaxone, ceftazidime	Broth microdilution	Disk diffusion	Disk diffusion or MICs with altered breakpoints[e]
Neisseria gonorrhoeae	Ceftriaxone, ciprofloxacin	Agar dilution	Disk diffusion	Not available
Neisseria meningitidis	Penicillin	Broth microdilution	Etest	Not available

[a]Broth microdilution methods are described in NCCLS document M7-A4 (48). Commercial methods that use this technique include Sceptor (BDMS), Sensititre (AcuMed), Pasco (Difco), MicroScan conventional panels, MicroTech, and MicroMedia.

[b]The oxacillin agar screen test is performed by inoculating a standardized amount of staphylococci onto a plate of Mueller-Hinton agar containing 6 μg/ml of oxacillin and 4% NaCl and incubating the plate for 24 h at 35°C.

[c]The vancomycin agar screen test is performed by inoculating a standardized amount of enterococci onto a plate of brain heart infusion agar containing 6 μg/ml of vancomycin and incubating the plate for 24 h at 35°C.

[d]Broth microdilution testing of pneumococci requires the addition of 2 to 5% lysed horse blood. Only selected commercial systems have FDA clearance for pneumococcal testing.

[e]The detection of ESBLs can be enhanced by using more sensitive screening breakpoints outlined in NCCLS documents M2-A6 and M7-A4.

intermediate, and resistant. Thus, physicians who suspect the presence of new resistant organisms in their hospitals should consult with the hospital's microbiologists regarding the optimal approach to identifying and testing of such organisms.

Responses to Antimicrobial Resistance

While resistance is increasing in many pathogens, the number of new antimicrobial agents approved for use in the United States has slowed. Thus, our ability to control outbreaks of infectious diseases through antimicrobial use alone has been diminishing. However, there are several new classes of antimicrobial agents, including everninomycins and oxazolidanones, which may be of value for therapy of several nosocomial pathogens. A recent report from the Hospital Infection Control Practices Advisory Committee on preventing the spread of vancomycin resistance (26) stresses the need for professional and public educational programs, enhanced microbiological surveillance, enhanced surveillance among patients, effective implementation of infection control procedures, and, perhaps most important, prudent use of antimicrobial agents for treatment and prophylaxis of infections.

Whether these recommendations can be generalized to aid in the control of other types of resistant organisms found in the hospital environment remains to be seen. Studies to validate the effectiveness of the guidelines in controlling the spread of vancomycin-resistant enterococci are in progress. The report also notes that our major surveillance resource in the United States for the detection of novel resistant organisms is the network of hospital microbiology laboratories, since these are the source of the data that feed into the NNIS and into other such programs. However, with the exception of *Mycobacterium tuberculosis*, drug-resistant *S. pneumoniae*, and *N. gonorrhoeae*, there are no national surveillance systems that systematically monitor resistance in community-acquired infections. Surveillance of penicillin resistance in pneumococci varies from state to state. Thus, it is up to infectious disease specialists, clinical microbiologists, pharmacists, and public health personnel to be vigilant for organisms with novel resistance patterns so that control measures can be effectively implemented. Emergence of drug-resistant organisms also has clear implications for vaccine and antimicrobial drug development priorities.

> *It is up to infectious disease specialists, clinical microbiologists, pharmacists, and public health personnel to be vigilant for organisms with novel resistance patterns*

Problems of infection due to resistant organisms require a combination of measures to ensure control (Table 15.2). However, these will have to be individualized to specific organism-antimicrobial pairs, specific health care institutions, and specific care settings.

The reservoir and mode of spread for important resistant organisms vary dramatically. For some organisms, like MRSA, the reservoir now is in some communities as well as in health care facilities. For others, like ESBL-containing gram-negative bacilli, acute care hospitals, especially intensive care units, are the main focus. Likewise, the mode of spread for MRSA seems closely linked to person-to-person spread, while gram-negative nonfermenting bacillary infections appear to be spread through liquids and respiratory therapy devices. Thus, one set of national guidelines for dealing with resistant organisms is unlikely to suffice for every type of resistance.

The setting in which resistant organisms are being encountered plays a strong role in design of control measures. For example, plans for control of resistance in long-term care facilities must be customized to the patients and types of care given in these facilities, where "strategies used in hospitals often are inapplicable" (53, 67). Guidelines for dealing with the home care setting will have to be adjusted in like fashion from place to place (37).

Finally, the approach to dealing with resistance is likely to vary not only from organism to organism but also from institution to institution and health care system to health care system. A pilot program that is part of a cooperative effort by the Rollins School of Public Health of Emory University and the Hospital Infections Program of the Centers for Disease Control and Prevention illustrates this point. Dubbed Project ICARE (Intensive Care Antimicrobial Resistance Epidemiology), the study involved eight hospitals participating in the NNIS system that reported additional information on antimicrobial resistance and antimicrobial use (4). Study of data on MRSA showed that antimicrobial use and resistance were closely linked in some but not all of the hospitals. In one site, problems with infection control leading to cross-infection appeared to be a major cause of resistance, while at another site, hospital levels of resistant organisms seemed to be due to a high prevalence of resistant isolates in the community. Thus, in deciding how to approach antimicrobial resistance, national or regional guidelines for preventing resistance will have to be modified to take into account local patterns, problems, and resources. Likewise, health care systems will need to consider their own policies, resources, and patient populations in interpreting the way that national guidelines are implemented in their own institutions, whether acute care, extended care, or ambulatory settings. For these reasons and others, "one size does not fit all," and guidelines, programs, or regulations designed to deal with resistance on a regional or national basis are not likely to be successful or cost-effective.

Summary

Resistance is an emerging problem in human medicine, and the effects of resistance are being noted on an ever-increasing scale. Whether it is treatment of nosocomial bacteremia in New York City or community-acquired dysentery in Central Africa, multiresistant organisms are diminishing our ability to control the spread of infectious diseases. Clearly, the rate at which resistant organisms develop is not solely a function of the use of antimicrobial agents in humans, but is also highly influenced by the use of these agents in veterinary medicine, animal husbandry, agriculture, and aquaculture, as has been emphasized at recent meetings sponsored by organizations such the as Rockefeller University (71) and the American Society for Microbiology (3) and in the report on bacterial resistance recently issued by the U.S. Office of Technology Assessment (74). We have entered an era where both physicians and patients must take on the responsibility to use antimicrobials wisely and judiciously. Just as in the days of the turn of the century when the public was an integral part of establishing quarantines for infectious diseases, now again the public's cooperation must be sought for this latest threat to public health. Most importantly, control strategies must be based on the underlying pathophysiology of resistance mechanisms discussed above if they are to have a chance for success.

Figure 15.1 Global map showing emergence of a number of antimicrobial-resistant organisms. The location does not necessarily represent the first resistant isolate of a particular species to be isolated, but indicates the widespread nature and geographic diversity of the antibiotic resistance problem. The *Vibrio cholerae*, *Shigella dysenteriae*, and *Salmonella typhi* strains were resistant to ampicillin, chloramphenicol, kanamycin, streptomycin, tetracycline, sulfonamides, and trimethoprim-sulfamethoxazole. The *Streptococcus pneumoniae* strains from South Africa were resistant to penicillin, chloramphenicol, tetracyclines, and trimethoprim-sulfamethoxazole.

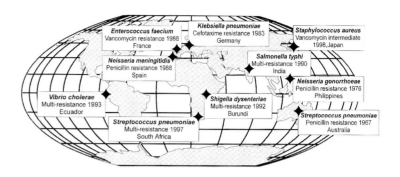

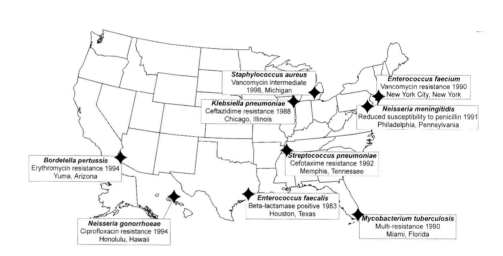

Figure 15.2 United States map showing emergence of a number of antimicrobial-resistant organisms. The location does not necessarily represent the first resistant isolate of a particular species to be isolated, but indicates the widespread nature and geographic diversity of the antibiotic resistance problem. The M. *tuberculosis* strain from Miami was resistant to isoniazid and rifampin and was variably resistant to other antimycobacterial agents such as ethambutol and ethionamide.

References

1. **Abraham, E. P., and E. Chain.** 1940. An enzyme from bacteria able to destroy penicillin. *Nature* **146:**837–839.

2. **Akiba, T., K. Koyama, Y. Ishiki, et al.** 1960. On the mechanism of the development of multiple drug resistant clones of *Shigella. Jpn. J. Microbiol.* **4:**219–222.

3. **American Society for Microbiology.** 1995. *Report of the ASM Task Force on Antibiotic Resistance.* American Society for Microbiology, Washington, D.C.

4. **Archibald, L., L. Phillips, D. Monnet, et al.** 1996. Antimicrobial resistance in isolates from inpatients and outpatients in the United States: the increasing importance of the intensive care unit. *Clin. Infect. Dis.* **24:**211–214.

5. **Berkelman, R., R. T. Bryan, M. T. Osterholm, J. W. LeDuc, and J. M. Hughes.** 1994. Infectious disease surveillance: a crumbling foundation. *Science* **264:**368–370.

6. **Burwen, D. R., S. N. Banerjee, and R. P. Gaynes.** 1994. Ceftazidime resistance among selected nosocomial gram-negative bacilli in the United States. *J. Infect. Dis.* **170:**1622–1625.

7. **Bush, K., G. A. Jacoby, and A. A. Medeiros.** 1995. A functional classification scheme for ß-lactamases and its correlation with molecular structure. *Antimicrob. Agents Chemother.* **39:**1211–1233.

8. **Centers for Disease Control and Prevention.** 1993. Nosocomial enterococci resistant to vancomycin—United States, 1989–1993. *Morbid. Mortal. Weekly Rep.* **42:**597–599.

9. **Centers for Disease Control and Prevention.** 1994. Addressing emerging infectious disease threats: a prevention strategy for the United States. Public Health Service, U.S. Department of Health and Human Services, Atlanta, Ga.

10. **Chetchotisakd, P., C. L. Phelps, and A. L. Hartstein.** 1994. Assessment of bacterial cross-transmission as a cause of infections in patients in intensive care units. *Clin. Infect. Dis.* **18:**929–937.

11. **Chow, J. W., M. J. Find, D. M. Shlaes, et al.** 1991. *Enterobacter* bacteremia: clinical features and emergence of antibiotic resistance during therapy. *Ann. Intern. Med.* **115:**585–590.

12. **Clewell, D. B., and C. Gawron-Burke.** 1986. Conjugative transposons and dissemination of antibiotic resistance in streptococci. *Ann. Rev. Microbiol.* **40:**635–659.

13. **Cohen, M.** 1992. Epidemiology of drug resistance: implications for a postantimicrobial era. *Science* **257:**1050–1055.

14. **Davies, J.** 1994. Inactivation of antibiotics and the dissemination of resistance genes. *Science* **264:**375–382.

15. **Davin-Regli, A., D. Monnet, P. Saux, C. Bosi, R. Charrel, A. Barthelemy, and C. Bollet.** 1996. Molecular epidemiology of *Enterobacter aerogenes* acquisition: one-year prospective study in two intensive care units. *J. Clin. Microbiol.* **34:**1474–1480.

16. **DeFlaun, M. F., and S. B. Levy.** 1991. Genes and their varied hosts, p. 1–32. *In* S. B. Levy and R. V. Miller (ed.), *Gene Transfer in the Environment.* McGraw-Hill Publishing, New York.

17. **Edmond, M. B., J. F. Ober, D. L. Weinbaum, M. A. Pfaller, T. Hwang, M. D. Sanford, and R. P. Wenzel.** 1995. Vancomycin-resistant *Enterococcus faecium* bacteremia: risk factors for infection. *Clin. Infect. Dis.* **20:**1126–1133.

18. **Elwell, L. P., J. deGraaff, D. Seibert, and S. Falkow.** 1975. Plasmid-linked ampicillin resistance in *Haemophilus influenzae* type b. *Infect. Immun.* **12:**404–410.

19. **Gardner, P., D. H. Smith, H. Beer, and R. Moellering.** 1970. Recovery of resistance factors from a drug-free community. *Lancet* **i**(641)**:**301.

20. **Gonzales, R., and M. Sande.** 1995. What will it take to stop physicians from prescribing antibiotics in acute bronchitis? *Lancet* **345:**665–666.

21. **Gootz, T. D.** 1990. Discovery and development of new antimicrobial agents. *Clin. Microbiol. Rev.* **3:**13–31.

22. **Hackbarth, C. J., and H. E Chambers.** 1989. Methicillin-resistant staphylococci: genetics and mechanisms of resistance. *Antimicrob. Agents Chemother.* **33:**991–994.

23. **Handwerger, S., B. Raucher, D. Altarac, J. Monka, S. Marchione, K. V. Singh, B. E. Murray, J. Wolff, and B. Walters.** 1993. Nosocomial outbreak due to *Enterococcus faecium* highly resistant to vancomycin, penicillin, and gentamicin. *Clin. Infect. Dis.* **16:**750–755.

24. **Hiramatsu, K., H. Hanaki, T. Ino, K. Yabuta, T. Oguri, and F. C. Tenover.** 1997. Methicillin-resistant *Staphylococcus aureus* clinical strain with reduced vancomycin susceptibility. *J. Antimicrob. Chemother.* **40:**135–136.

25. **Hofmann, J., M. S. Cetron, M. M. Farley, W. S. Baughman, R. R. Facklam, J. A. Elliott, K. A. Deaver, and R. F. Breiman.** 1995. The prevalence of drug-resistant *Streptococcus pneumoniae* in Atlanta. *N. Engl. J. Med.* **333:**481–486.

26. **Hospital Infection Control Practices Advisory Committee.** 1995. Recommendations for preventing the spread of vancomycin resistance. *Infect. Control Hosp. Epidemiol.* **16:**105–113.

27. **Infante-Rivard, C., and A. Fernandez.** 1993. Otitis media in children: frequency, risk factors, and research avenues. *Epidemiol. Rev.* **15:**444–465.

28. **Jacoby, G. A., and A. A. Medeiros.** 1991. More extended-spectrum beta-lactamases. *Antimicrob. Agents Chemother.* **35:**1697–1704.

29. **Jernigan, J. A., M. A. Clemence, G. A. Stott, et al.** 1995. Control of methicillin-resistant *Staphylococcus aureus* at a university hospital: one decade later. *Infect. Control Hosp. Epidemiol.* **16:**686–696.

30. **Katsanis, G. P., J. Spargo, M. J. Ferraro, L. Sutton, and G. A. Jacoby.** 1994. Detection of *Klebsiella pneumoniae* and *Escherichia coli* strains producing extended-spectrum ß-lactamases. *J. Clin. Microbiol.* **32:**691–696.

31. **Kaufhold, A., A. Podbielski, T. Horaud, and P. Ferrieri.** 1992. Identical genes confer high-level resistance to gentamicin upon *Enterococcus faecalis*, *Enterococcus faecium*, and *Staphylococcus aureus*. *Antimicrob. Agents Chemother.* **36:**1215–1218.

32. **Kirby, W. M. M.** 1944. Extraction of a highly potent penicillin inactivator from penicillin resistant staphylococci. *Science* **99:**452–455.

33. **Klugman, K.** 1990. Pneumococcal resistance to antibiotics. *Clin. Microbiol. Rev.* **3:**171–196.

34. **Knothe, H., P. Shah, V. Krcmery, M. Antal, and S. Mitsuhashi.** 1983. Transferable resistance to cefotaxime, cefoxitin, cefamandole, and cefuroxime in clinical isolates of *Klebsiella pneumoniae* and *Serratia marcescens*. *Infection* **11:**315–317.

35. **Leclercq, R., and P. Courvalin.** 1997. Resistance to glycopeptides in enterococci. *Clin. Infect. Dis.* **24:**545–556.

36. **Lederberg, J., R. E. Shope, and S. C. Oaks, Jr. (ed.).** 1992. *Emerging Infections: Microbial Threats to Health in the United States.* National Academy Press, Washington, D.C.

37. **Lorenzen, A. N., and D. J. Itkin.** 1992. Surveillance of infection in home care. *Am. J. Infect. Control* **20:**326–329.

38. **Luber, A. D., R. A. Jacobs, M. Jordan, et al.** 1996. Relative importance of oral versus intravenous vancomycin exposure in the development of vancomycin-resistant enterococci. *J. Infect. Dis.* **173:**1292–1294.

39. **Lyytikäinen, O., S. Kõljalg, M. Härmä, and J. Vuopio-Varkila.** 1995. Outbreak caused by two multi-resistant *Acinetobacter baumannii* clones in a burns unit: emergence of resistance to imipenem. *J. Hosp. Infect.* **31:**41–54.

40. **McCaig, L. F., and J. M. Hughes.** 1995. Trends in antimicrobial drug prescribing among office-based physicians in the United States. *JAMA* **273:**214–219.

41. **McGowan, J. E., Jr.** 1983. Antimicrobial resistance in hospital organisms and its relation to antibiotic use. *Rev. Infect. Dis.* **5:**1033–1048.

42. **McGowan, J. E., Jr., and F. C. Tenover.** 1997. Control of antimicrobial resistance in the health care system. *Infect. Dis. Clin. North Am.* **11:**297–311.

43. **Meyer, K. S., C. Urban, J. A. Eagan, B. J. Berger, and J. J. Rahal.** 1993. Nosocomial outbreak of *Klebsiella* infection resistant to late-generation cephalosporins. *Ann. Intern. Med.* **119:**353–358.

44. **Montecalvo, M. A., H. Horowitz, C. Gedris, C. Carbonaro, F. C. Tenover, A. Issah, P. Cook, and G. P. Wormser.** 1994. Outbreak of vancomycin-, ampicillin-, and aminoglycoside-resistant *Enterococcus faecium* bacteremia in an adult oncology unit. *Antimicrob. Agents Chemother.* **38:**1363–1367.

45. **Murray, B. E.** 1991. New aspects of antimicrobial resistance and the resulting therapeutic dilemmas. *J. Infect. Dis.* **163:**1185–1194.

46. **Murray, B. E.** 1997. Vancomycin-resistant enterococci. *Am. J. Med.* **102:**284–293.

47. **Murray, B. E., B. Mederski-Samoraj, S. K. Foster, J. L. Brunton, and P. Harford.** 1986. In vitro studies of plasmid-mediated penicillinase from *Streptococcus faecalis* suggest a staphylococcal origin. *J. Clin. Invest.* **77:**289–293.

48. **National Committee for Clinical Laboratory Standards.** 1997. *Methods for Dilution Antimicrobial Susceptibility Tests for Bacteria That Grow Aerobically,* 4th ed. Approved standard M7-A4. National Committee for Clinical Laboratory Standards, Wayne, Pa.

49. **Navarro, F., and P. Courvalin.** 1994. Analysis of genes encoding D-alanine-D-alanine ligase-related enzymes in *Enterococcus casseliflavus* and *Enterococcus flavescens. Antimicrob. Agents Chemother.* **38:**1788–1793.

50. **Neu, H. C.** 1982. The new beta-lactamase-stable cephalosporins. *Ann. Intern. Med.* **97:**408–419.

51. **Neu, H. C.** 1990. Quinolones: an overview. *Diag. Microbiol. Infect. Dis.* **13:**195–196.

52. **Neu, H. C.** 1992. The crisis in antibiotic resistance. *Science* **257:**1064–1073.

53. **Nicolle, L. E., D. Bentley, R. Garibaldi, et al.** 1996. SHEA position paper: antimicrobial use in long-term-care facilities. *Infect. Control Hosp. Epidemiol.* **17:**119–128.

54. **Noble, W. C., Z. Virani, and R. G. A. Cree.** 1992. Co-transfer of vancomycin and other resistance genes from *Enterococcus faecalis* NCTC 12201 to *Staphylococcus aureus*. FEMS *Microbiol. Lett.* **93:**195–198.

55. **Ounissi, H., E. Derlot, C. Carlier, and P. Courvalin.** 1990. Gene homogeneity of aminoglycoside-modifying enzymes in gram-positive cocci. *Antimicrob. Agents Chemother.* **34:**2164–2168.

56. **Phillipon, A., R. Labia, and G. Jacoby.** 1989. Extended-spectrum ß-lactamases. *Antimicrob. Agents Chemother.* **33:**1131–1136.

57. **Phillips, I.** 1976. Beta-lactamase producing penicillin-resistant gonococcus. *Lancet* **ii:**656–657.

58. **Reichler, M. R., A. A. Allphin, R. F. Breiman, J. R. Schreiber, J. E. Arnold, L. K. McDougal, R. R. Facklam, B. Boxerbaum, D. May, R. O. Walton, et al.** 1992. The spread of multiply resistant *Streptococcus pneumoniae* at a day care center in Ohio. *J. Infect. Dis.* **166:**1346–1353.

59. **Rice, L. B., S. H. Willey, G. A. Papanicolaou, A. A. Medeiros, G. M. Eliopoulos, R. C. Moellering, Jr., and G. A. Jacoby.** 1990. Outbreak of ceftazidime resistance caused by extended-spectrum ß-lactamases at a Massachusetts chronic-care facility. *Antimicrob. Agents Chemother.* **34:**2193–2199.

60. **Ries, A. A., J. G. Wells, D. Olivola, M. Ntakibirora, S. Nyandwi, M. Ntibakivayo, C. B. Ivey, K. D. Greene, F. C. Tenover, S. P. Wahlquist, et al.** 1994. Epidemic *Shigella dysenteriae* type 1 in Burundi: pan-resistance and implications for prevention. *J. Infect. Dis.* **169:**1035–1041.

61. **Rowe, P. M.** 1996. Preparing for battle against vancomycin resistance. *Lancet* **347:**252.

62. **Roy, C., C. Segura, M. Tirado, R. Reig, M. Hermida, D. Teruel, and A. Foz.** 1985. Frequency of plasmid-determined beta-lactamases in 680 consecutively isolated strains of *Enterobacteriaceae*. *Eur. J. Clin. Microbiol.* **4:**146–147.

63. **Sanders, C. C., and B. Wiedemann.** 1988. Conference summary. *Rev. Infect. Dis.* **10:**679–682.

64. **Simpson, I. N., J. Finlay, D. J. Winstanley, N. Dewhurst, J. W. Nelson, S. L. Butler, and J. R. Govan.** 1994. Multi-resistance isolates possessing chacteristics of both *Burkholderia* (*Pseudomonas*) *cepacia* and *Burkholderia gladioli* from patients with cystic fibrosis. *J. Antimicrob. Chemother.* **34:**353–361.

65. **Sloas, M. M., F. F. Barrett, P. J. Chesney, B. K. English, B. C. Hill, F. C. Tenover, and R. J. Leggiadro.** 1992. Cephalosporin treatment failure in penicillin- and cephalosporin-resistant *Streptococcus pneumoniae* meningitis. *Pediatr. Infect. Dis. J.* **11:**662–666.

66. **Sougakoff, W., S. Goussard, G. Gerbaud, and P. Courvalin.** 1988. Plasmid-mediated resistance to third generation cephalosporins caused by point mutations in TEM-type penicillinase genes. *Rev. Infect. Dis.* **10:**879–884.

67. **Strasbaugh, L. J., K. B. Crossley, B. A. Nurse, and L. D. Thrupp.** 1996. SHEA position paper: antimicrobial resistance in long-term care facilities. *Infect.Control Hosp. Epidemiol.* **17:**129–140.

68. **Swenson, J. M., N. C. Clark, M. J. Ferraro, D. F. Sahm, G. Doern, M. A. Pfaller, L. B. Reller, M. P. Weinstein, R. J. Zabransky, and F. C. Tenover.** 1994. Development of a standardized screening method for detection of vancomycin-resistant enterococci. *J. Clin. Microbiol.* **32:**1700–1704.

69. **Tenover, F. C.** 1991. Novel and emerging mechanisms of antimicrobial resistance in nosocomial pathogens. *Am. J. Med.* **91**(Suppl. B)**:**76S–81S.

70. **Tenover, F. C., J. M. Swenson, C. M. O'Hara, and S. A. Stocker.** 1995. Ability of commercial and reference antimicrobial susceptibility testing methods to detect vancomycin resistance in enterococci. *J. Clin. Microbiol.* **33:**1524–1527.

71. **Tomasz, A.** 1994. Multiple-antibiotic-resistant pathogenic bacteria: a report on the Rockefeller University Workshop. *N. Engl. J. Med.* **330:**1247–1251.

72. **Travis, T.** 1994. Reviving the antibiotic miracle? *Science* **264:**360–362.

73. **Trieu-Cuot, P., G. Gerbaud, T. Lambert, and P. Courvalin.** 1985. In vivo transfer of genetic information between gram-negative and gram-positive bacteria. *EMBO J.* **4:**3583–3587.

74. **U.S. Congress, Office of Technology Assessment.** 1995. *Impacts of Antibiotic Resistant Bacteria*, OTA-H-629, September. U.S. Government Printing Office, Washington, D.C.

75. **Williams, R. J.** 1988. Epidemiology of antibiotic resistance in gram-negative bacteria. *J. Hosp. Infect.* **11**(Suppl. A)**:**130–134.

chapter 16

Emerging Infectious Agents and the Forensic Pathologist: The New Mexico Model[†]

Kurt B. Nolte, Gary L. Simpson, and R. Gibson Parrish

On May 14, 1993, an investigator for the New Mexico Office of the Medical Investigator was notified of the sudden death of a 19-year-old man from a rural New Mexico community. The man had collapsed while en route to his fiancee's funeral. Further investigation revealed that the young couple died after strikingly similar illnesses characterized by flulike symptoms including fever, chills, and body aches, followed by the abrupt onset of cough and shortness of breath. Worried about the potential diagnosis of plague, the investigator arranged for immediate autopsies to be performed on both bodies that evening. The prosecting forensic pathologist was struck by the similar autopsy findings in the two individuals and those of another young woman examined approximately 1 month earlier, who had died with the same symptoms. The pathologist notified the New Mexico Department of Health that evening of an

Kurt B. Nolte, Office of the Medical Investigator, University of New Mexico School of Medicine, 700 Camino de Salud, Albuquerque, NM 87131-5091. **Gary L. Simpson,** Public Health Division, New Mexico Department of Health, 1190 St. Francis Drive, Santa Fe, NM 87502. **R. Gibson Parrish,** Division of Environmental Hazards and Health Effects, National Center for Environmental Health, Centers for Disease Control and Prevention, Mailstop F-35, 4770 Buford Highway, N.E., Atlanta, GA 30341-3714.

[†]Reprinted with permission from *Arch. Pathol. Lab. Med.* **120:**125–128, 1996.

Pathology of Emerging Infections 2
Edited by Ann Marie Nelson and C. Robert Horsburgh, Jr.
© 1998 American Society for Microbiology, Washington, D.C.

apparent cluster of fatal respiratory disease. In the following days, many more cases throughout the southwestern United States were recognized by clinicians and pathologists (4). After a rapid investigation involving the cooperation of several different state and federal agencies, the hantavirus pulmonary syndrome was recognized and described (11, 19). A well-organized and vigilant statewide medical examiner system was a critical element in the discovery of this disease.

At first glance, medicolegal death investigation systems may not seem relevant to infectious disease surveillance. In most jurisdictions, forensic pathologists employed as medical examiners, or pathologists contracted by coroners, are authorized by legislated statute to investigate deaths that are violent, sudden, suspicious, unexplained, or unnatural (9). These statutes often direct the pathologist to determine the cause of death (disease or injury initiating the fatal sequence of events), manner of death (circumstances under which the death occurred, i.e., natural versus homicide, suicide, or accident), and the condition of the body.

> *Not surprisingly, most death investigation systems have been biased toward the investigation of violent deaths*

Not surprisingly, most death investigation systems have been biased toward the investigation of violent deaths. However, natural deaths occurring suddenly, unexplained deaths, and deaths of public health importance have often come under the scrutiny of forensic pathologists. These deaths frequently involve infectious diseases (18). Historically, however, forensic pathologists have been satisfied with general pathologic diagnoses rather than organism-specific diagnoses in these cases. For example, deaths are classified as lobar pneumonia rather than pneumococcal pneumonia. Often, the necessary diagnostic tests to achieve an organism-specific diagnosis, such as cultures, electron microscopy, or immunohistochemistry, are not performed. Unfortunately, limitations such as these impair the usefulness of medicolegal death investigation systems in recognizing emerging infections.

Infectious diseases are considered to be "emerging" when their incidence in humans has increased within the past 20 years or threatens to increase in the near future (14). Infectious diseases may emerge because of changes in or evolution of existing organisms, the spread of known organisms to new areas or populations, or the occurrence of previously unrecognized infections in areas undergoing environmental changes. Known infections may also reemerge after a decline in incidence (5, 14). In addition to the hantavirus outbreak, in recent years the New Mexico Office of the Medical Investigator has identified an outbreak of fatal pneumococcal disease in a day care setting (7) and has participated in the investigation of an outbreak of fatal meningococcal disease. Other resurgent and important infections not infrequently recognized at autopsy in this state include tuberculosis and plague.

Recognition of the importance of early infectious disease detection has resulted in the creation of a New Mexico infectious disease death-review team. This group meets quarterly to examine all medical examiner autopsies in which an infection has been demonstrated or is suspected of having caused or contributed to the death, or in which a significant incidental infection is found. The working group comprises the disciplines of infectious diseases, pulmonary medicine, forensic and clinical pathology, clinical microbiology, molecular diagnostics, epidemiology, and public health. Participants also represent a diverse array of academic, public, and private organizations and institutions. The collaborative nature of this working group not only broadens the context of medical review and discussion, but also facilitates the commitment of organizational and institutional resources for more extensive case investigations.

The focus of the working group process is (i) to identify notable pathogens, unusual clinical or pathologic syndromes, or significant epidemiologic settings that merit more extensive investigation and (ii) to monitor certain sentinel populations (such as intravenous drug users, chronic alcoholics, immunocompromised individuals, and children under the age of 2 years) that have been associated with emerging and/or reemerging infectious diseases. Intravenous drug abusers are clearly linked with AIDS and other infections. Alcoholics have an increased incidence of pulmonary infections, including tuberculosis (1). Children under the age of 2 years serve as sentinels for vaccine-preventable diseases (7). Preliminary data generated by this group indicate that approximately 25% of natural disease death cases autopsied at the New Mexico Office of the Medical Investigator are a consequence of infections. Additionally, a review of 10 years of autopsy records revealed that fatal myocarditis, a relatively rare antemortem clinical diagnosis, occurred at 50% of the frequency of fatal meningitis cases.

It should be emphasized that the New Mexico medical examiner system is a centralized, academically based, forensic pathology resource. The New Mexico Office of the Medical Investigator is a statewide medical examiners office located at the University of New Mexico School of Medicine in Albuquerque. It was founded in 1972 when the state changed from a coroner to a medical examiner system. This nonpolitical office is overseen by a Board of Medical Investigators composed of the Dean of the School of Medicine, the Chief of the New Mexico State Police, the Secretary of the New Mexico Department of Health, and the President of the New Mexico Board of Thanatopractice. A Chief Medical Investigator heads a staff of five board-certified forensic pathologists, seven central office investigators, and approximately 130 field investigators, as well as other technical and support staff. Uniquely, all of the forensic pathologists have joint appointments and responsibilities within the School of Medicine. In addition to the forensic autopsy service, the office administers the University Hospital autopsy service in the same facility. The office trains two or three forensic pathology fellows per year, and each pathology resident is required to rotate through the office for 2 months of autopsy pathology and 3 months of forensic pathology training. The close ties between the office and the university promote collaboration, research, and consultation.

All deaths fitting legislated criteria and occurring within the state are reported to a single office. The office investigates over 4,100 of the 12,000 deaths per year in New Mexico and performs approximately 1,400 autopsies per year. The autopsy population in 1994 included an increased representation of several sentinel groups, including children under age 2 years (7%), alcoholics (greater than 7%), intravenous drug abusers (greater

The New Mexico medical examiner system is a centralized, academically based, forensic pathology resource

than 5%), and AIDS patients (1.3%). All autopsies are performed in the central facility at the University of New Mexico School of Medicine. The public health benefits of this system are significant. Because of its organizational structure, the system permits statewide, population-based surveillance of infectious disease-associated deaths with a consistent degree of sensitivity and specificity. The result is a surveillance system that can detect emerging and reemerging infectious diseases as well as known, reportable infections of public health significance. Findings of the Office of the Medical Investigator are reported in a comprehensive autopsy report, which is maintained in a computerized database. The quality of data processing allows for both retrospective surveys and prospective coding to address epidemiologic and other research issues. The strong academic affiliation of the office with the University of New Mexico School of Medicine supports and promotes consultation and collaboration, enhancing both diagnostic accuracy and the utilization of data for scholarly work.

Most states, however, do not have such a centralized, academically based, forensic pathology system for the investigation of deaths. In fact, in 31 states the investigation of deaths and the determination of the cause and manner of death are the responsibility of a local official, usually a county or district-based coroner or medical examiner (9). While the investigation of deaths in the remaining 19 states and the District of Columbia is the responsibility of a state medical examiner's office, few of these offices have close academic affiliations, and autopsies in most states are not performed at a single central facility. In addition, the qualifications of medical examiners and coroners vary considerably. Most coroners are not required to have any medical training, and many medical examiners are not required to have any forensic training (9). While these organizational and personnel considerations alone do not mean that deaths will be inadequately investigated, they do not provide an optimal environment for identifying the spectrum of infectious disease deaths.

The statutes in most states require the investigation of similar types of deaths. However, the reporting of these deaths, including those potentially caused by emerging infectious agents, to the medical examiner or coroner is notoriously incomplete. Even deaths caused by injuries and violence, which are reportable in virtually all states, are incompletely reported (10). Once reported, most deaths are initially investigated by a lay investigator, who may lack the training to recognize deaths possibly caused by infectious agents. Furthermore, the extent of the investigation, including whether an autopsy is conducted and its extent, varies by jurisdiction. For example, the autopsy rate for deaths due to blunt and penetrating trauma, even when such trauma results in homicide, varies considerably from state to state (20). This is often a result of the availability of pathologists and adequate autopsy facilities and laboratory support, which in turn are dependent on the financial resources of the office.

An autopsy on an infectious death case does not necessarily guarantee that an infectious organism will be identified. To make organism-specific diagnoses, autopsy pathologists often require ancillary tests beyond gross and

In 31 states the investigation of deaths and the determination of the cause and manner of death are the responsibility of a local official

histologic evaluation. The most commonly used procedure is a culture of body fluids and tissue. However, studies have demonstrated that the collection and interpretation of postmortem cultures are fraught with difficulties, including bacterial contamination and postmortem overgrowth (24). Other techniques used to identify infectious agents have included electron microscopy and serology. However, searching for organisms with the electron microscope can be painstaking and dependent on tissue preservation, and serologically detectable immune responses to infectious agents may not yet have occurred at the time of death.

Recent advances in molecular biology have created an arsenal of highly specific techniques to identify infectious agents in autopsy tissues. Immunohistochemical techniques can identify specific antigens from pathogenic agents in formalin-fixed, paraffin-embedded tissue. Organisms detectable by this process include herpes simplex virus, hepatitis B virus, measles virus, *Legionella* spp., group B streptococci, influenza virus, and mycobacteria (21). Immunohistochemical methods using antiserum to hantaviral nucleocapsid antigen were critical to the early understanding of hantavirus pulmonary syndrome (25). Nucleic acid probes can be used on a variety of fresh, frozen, and formalin-fixed autopsy tissues, as well as on clinical specimens, to identify both known and unknown infectious agents including viruses, bacteria, and parasites. In situ hybridization has extended the reach of diagnostic assays to archived paraffin blocks (26). Unfortunately, a large number of forensic pathologists remain unaware of these techniques or do not have access to the technology; consequently, appropriate specimens are not retained at autopsy. If an infectious disease process is suspected or if a death is unexplained, prosecting pathologists should consider retaining serum, blood, and frozen tissues in addition to obtaining standard cultures. It is especially important that representative samples of all major organs be embedded and saved as paraffin blocks for further histologic, immunologic, and molecular testing. These tissues should be kept a minimum amount of time in formalin prior to processing (optimally less than 24 h) to avoid antigenic or nucleic acid degradation. Medical examiners' offices that can maintain tissue banks of archived specimens combined with computerized retrievable autopsy records can be a valuable source of information when new infectious agents emerge.

If an infectious disease process is suspected or if a death is unexplained, prosecting pathologists should consider retaining serum, blood, and frozen tissues

Directing pathologists and forensic pathologists to search for emerging infections is not without danger. It is important to recognize that autopsy has long been identified as a procedure that carries with it the risk of infectious disease transmission, for prosectors as well as for observers and other individuals in close proximity. Infections have been transmitted at autopsy by both direct cutaneous inoculation and aerosolization. For example, pathologists have died from streptococcal sepsis as a result of minor trauma sustained during the performance of autopsies on individuals with the same disease (13). Other infections that can be transmitted by direct inoculation include tuberculosis, blastomycosis, AIDS, hepatitis B, rabies, and some of the viral hemorrhagic fevers (2, 3, 8, 12, 16). The prototypical organism transmitted by autopsy aerosols is *Mycobacterium tuberculosis*. Historically, large segments of medical school classes would become tuberculin positive after the portion of their curriculum involving autopsy exposure (17). In recent years, autopsy-transmitted outbreaks of tuberculosis have occurred in the Syracuse Medical Examiner's Office (23), the University of Arkansas School of Medicine, the University of Health Sciences/Chicago Medical School, and the Los Angeles Coroner's Office (Associated Press of Los Angeles, August 9, 1995) (6, 15, 22). The Syracuse outbreak involved multidrug-resistant tuberculosis (23). Other infections that can be transmitted by autopsy aerosols include plague, rabies, anthrax, and meningococcemia (8).

Unfortunately, most medical examiners' facilities, and indeed most autopsy facilities, in the United States are not constructed to mitigate these risks. Many medical examiners' offices are situated within aging facilities, often with shared ventilation between prosecting and administrative space. Most facilities barely meet biosafety level 2 standards. Although precautions have been promulgated to prevent the transmission of both blood-borne and aerosolized pathogens (3, 6), many forensic pathologists have been slow to come into compliance. The hantavirus outbreak focused the New Mexico office on issues of biosafety. An isolation autopsy room was altered so that the air is now exhausted through a high-efficiency particulate air filter. Power-assisted personal respirators were purchased to achieve biosafety level 3 standards. To handle sporadic and generalized infectious outbreaks in the future, we need to have a better-prepared infrastructure. Funding should be made available to bring autopsy facilities into compliance with accepted public health standards (3, 6, 8). These facilities should be able to function at biosafety level 3 and should provide protection against aerosolized pathogens.

In summary, several factors influence how well deaths from possible emerging infections are recognized. These include (i) the ability of clinicians and police to identify possible cases and to refer them to the medical examiner's or coroner's office; (ii) the level of training and experience of medical examiners, coroners, and their deputies, including lay investigators; (iii) the quality of the resources and facilities necessary for a thorough postmortem examination of suspicious deaths and the protection of autopsy and other personnel from infectious agents; (iv) the ability to easily search written and computerized records of postmortem findings; and (v) the degree to which the medical examiner reports suspicious deaths to appropriate public health agencies for further investigation and surveillance.

To address emerging infectious diseases, the Centers for Disease Control and Prevention has developed a strategic plan that includes improving surveillance, applied research, prevention and control, and infrastructure (5). Medicolegal death investigation systems can help fulfill these goals by attempting to achieve organism-specific diagnoses in deaths being examined; closely scrutinizing sentinel groups such as alcoholics and intravenous drug users; computerizing data and organizing infectious disease data of epidemiologic relevance; conducting and assisting with research that enhances the identification of infectious organisms in autopsy tissues; and developing comprehensive autopsy protocols that include saving tissue for more sophis-

> *To handle sporadic and generalized infectious outbreaks in the future, we need to have a better-prepared infrastructure*

ticated molecular diagnostic tests. Clearly, the infrastructure (including the organization and staffing of medicolegal death investigation offices and the biosafety engineering aspects of autopsy facilities that prevent the transmission of infectious pathogens) will need to change. For our colleagues who practice in undersupported public service agencies, this will represent a major challenge.

Acknowledgments

We thank James L. Luke, Ross E. Zumwalt, and Bronwyn E. Wilson for their editorial comments and direction.

References

1. **Carpenter, J. L., and D. Y. Huang.** 1991. Community-acquired pulmonary infections in a public municipal hospital in the 1980s. *South. Med. J.* **84:**299–306.

2. **Centers for Disease Control.** 1988. Management of patients with suspected viral hemorrhagic fever. *Morbid. Mortal. Weekly Rep.* **37**(Suppl. S-3)**:**1–15.

3. **Centers for Disease Control.** 1989. Guidelines for prevention of transmission of human immunodeficiency virus and hepatitis B virus to health-care and public safety workers. *Morbid. Mortal. Weekly Rep.* **38**(Suppl. S-6)**:**1–37.

4. **Centers for Disease Control and Prevention.** 1993. Outbreak of acute illness: southwestern United States, 1993. *Morbid. Mortal. Weekly Rep.* **42:**421–424.

5. **Centers for Disease Control and Prevention.** 1994. *Addressing Emerging Infectious Disease Threats: a Prevention Strategy for the United States.* Centers for Disease Control and Prevention, Atlanta.

6. **Centers for Disease Control and Prevention.** 1994. Guidelines for preventing the transmission of *Mycobacterium tuberculosis* in health-care facilities, 1994. *Morbid. Mortal. Weekly Rep.* **43**(RR-13)**:**1–132.

7. **Centers for Disease Control and Prevention.** 1995. Hemorrhage and shock associated with invasive pneumococcal infection in healthy infants and children: New Mexico, 1993–1994. *Morbid. Mortal. Weekly Rep.* **43:**949–952.

8. **Centers for Disease Control and Prevention/National Institutes of Health.** 1993. *Biosafety in Microbiological and Biomedical Laboratories*, 3rd ed. Department of Health and Human Services publication (CDC) 938395. Centers for Disease Control and Prevention, Atlanta.

9. **Combs, D. L., R. G. Parrish, and R. Ing.** 1992. *Death Investigation in the United States and Canada, 1992.* Centers for Disease Control and Prevention, Atlanta.

10. **Dijkhuis, H., C. Zwerling, G. Parrish, T. Bennett, and H. C. Kemper.** 1994. Medical examiner data in injury surveillance: a comparison with death certificates. *Am. J. Epidemiol.* **139:**637–643.

11. **Duchin, J. S., F. T. Koster, C. J. Peters, G. L. Simpson, B. Tempest, S. R. Zaki, T. G. Ksiazek, P. E. Rollin, S. Nichol, and E. T. Umland.** 1994. Hantavirus pulmonary syndrome: a clinical description of 17 patients with a newly recognized disease. *N. Engl. J. Med.* **330:**949–955.

12. **Goette, D. K., K. W. Jacobson, and R. D. Doty.** 1978. Primary inoculation tuberculosis of the skin (prosectors paronychia). *Arch. Dermatol.* **114:**567–569.

13. **Hawkey, P. M., S. J. Pedler, and P. J. Southall.** 1980. *Streptococcus pyogenes:* a forgotten occupational hazard in the mortuary. *Br. Med. J.* **281:**1058.

14. **Institute of Medicine.** 1992. *Emerging Infections: Microbial Threats to Health in the United States.* National Academy Press, Washington, D.C.

15. **Kantor, H. S., R. Poblete, and S. L. Pusateri.** 1988. Nosocomial transmission of tuberculosis from unsuspected disease. *Am. J. Med.* **84:**833–837.

16. **Larson, D. M., M. R. Eckman, R. L. Alber, and V. G. Goldschmidt.** 1983. Primary cutaneous (inoculation) blastomycosis: an occupational hazard to pathologists. *Am. J. Clin. Pathol.* **79:**253–255.

17. **Meade, G. M.** 1948. Prevention of primary tuberculosis infections in medical students: the autopsy as source of primary infection. *Am. Rev. Tuberc.* **58:**675–683.

18. **Neuspiel, D. R., and L. H. Kuller.** 1985. Sudden and unexpected natural death in childhood and adolescence. *JAMA* **254:**1321–1325.

19. **Nolte, K. B., R. M. Feddersen, K. Foucar, S. R. Zaki, F. T. Koster, D. Madar, T. L. Merlin, P. J. McFeeley, E. T. Umland, and R. E. Zumwalt.** 1995. Hantavirus pulmonary syndrome in the United States: a pathological description of a disease caused by a new agent. *Hum. Pathol.* **26:**110–120.

20. **Pollock, D. A., J. M. O'Neil, R. G. Parrish, D. L. Combs, and J. L. Annest.** 1993. Temporal and geographic trends in the autopsy frequency of blunt and penetrating trauma deaths in the United States. *JAMA* **269:**1525–1531.

21. **Taylor, C. R.** 1994. Principles of immunomicroscopy, p. 1-20. *In* C. R. Taylor (ed.), *Immunomicroscopy: a Diagnostic Tool for the Surgical Pathologist*, 2nd ed. W. B. Saunders Co., Philadelphia.

22. **Templeton, G. L., L. A. Illing, L. Young, D. Cave, W. W. Stead, and J. H. Bates.** 1995. The risk for transmission of *Mycobacterium tuberculosis* at the bedside and during autopsy. *Ann. Intern. Med.* **122:**922–925.

23. **Ussery, X. T., J. A. Bierman, S. E. Valway, T. A. Seitz, G. T. DiFerdinando, Jr., and S. M. Ostroff.** 1995. Transmission of multidrug-resistant *Mycobacterium tuberculosis* among persons exposed in a medical examiner's office, New York. *Infect. Control Hosp. Epidemiol.* **16:**160–165.

24. **Wilson, S. J., M. L. Wilson, and L. B. Reller.** 1993. Diagnostic utility of postmortem blood cultures. *Arch. Pathol. Lab. Med.* **117:**986–988.

25. **Zaki, S. R., P. W. Greer, L. M. Coffield, C. S. Goldsmith, K. B. Nolte, K. Foucar, R. M. Feddersen, R. E. Zumwalt, G. L. Miller, and A. S. Khan.** 1995. Hantavirus pulmonary syndrome: pathogenesis of an emerging infectious disease. *Am. J. Pathol.* **146:**552–579.

26. **Zaki, S. R., and A. M. Marty.** 1995. New technology for the diagnosis of infectious disease, p. 127–154. *In* W. Doerr and G. Seifert (ed.), *Tropical Pathology.* Springer-Verlag, Berlin.

chapter 17

Bovine Spongiform Encephalopathy

Corrie Brown

Bovine spongiform encephalopathy (BSE) is an emerging disease of cattle that was first reported in 1987 (36) and captured the attention of regulatory agencies around the world. Nine years later, after an apparent cross-species jump from cattle to humans (42), it became an intense interest for human health authorities and the general public as well, with the specter of a potential food-borne epidemic of dementia.

BSE is a recent addition to the group of diseases known as transmissible spongiform encephalopathies (TSEs). Also known as prion diseases, all of these maladies are characterized by progressive dementia and the presence of characteristic vacuolar changes in histologic sections of brain.

The first TSE reported was scrapie of sheep in 1772 (29). The transmissibility of scrapie was inadvertently confirmed through a mass vaccination of sheep against louping ill, using formalin-treated suspensions of ovine brain. Investigations of kuru, an unusual progressive central nervous system disorder

Corrie Brown, Department of Veterinary Pathology, College of Veterinary Medicine, The University of Georgia, D.W. Brooks Drive, Athens, GA 30602-7388.

Pathology of Emerging Infections 2
Edited by Ann Marie Nelson and C. Robert Horsburgh, Jr.
© 1998 American Society for Microbiology, Washington, D.C.

among the Fore Highlanders in New Guinea, showed it had remarkable similarity to scrapie, prompting Bill Hadlow, a veterinary pathologist familiar with scrapie, to suggest its transmissible nature (17). Carleton Gajdusek later won the Nobel prize for uncovering the cause and transmissibility of kuru. Creutzfeldt-Jakob disease (CJD), a clinical entity among humans, was also classified as a spongiform encephalopathy, based on pathologic similarities. Other less common spongiform encephalopathies of humans include Gerstmann-Straussler-Scheinker disease and fatal familial insomnia. Transmissible mink encephalopathy, a disease of ranch-reared mink, was reported by Hartsough and Burger (19). Naturally occurring spongiform encephalopathies have been reported in captive mule deer (*Odocoileus hemionus hemionus*) (43) and Rocky Mountain elk (*Cervus elaphus nelsoni*) (44). Since the description of BSE, there has been a heightened awareness of spongiform encephalopathies, with increased reporting in various species.

Pathogenesis

The TSEs are highly unusual in their causation. Several theories have been advanced to account for the etiology. At first, they were believed to be caused by a conventional virus. However, the agents are extremely resistant to physical and chemical inactivation. Next, a virino theory was proposed, which postulated that the agent was a strand of nucleic acid surrounded by a highly resistant protein coat. This theory is now being discredited because of the failure to find the identifying nucleic acid within affected tissue (31). A revolutionary idea concerned the possibility that TSEs were caused by an abnormal form of a normal brain protein. This abnormal form is termed *proteinaceous infectious particle*, which has been shorted to *prion* (31). There is a cellular prion protein (PrP), designated PrP^{sen}, which is a normal, host-encoded glycoprotein found on the surface membrane of cells in brain and other tissues. This PrP^{sen} is converted to PrP^{res}, a protease-resistant isoform, either through interaction of PrP^{res} with PrP^{sen} (infectious cases) or through a spontaneous or genetically determined catalytic conversion of PrP^{sen} to PrP^{res} (32). These posttranslationally modified PrP^{res} proteins are very resistant to degradation and accumulate in neurons, causing cell damage and death (32). Often the PrP^{res} molecules aggregate into β-sheet conformation, creating plaques (11). All spongiform encephalopathies are now thought to be due to accumulation of PrP^{res} and resulting neuronal degeneration.

A revolutionary idea concerned the possibility that TSEs were caused by an abnormal form of a normal brain protein

Epidemiology

The first record of BSE was the description of a novel histopathologic encephalopathy of cattle in 1987 (36). By examining clinical records from a cluster of these unusual cases it was determined that the first clinical signs referable to the new entity were observed in April 1985. The authors designated a provisional appellation of "bovine spongiform encephalopathy" to characterize this syndrome (36). Within months, the number of cases expanded considerably, generating widespread concern.

The earliest epidemiologic studies proposed that the pattern of BSE was consistent with an extended common-source epidemic (41), with the conclusion that cattle were exposed to a transmissible agent via feedstuffs. Meat and bonemeal were suggested as the vehicle of infection (41).

Further epidemiologic studies implicated that exposure occurred in 1981–1982, concurrent with the cessation of the hydrocarbon solvent extraction of fat from meat and bonemeal (40). The hydrocarbons which function as organic solvents used in the extraction procedures were known to decrease the infectivity of scrapie-infected mouse brains (21). Also, the solvent extraction process included the application of steam heat, which theoretically would decrease the titer of any TSE agent. Removal of both the hydrocarbons and the moist heat treatment perhaps resulted in a TSE dose surviving in the meat and bonemeal.

As noted above, the earliest cases were recorded in 1987. The disease became reportable in June of 1988, and in July of 1988 the feeding of ruminant-derived protein to ruminants was banned (38). An almost exponential increase in the number of cases was seen between the middle of 1989 and early 1993 (Fig. 17.1) (38). The peak period was January 1993, with almost 1,000 new cases diagnosed per week (2). The reasons for the increase in cases subsequent to the feeding ban are related to the long incubation period of the disease and the recycling of infective material from cattle prior to the ban (38). It is estimated that infective material from cattle would have contaminated ruminant protein supplements as early as 1984–1985 (38). Another reason for the increase subsequent to the feeding ban may have been the lack of stringent enforcement of the ban. Although a feeding ban was instituted, farmers were not subsidized for any outdated material already on hand, and it is believed that some continued to use the contaminated supplement (39). Most cases in England have occurred in dairy cows 3 to 6 years of age (2). In contrast to some of the other spongiform encephalopathies, notably scrapie in sheep, there does not seem to be any genetic susceptibility to the disease in cattle (22), with an equal susceptibility among cohorts (38). Subsequent to 1993, the number of cases seen per year began to decline (38). A concern that emerged was the presence of BSE in numerous animals born after the feeding ban. Close examination of these cases indicated that most or all were fed feedstuffs manufactured prior to July 1988 (39). Maternal transmission is thought to be minimal, probably on the order of 1% (2).

From November 1986 until November 1996, approximately 164,600 head of cattle in 34,000 herds were diagnosed with BSE in Great Britain (Fig. 17.1) (2). Subsequent to its appearance in the U.K., BSE has now been reported from a number of countries, including Denmark, the Falkland Islands, Oman, France, Portugal, Republic of Ireland, Italy, Germany, Switzerland, and Canada (3, 6). To date, all cases have been linked to cattle imported from the U.K. or imported feedstuffs.

Active and vigorous surveillance in the United States has failed to unearth any cases of BSE in this country (2, 9). The importation of cattle to the United States from Great Britain was banned in 1989. Between 1981 and 1989, 499 head of cattle were imported to the United States. These

An almost exponential increase in the number of BSE cases was seen between the middle of 1989 and early 1993

cattle have been monitored for signs of disease. After the proposed link of BSE with a disease of humans in 1996, an effort was made to purchase and destroy all of these cattle, with histologic examination of brain to detect any incipient lesions of BSE. Fewer than 25 of these British-origin cattle remain in the United States today. The U.S. Department of Agriculture maintains active monitoring of the health and movement of these remaining British cattle.

Since the initial reporting of BSE, spongiform encephalopathies have been reported sporadically in a number of exotic species in zoos, including nyala (*Tragelaphus angasi*) (24), gemsbok (*Oryx gazella*) (24), eland (*Taurotragus oryx*) (13), Arabian oryx (*Oryx leucoryx*) (25), greater kudu (*Tragelaphus strepsiceros*) (25), cheetah (*Acinonyx jubatus*) (30), and puma (*Felis concolor*) (45). In addition, spongiform encephalopathy has been documented in over 70 domestic cats (*Felis domesticus*) in Great Britain (2, 47). The source of all of these cases is believed to be BSE-contaminated feed material, specifically meat and bonemeal.

Clinical Features

There is a strong correlation between characteristic neurologic clinical signs and the histologic confirmation of BSE. The most common clinical sign reported is increased nervousness or apprehension (41). This apprehension is characterized by a reluctance to enter the milking parlor and separation from the rest of the herd at pasture. Animals are hyperesthetic, responding in an exaggerated way to sound or touch (36), often with very vigorous kicking in response to manipulation in the milking parlor. Excessive ear twitching and nose licking are reported frequently. Postural changes, including rear limb ataxia, tremors, and kyphosis, or a "roach back" appearance, are commonly seen (9, 46). Rapid weight loss occurs despite no decrease in appetite. Ataxia progresses to severe incoordination, paresis, and paralysis (8, 44). The clinical course is progressive, and slaughter usually occurs between 1 and 6 months from the onset of the first clinical signs (36).

The most common clinical sign reported is increased nervousness or apprehension

Public Health Implications of BSE

A surveillance unit was assembled in the U.K. in 1990 specifically for the purpose of identifying any increase in human TSEs. In March of 1996, this unit reported 10 cases, identified over a 10-month period, with an unusual clinicopathologic signature that merited public health attention (42). These new cases were designated variant CJD (vCJD) and differed from the previously seen CJD in that they all occurred in individuals less than 45 years of age and had a prolonged clinical course averaging 13 months, often including behavioral changes. In contrast, previously documented, or sporadic, CJD occurs most frequently in individuals over 60 years of age and is a rapidly progressive dementia, with myoclonus, cortical blindness, and death within 6 months of onset. Also, these new cases of vCJD had neuropathologic changes distinct from previously described CJD. Specifically, there were extensive PrP plaques affecting both brain stem and cerebral cortex. The PrP plaques are seen in only 10% of sporadic CJD cases and are usually localized to the cerebellum (23, 42). As of July 1997, 20 cases of vCJD were reported, with all in the U.K. except for one case in France (16). In October 1997, two new studies underscored the relatedness of BSE and vCJD. Inoculation into mice resulted in identical patterns of brain pathology (5), and glycoform profiles of prion protein from each disease were indistinguishable (20).

Origin of BSE

Initial epidemiologic studies implicated a common-source epidemic as the underlying reason for the emergence of BSE, with the scrapie agent being strongly incriminated.

Experiments undertaken to determine if the scrapie agent, when introduced into cattle, would produce a clinicopathologic syndrome of BSE, have produced inconclusive results regarding BSE's origin. Calves inoculated via multiple routes with cerebral homogenates from either sheep or goats affected by scrapie developed neurologic disease characterized primarily by ataxia, without the hyperexcitability or apprehension that is so characteristic of the BSE disease. Neurohistologic changes were subtle and consistent with scrapie, namely, moderate astrocytosis and a few vacuolated neurons. Vacuolar change in the neuropil, which is considered the most characteristic change in BSE, was negligible in these animals (7). Intracerebral inoculation of 18 newborn calves with a brain suspension made from nine sheep with scrapie resulted in clinical disease within 18 months. Clinical signs were predominantly incoordination and posterior weakness. Unlike cattle with BSE, these animals had decreased tactile and auditory sensory perceptions. Brain lesions were inconsistent and subtle, with little difference compared to normal control brains (8).

BSE has been transmitted to numerous species experimentally, including mice (15), sheep (14), mink (33), pigs (10), and monkeys (4, 26). Inoculation into sheep resulted in clinical disease, with infectivity confirmed in both brain and spleen (14). Both oral and intracerebral inoculation of BSE-affected brain homogenates into mink resulted in clinical disease. The clinicopathologic pattern was distinct from the previously reported transmissible mink encephalopathy (19, 33). Intracerebral inoculation of marmosets with either BSE- or scrapie-affected brain homogenates resulted in clinical disease and spongiform neurohistopathologic changes (4). Cynomolgus macaques inoculated intracerebrally with a BSE brain suspension developed depression, edginess, truncal ataxia, and tremors 150 weeks after inoculation (26). The neurohistopathology consisted of numerous plaques, indistinguishable from the florid plaques described in vCJD (42). Consequently, the BSE "signature" in cynomolgus macaques is identical to vCJD in humans. Inoculation of a TSE into mice gives a specific "lesion profile," which is used to type strains. When subjected to this analysis, the seven known strains of BSE were shown to be indistinguishable from feline spongiform encephalopathy, spongiform

BSE has been transmitted to numerous species experimentally

encephalopathy of zoo antelopes, and vCJD. The BSE lesion profiles were distinct from those of sporadic CJD and scrapie (1).

Many investigators conclude that the origin of BSE may be an as yet unidentified strain of scrapie, or that it may have originated from the TSE of another species that contaminated meat and bonemeal.

Treatment

BSE is a progressive condition. There is no treatment.

Prevention

The only prevention is to ensure that cattle are not allowed to consume any recycled protein from animals suffering from a TSE.

Diagnosis

The diagnosis of BSE rests on histopathologic confirmation of characteristic lesions

The diagnosis of BSE rests on histopathologic confirmation of characteristic lesions. There are no gross abnormalities in BSE-affected brains. Histologic lesions are usually bilateral and symmetrical and consist of vacuolar and other degenerative changes in the gray matter. The most remarkable feature is vacuolation of the neuropil, the so-called spongiform change (Fig. 17.2). Vacuoles may also be present in neuronal perikarya (Fig. 17.3). Occasional solitary necrotic neurons or shrunken basophilic neurons may be observed (38). Some gemistocytic astrocytes or mild gliosis (9) may be seen as well. Examination of a single section of the medulla oblongata at the level of the obex is sufficient for rendering a diagnosis (34). This is because this area contains the solitary tract nucleus and the spinal tract nucleus of the trigeminal areas, two preferential sites for BSE changes to appear. Other sites to examine include the caudal cerebellar peduncle and mesencephalon (9). Vacuolation of the red nucleus and oculomotor nucleus occurs in clinically normal cattle and should be regarded as an incidental finding (9, 35).

Ancillary diagnostic tests involve fibril detection by electron microscopy (37) or PrP detection by Western blot (immunoblot) (12) or immunohistochemistry (18, 28). Both Western blot and immunohistochemistry utilize antibodies to the scrapie-associated fibrils.

Ultrastructurally, the spongiform change has been shown to consist of membrane-bound spaces within neuronal processes, mainly dendrites (27). The spaces, or vacuoles, contain abundant curled membranes and amorphous material. The curled membranes may be the ultrastructural equivalent of prion protein. Dystrophic axons contain accumulations of electron-dense material, including neurofilaments and mitochondria (27, 38). These axonal changes are thought to be the result of impaired axoplasmic transport, perhaps due to accumulation of abnormal prion protein and general hindrance of neuronal function.

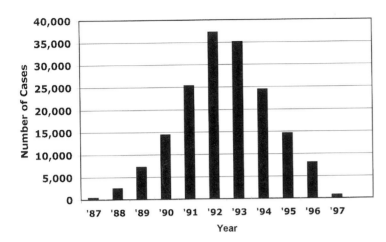

Figure 17.1   BSE cases diagnosed in cattle in the U.K.

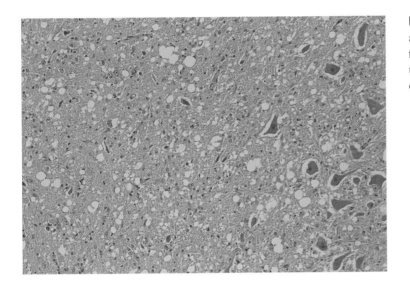

Figure 17.2   Vacuolation of the neuropil seen in a cross section of the medulla taken at the obex from a BSE-affected cow. This is the most characteristic lesion seen with BSE. Hematoxylin and eosin stain.

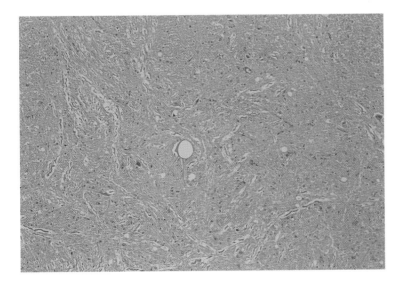

Figure 17.3   Vacuolation within neuronal perikaryon, medulla, BSE-affected cow. Hematoxylin and eosin stain.

References

1. **Almond, J.** 1997. The UK epidemic of BSE: is it a threat to human health? *In Conference on Emerging Infections.* Harvard School of Public Health, Boston.

2. **Anonymous.** 1997. *BSE Fact Sheet.* U.S. Department of Agriculture, Washington, D.C.

3. **Anonymous.** 1996. *Bovine Spongiform Encephalopathy (BSE).* Fact Sheet N113, March. World Health Organization, Geneva.

4. **Baker, H. F., R. M. Ridley, and G. A. H. Wells.** 1993. Experimental transmission of BSE and scrapie to the common marmoset. *Vet. Rec.* **132:**403–406.

5. **Bruce, M. E., R. G. Will, J. W. Ironside, I. McConnell, D. Drummond, A. Suttie, L. McCardle, A. Chree, J. Hope, C. Birkett, S. Cousens, H. Fraser, and C. J. Bostock.** 1997. Transmission to mice indicates that "new variant" CJD is caused by the BSE agent. *Nature* **389:**498–501.

6. **Chen, S. S., K. M. Charlton, A. V. Balachandran, B. P. O'Connor, and C. C. Jenson.** 1996. Bovine spongiform encephalopathy identified in a cow imported to Canada from the United Kingdom: a case report. *Can. Vet. J.* **37:**38–40.

7. **Clark, W. W., J. L. Hourrigan, and W. J. Hadlow.** 1995. Encephalopathy in cattle experimentally infected with the scrapie agent. *Am. J. Vet. Res.* **56:**606–612.

8. **Cutlip, R. C., J. M. Miller, R. E. Race, A. L. Jenny, J. B. Katz, H. D. Lehmkuhl, B. M. DeBey, and M. M. Robinson.** 1994. Intracerebral transmission of scrapie to cattle. *J. Infect. Dis.* **169:**814–820.

9. **Davis, A. J., A. L. Jenny, and L. D. Miller.** 1991. Diagnostic characteristics of bovine spongiform encephalopathy. *J. Vet. Diag. Invest.* **3:**266–271.

10. **Dawson, M., G. A. H. Wells, B. N. J. Parker, and A. C. Scott.** 1990. Primary parenteral transmission of bovine spongiform encephalopathy to the pig. *Vet. Rec.* **127:**338.

11. **DeArmond, S. J., and S. B. Prusiner.** 1996. Transgenetics and neuropathology of prion diseases, p. 125–132. *In* S. B. Prusiner (ed.), *Prions Prions Prions.* Springer-Verlag, New York.

12. **Farquhar, C. F., R. A. Somerville, and L. A. Ritchie.** 1989. Post-mortem immunodiagnosis of scrapie and bovine spongiform encephalopathy. *J. Virol. Methods* **24:**215–222.

13. **Fleetwood, A. J., and C. W. Furley.** 1990. Spongiform encephalopathy in an eland. *Vet. Rec.* **126:**408–409.

14. **Foster, J. D., M. Bruce, I. McConnell, A. Chree, and H. Fraser.** 1996. Detection of BSE infectivity in brain and spleen of experimentally infected sheep. *Vet. Rec.* **138:**546–548.

15. **Fraser, H., I. McConnell, G. A. H. Wells, and M. Dawson.** 1988. Transmission of bovine spongiform encephalopathy to mice. *Vet. Rec.* **123:**472.

16. **Gomez, T.** 1997. APHIS-USDA Liaison with CDC, July. Personal communication.

17. **Hadlow, W. J.** 1959. Scrapie and kuru. *Lancet* **ii:**289.

18. **Haritani, M., Y. I. Spencer, and G. A. H. Wells.** 1994. Hydrated autoclave pretreatment enhancement of prion protein immunoreactivity in formalin-fixed bovine spongiform encephalopathy-affected brain. *Acta Neuropathol.* **87:**86–90.

19. **Hartsough, G. R., and D. Burger.** 1965. Encephalopathy of mink. I. Epizootiologic and clinical observations. *J. Infect. Dis.* **115:**387–392.

20. **Hill, A. F., M. Desbruslais, S. Joiner, K. C. L. Sidle, L. J. Doey, P. Lantos, I. Gowland, and J. Collinge.** 1997. The same prion strain causes vCJD and BSE. *Nature* **389:**448–450.

21. **Hunter, G. D., R. H. Kimberlin, G. C. Millson, and R. A. Gibbons.** 1971. An experimental examination of the scrapie agent in cell membrane mixtures. I. Stability and physicochemical properties of the scrapie agent. *J. Comp. Pathol.* **81:**23–32.

22. **Hunter, N., W. Goldmann, G. Smith, and J. Hope.** 1994. Frequencies of PrP gene variants in healthy cattle and cattle with BSE in Scotland. *Vet. Rec.* **135:**400–403.

23. **Ironside, J. W.** 1996. Review: Creutzfeldt-Jakob disease. *Brain Pathol.* **6:**379–388.

24. **Jeffrey, M., and G. A. H. Wells.** 1988. Spongiform encephalopathy in a nyala (*Tragelaphus angasi*). *Vet. Pathol.* **25:**398–399.

25. **Kirkwood, J. K., G. A. H. Wells, J. W. Wilesmith, A. A. Cunningham, and S. I. Jackson.** 1990. Spongiform encephalopathy in an Arabian oryx (*Oryx leucoryx*) and a greater kudu (*Tragelaphus strepsiceros*). *Vet. Rec.* **127:**418–420.

26. **Lasmézas, C. I., J.-P. Deslys, R. Demalmay, K. T. Adjou, F. Lamoury, D. Dormont, O. Robain, J. W. Ironside, and J.-J. Hauw.** 1996. BSE transmission to macaques. *Nature* **381:**743–744.

27. **Liberski, P. P., R. Yanagihara, G. A. H. Wells, C. J. Gibbs, Jr., and D. C. Gajdusek.** 1992. Comparative ultrastructural neuropathology of naturally occurring bovine spongiform encephalopathy and experimentally induced scrapie and Creutzfeldt-Jakob disease. *J. Comp. Pathol.* **106:**361–381.

28. **McBride, P. A., M. E. Bruce, and H. Fraser.** 1988. Immunostaining of scrapie cerebral amyloid plaques with antisera raised to scrapie-associated fibrils (SAF). *Neuropathol. Appl. Neurobiol.* **14:**325–336.

29. **Parry, H. B.** 1983. Recorded occurrences of scrapie from 1750, p. 31–59. *In* D. R. Oppenheimer (ed.), *Scrapie Disease in Sheep.* Academic Press, London.

30. **Peet, R. L., and J. M. Duran.** 1992. Spongiform encephalopathy in an imported cheetah (*Acinonyx jubatus*). *Aust. Vet. J.* **69:**171.

31. **Prusiner, S. B.** 1982. Novel proteinaceous infectious particles cause scrapie. *Science* **216:**136–144.

32. **Prusiner, S. B.** 1991. Molecular biology of prion disease. *Science* **252:**1511–1522.

33. **Robinson, M. M., W. J. Hadlow, T. P. Huff, G. A. H. Wells, M. Dawson, R. F. Marsh, and J. R. Gorham.** 1994. Experimental infection of mink with bovine spongiform encephalopathy. *J. Gen. Virol.* **75:**2151–2155.

34. **Wells, G. A. H., R. D. Hancock, W. A. Cooley, M. S. Richards, R. J. Higgins, and G. P. David.** 1989. Bovine spongiform encephalopathy: diagnostic significance of vacuolar changes in selected nuclei of the medulla oblongata. *Vet. Rec.* **125:**521–524.

35. **Wells, G. A., and I. S. McGill.** 1992. Recently described scrapie-like encephalopathies of animals: case definitions. *Res. Vet. Sci.* **53:**1–10.

36. **Wells, G. A. H., A. C. Scott, C. T. Johnson, R. F. Gunning, R. D. Hancock, M. Jeffrey, M. Dawson, and R. Bradley.** 1987. A novel progressive spongiform encephalopathy in cattle. *Vet. Rec.* **121:**419–420.

37. **Wells, G. A. H., A. C. Scott, J. W. Wilesmith, M. M. Simmons, and D. Matthews.** 1994. Correlation between the results of a histopathological examination and the detection of abnormal brain fibrils in the diagnosis of bovine spongiform encephalopathy. *Res. Vet. Sci.* **56:**346–351.

38. **Wells, G. A. H., and J. W. Wilesmith.** 1995. The neuropathology and epidemiology of bovine spongiform encephalopathy. *Brain Pathol.* **5:**91–103.

39. **Wilesmith, J. W., and J. B. M. Ryan.** 1993. Bovine spongiform encephalopathy: observations on the incidence in 1992. *Vet. Rec.* **132:**300–301.

40. **Wilesmith, J. W., J. B. M. Ryan, and M. J. Atkinson.** 1991. Bovine spongiform encephalopathy: epidemiological studies on the origin. *Vet. Rec.* **128:**199–203.

41. **Wilesmith, J. W., G. A. H. Wells, M. P. Cranwell, and J. B. M. Ryan.** 1988. Bovine spongiform encephalopathy: epidemiological studies. *Vet. Rec.* **123:**638–644.

42. **Will, R. G., J. W. Ironside, M. Zeidler, S. Cousens, K. Estebeiro, A. Alperovitch, S. Poser, M. Pocchiari, A. Hofman, and P. G. Smith.** 1996. A new variant of Creutzfeldt-Jakob disease in the UK. *Lancet* **347:**921–925.

43. **Williams, E. S., and S. Young.** 1980. Chronic wasting disease of captive mule deer: a spongiform encephalopathy. *J. Wildlife Dis.* **16:**89–98.

44. **Williams, E. S., and S. Young.** 1982. Spongiform encephalopathy of Rocky Mountain elk. *J. Wildlife Dis.* **18:**465–472.

45. **Willoughby, K., D. F. Kelly, D. G. Lyon, and G. A. H. Wells.** 1992. Spongiform encephalopathy in a captive puma (*Felis concolor*). *Vet. Rec.* **131:**431–434.

46. **Winter, M. H., B. M. Aldridge, P. R. Scott, and M. Clark.** 1989. Occurrence of 14 cases of bovine spongiform encephalopathy in a closed dairy herd. *Br. Vet. J.* **145:**191–194.

47. **Wyatt, J. M., G. R. Pearson, T. N. Smerdon, T. J. Gruffydd-Jones, G. A. H. Wells, and J. W. Wilesmith.** 1991. Naturally occurring scrapie-like spongiform encephalopathy in five domestic cats. *Vet. Rec.* **129:**233–236.

chapter 18

Emerging Infections in Captive Wildlife

Tracey S. McNamara

There have been dramatic changes in the zoo field in the past 100 years. Some, such as the spectacular naturalistic settings currently found in most zoos, can be appreciated by even the casual visitor. However, the most impressive part of any zoo is never seen by the general public: the behind-the-scenes activities of dedicated professionals working on behalf of conservation. Given the special nature of the animals and the rarity of many species found in zoological collections, providing for their health and well-being can present a challenge to caretakers. To fully understand the nature of this task, an introduction to the "new zoo" is warranted.

Species Survival Plans: The Big Picture

The American Zoo and Aquarium Association (AZA) sets the guidelines for today's zoos. Accreditation inspections ensure that members adhere to the stringent guidelines that are part of the accreditation process.

Tracey S. McNamara, Department of Pathology, Wildlife Conservation Society, 2300 Southern Boulevard, Bronx, NY 10460.

Pathology of Emerging Infections 2
Edited by Ann Marie Nelson and C. Robert Horsburgh, Jr.
© 1998 American Society for Microbiology, Washington, D.C.

What few people realize is that the mission of their local zoo extends far beyond its perimeter fence

There are currently 184 accredited zoos in North America. On a day-to-day basis, these institutions strive to inspire the public to care about wild animals and their environment. What few people realize is that the mission of their local zoo extends far beyond its perimeter fence. Through a group of AZA-sponsored management strategies known as the Special Survival Plan (SSP) Program, zoos and aquariums work cooperatively to ensure the survival of selected wildlife species around the world. The mission of the SSP program is to:

- organize scientifically managed captive breeding programs for selected wildlife as a hedge against extinction
- cooperate with other institutions and agencies to ensure integrated conservation strategies
- increase public awareness of wildlife conservation issues, including development and implementation of education strategies at our member institutions and in the field, as appropriate
- conduct basic and applied research to contribute to our knowledge of various species
- train wildlife and zoo professionals
- develop and test various technologies relevant to field conservation
- reintroduce captive-bred wildlife into restored or secure habitats as appropriate and necessary (1)

SSP programs allow zoos to actively manage their collections for genetically diverse and demographically stable self-sustaining populations of rare and endangered species. There are currently 87 SSPs covering about 125 individual species, such as the West African lowland gorilla, the Bali mynah, and the Chinese alligator. In addition to captive breeding recommendations, the SSP programs also provide participants with standardized husbandry and health guidelines based on the best available information.

The Role of Zoo Veterinarians

As zoos have evolved, so too has the role of the veterinarian. In the past, many medical procedures were performed by non-veterinary staff. Today, most accredited zoos employ full- or part-time veterinarians. This specialized area of veterinary medicine is now a boarded specialty (The American College of Zoological Medicine), and formal training internships and residencies are available in nine veterinary institutions in the United States. It is not unusual to find zoo veterinarians using advanced technologies like magnetic resonance imagery, computed tomography, ultrasonography, endoscopy, and mammography on their zoo patients in the effort to provide them with the best of medical care.

In spite of all of these advances, every now and then the conservation community is reminded, in rather dramatic terms, of just how much remains to be learned. The outbreak of a novel morbillivirus in pinnipeds (3) and cetaceans (4) caused massive die-offs of animals and public alarm. The crossover of canine distemper virus into lions in the Serengeti (2) was yet another reminder of the mind-boggling number of variables that must be addressed in modern conservation programs. When a serious viral problem was detected in captive golden lion tamarins scheduled to be released in Brazil as part of an SSP program, the entire concept of the safety of mixing captive and free-ranging populations came under intensive review. At the International Conference on Implications of Infectious Disease for Captive Propagation and Reintroduction of Threatened Species held in Oakland, California, on 11–13 November 1992 (6), participants concluded that the conservation community lacked sufficient information on the incidence, distribution, and risks of disease in both captive and free-ranging populations and called for increased emphasis on the development of diagnostic technology and the collection of standardized data.

Much of the desired information could be obtained through systematic necropsy evaluations of captive and free-ranging wildlife. Some of the most successful SSPs (e.g., black rhinoceros, golden lion tamarin, and cheetah) have been those where thorough pathological studies have been incorporated into management protocols.

Unfortunately, while most SSPs have veterinary advisors, only a handful of veterinary pathologists are involved in the zoo field. In fact, of the 184 accredited zoos, only 4 have long-established pathology departments! These are the National Zoo in Washington, D.C., the San Diego Zoological Society, the Philadelphia Zoological Society, and the Wildlife Conservation Society (Bronx Zoo). More recently, programs have been developed at the St. Louis Zoological Society and in Chicago at the Lincoln Park Zoo, Brookfield Zoo, and the Shedd Aquarium. Lacking the budgetary wherewithal to hire full-time pathologists on their own, the latter three institutions pooled their resources to support a full-time pathologist and residency program.

With the exception of these institutions, other zoos lack the finances to pay for in-house pathology services. In most cases, necropsies are performed by clinical veterinarians with minimal training in pathology, and selected tissues are mailed out to local diagnostic laboratories or universities, resulting in delayed diagnoses of variable quality.

"Zoo Pathology": A New Frontier

When one considers the zoo setting, this lack of rapid and accurate diagnostic service is alarming. Zoo animals are managed in herds, flocks, or breeding pairs, where disease in one individual may rapidly spread to others in the group. As many zoos like to keep a variety of species together for exhibit purposes, animals also run the risk of interspecies disease transmission. The threat of inadvertently introduced disease is a constant issue, as most zoos are found in large urban parks where skunks, raccoons, and other feral wildlife may come into contact with zoo animals in spite of the most intensive pest control programs. And, while veterinarians may be able to protect domestic species from known disease threats through the use of an arsenal of antimicrobial agents and vaccines, the same cannot be said of zoo species, as drugs developed for domestic animals may not protect, or may even cause disease in wildlife.

[The] lack of rapid and accurate diagnostic service is alarming

Considering all these factors, a compelling argument can be made for the absolute necessity of increasing rapid diagnostic pathology service to zoological collections. Given the small numbers of these rare and endangered animals, can we afford to lose even one to an otherwise preventable disease simply because it was not detected?

There will be no quick solution to this problem. Zoos are nonprofit organizations, and it is highly unlikely the majority of them will ever be capable of financing the pathology service they so desperately need. What then of the veterinary colleges found throughout the country? Many of them are in close proximity to a number of smaller zoos. Could they not provide some of the necessary resources and expertise?

Such a sharing of resources could be of significant advantage, as zoos and universities have much to offer one another. Zoological medicine is an increasingly popular career path for graduating veterinarians, and students would benefit by the incorporation of information on "nontraditional" species in the veterinary curriculum. Even if individual instructors have no interest whatsoever in conservation issues, zoos can provide them with a wealth of comparative teaching materials. Zoo species would benefit indirectly from any additional information gained from basic studies done in university settings.

This partnership may be difficult to cultivate, however. While veterinarians enjoy the reputation of caring for "all creatures great and small," George Orwell's quote, "All animals are created equal, but some animals are more equal than others" (5), is perhaps more accurate. The reality is that nondomestic species have never received the same attention as domestic dogs, cats, horses, chickens, or swine. Some would argue that, given the extraordinary expansion of the field of veterinary medicine in the past 40 years, it would be impossible to cram anything further into the curriculum. Yet there is an inherent lack of logic in the assumption that one can freely extrapolate what is currently known about domestic species and apply it to the myriad of species found in zoological collections. Does it not stand to reason that exotic species might have their own unique set of disease problems, as is true of the dog, mouse, and cow?

They do. In fact, with some effort, one can find quite a bit of information on the disease problems of exotic species. However, this information is not yet readily available to all veterinary diagnostic pathologists. Efforts are under way to create formalized training materials in this area of expertise and make them universally accessible via interlibrary loan and/or electronic media.

In short, zoo pathologists hope to take the "exotic" out of exotics. Until this can be accomplished, "routine" diagnostic pathology service will not be available to the zoo community and the animals in their care. Consequently, diseases will continue to "emerge" in zoo animals for some time to come, not necessarily because they are, indeed, "new" diseases, but because it is the first time someone took the trouble to stop and look.

Nondomestic species have never received the same attention as domestic dogs, cats, horses, chickens, or swine

References

1. **American Zoo and Aquarium Association.** 1997. About Species Survival Plan. Http://www.aza.org/aza/ssp/aboutssp.html.

2. **Anonymous.** 1994. Serengeti's big cats going to the dogs. *Science* **264:**1664.

3. **Kennedy, S., J. A. Smyth, P. F. Cush, P. Duignan, M. Platten, S. J. McCullough, and G. M. Allan.** 1989. Histopathologic and immunocytochemical studies of distemper in seals. *Vet. Pathol.* **26:**97–103.

4. **Kennedy, S., J. A. Smyth, P. F. Cush, M. McAliskey, S. J. McCullough, and B. K. Rima.** 1991. Histopathologic and immunocytochemical studies of distemper in harbor porpoises. *Vet. Pathol.* **28:**107.

5. **Orwell, G.** 1995. *Animal Farm,* 50th Anniversary Edition, p. 149. Harcourt, Brace & Company, New York.

6. **Wolff, P. L., and U. S. Seal.** 1993. Implications of infectious disease for captive propagation and reintroduction of threatened species. *J. Zoo Wildlife Med.* **24(3):**229–230.

Index